Quarter Librar~ ~s metropolitan university
this item

Omega–3 Fatty Acids, the Brain and Retina

World Review of Nutrition and Dietetics

Vol. 99

Series Editor

Artemis P. Simopoulos

The Center for Genetics, Nutrition and Health, Washington, D.C., USA

Omega–3 Fatty Acids, the Brain and Retina

Volume Editors

Artemis P. Simopoulos

The Center for Genetics, Nutrition and Health, Washington, D.C., USA

Nicolas G. Bazan

New Orleans Louisiana State University Health Sciences Center

20 figures and 19 tables, 2009

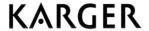 Basel · Freiburg · Paris · London · New York · Bangalore ·
Bangkok · Shanghai · Singapore · Tokyo · Sydney

Artemis P. Simopoulos
The Center for Genetics
Nutrition and Health
Washington, D.C., USA

Nicolas G. Bazan
Neuroscience Center of Excellence
and Department of Opthalmology
Louisiana State University
Health Sciences Center
New Orleans, USA

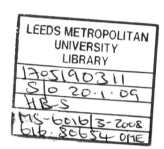
Library of Congress Cataloging-in-Publication Data

Omega-3 fatty acids, the brain, and retina / volume editors, Artemis P.
Simopoulos, Nicolas G. Bazan.
     p. ; cm. – (World review of nutrition and dietetics ; v. 99)
  Includes bibliographical references and indexes.
  ISBN 978–3–8055–9019–8 (hard cover : alk. paper)
  1. Nervous system–Degeneration–Molecular aspects.   2. Omega-3 fatty
acids–Physiological effect.   3. Retina–Pathophysiology.   I. Simopoulos,
Artemis P., 1933–   II. Bazán, Nicolás G.   III. Series.
  [DNLM: 1. Brain Diseases–metabolism.   2. Brain Chemistry.   3. Fatty
Acids, Omega-3–physiology.   4. Retina–chemistry. W1 WO898 v.99 2009 / WL
348 O55 2009]
  RC394.D35O64 2009
  616.80654–dc22
                                                                2008045444

Bibliographic Indices. This publication is listed in bibliographic services, including Current Contents® and PubMed/MEDLINE.

© Copyright 2009 by S. Karger AG, P.O. Box, CH–4009 Basel (Switzerland)
www.karger.com
Printed in Switzerland on acid-free and non-aging paper (ISO 9706) by Reinhardt Druck, Basel
ISSN 0084–2230
ISBN 978–3–8055–9019–8
e-ISBN 978–3–8055–9020–4

Contents

Preface

Research on omega–3 fatty acids has expanded enormously over the past 10 years. Beginning with the mid 1970s, most of the research focused on the role of omega–3 fatty acids in the secondary prevention of cardiovascular disease. Epidemiological observations, animal studies, clinical intervention studies, and studies at the molecular level firmly established the importance of omega–3 fatty acids, in the prevention and management of cardiovascular disease. Furthermore, studies on the mechanisms and the need to balance the omega–6 to the omega–3 ratio for homeostasis and normal development have been carried out at the molecular level and in transgenic animals using lipidomics and informatics. It is now accepted that docosahexaenoic acid (DHA) and arachidonic acid (AA) are essential for brain development during pregnancy, lactation and throughout the life cycle. Recently, studies on brain and retinal function as well as mental health have dominated the field. That DHA can affect brain function and behavior is no longer controversial. The studies on age-related macular degeneration (AMD) given supplemental DHA have revealed significant interactions between DHA and genetic variants. In animal experiments, deficiencies in DHA show impairments in cognitive development correctable by its repletion. Furthermore, the consumption of DHA or fish oil by humans slows cognitive decline in the aged and in subjects with early Alzheimer's disease (AD) and promotes mental development in infants. Over 60 countries worldwide have supplemented infant formula with DHA and AA, yet the Food and Nutrition Board of the Institute of Medicine has not determined the nutritional requirement of DHA.

There have been a number of volumes in the series of the *World Review of Nutrition and Dietetics* (WRND) on various aspects of omega–6 and omega–3 essential fatty acids (EFA) beginning with Volume 66: Health Effects of Omega–3 Polyunsaturated Fatty Acids in Seafoods, published in 1991, which truly established the field. It was followed by Volume 75: Fatty Acids and Lipids: Biological Aspects, published in 1994.

Volume 83: The Return of Omega-3 Fatty Acids into the Food Supply I. Land-Based Animal Food Products and Their Health Effects, published in 1998. Volume 88: Fatty Acids and Lipids – New Findings, published in 2001. Volume 92: Omega–6/Omega–3 Essential Fatty Acid Ratio: The Scientific Evidence, published in 2003. The present volume 99: Omega–3 Fatty Acids, the Brain and Retina is the sixth in the series, published in 2008.

The volume begins with the paper by Artemis P. Simopoulos on 'Omega–6/Omega–3 Essential Fatty Acids: Biological Effects' which sets the stage for what follows. Dr. Simopoulos emphasizes the changes that have taken place in the food supply that led to high intake of omega–6 and low intake of omega–3 fatty acids, particularly the last 50 years, and the biological effects of the resulting imbalanced omega–6/omega–3 ratio. Major advances have taken place in the concepts of inflammation and proresolution of new lipid mediators, lipoxins, resolvins and protectins discovered by using new approaches mainly lipidomics and informatics. Finally the paper provides an overview of mental illness and eye disease that are presented in detail in the papers that follow.

A number of epidemiological studies across populations have clearly shown an inverse relationship between fish intake and depression, as well as cognitive dysfunction in elderly populations. Animal experiments deficient in DHA have shown deficits in learning and memory. In some studies in Finland and Japan where the fish intake is already high, such inverse relationships have not been seen consistently. But in the majority of studies the data are consistent between low fish intake and prevalence of major depression. For example, prevalence rates of major depression are 50 times higher among countries with little seafood consumption compared to countries with the highest consumption. Furthermore, at autopsy the concentration of DHA is 30% lower in the dorsolateral prefrontal cortex of subjects with major depression. Of interest is the fact that three meta-analyses have reported robust treatment effect sizes for omega–3 long-chain fatty acids that are larger than those reported for most antidepressant pharmaceuticals. Clinical intervention studies have generated data that impulsive violence, post-traumatic stress disorders, personality and substance abuse disorders may be prevented or treated using appropriate amounts of omega–3 fatty acids.

Dr. Hibbeln in his paper 'Depression, Suicide and Deficiencies of Omega–3 Essential Fatty Acids in Modern Diets' reviews the studies of major depression including the ecological and epidemiological aspects, intervention studies, as well as the data on tissue composition. Dr. Hibbeln concludes that a strong and consistent body of data from ecological, epidemiological, case-control tissue compositional studies and randomized placebo-controlled trials indicate that low seafood consumption, omega–3 intake and body compositional status are linked to greater risks for significant depressive symptoms. This body of data is evaluated in light of the Hill Criteria for assessing causality. While substantial work needs to be conducted in the study of omega–3 deficiencies and increased suicide risk, current data suggests an apparent beneficial effect. Religious dietary practices followed for centuries are remarkably consistent with current dietary recommendations issued by international scientific bodies. Modern diets increase the likelihood of omega–3 deficiencies, perhaps manifested as depressive symptoms and self-destructive behaviors.

In the next paper, 'Application of Serial Structural Magnetic Resonance Imaging Analysis and Proton and 31-Phosphorus Magnetic Resonance Spectroscopy to the Investigation of Cerebral Fatty Acids in Major Depressive Disorder, Huntington's Disease (Chorea), and Myalgic Encephalomyelitis (Chronic Fatigue Syndrome), and in Forensic Patients with Schizophrenia Who Have Seriously and Violently Offended', Dr. Puri et al. describe recent advances in the analysis of serial magnetic resonance structural cerebral scans and in the use of proton neurospectroscopy and 31-phosphorus neurospectroscopy. The authors show how these technologies can be applied to further our understanding of the role played by lipids in the pathophysiology of major neurologic and psychiatric disorders, including major depressive disorder, Huntington's disease (Huntington's chorea), myalgic encephalomyelitis (chronic fatigue syndrome), and schizophrenia and how these techniques may be employed to study the cerebral effects of nutritional supplementation in these and related disorders.

Major discoveries have taken place on the function of neuroprotectin D1 (NPD1) which is produced from DHA. Drs Niemoller et al. present the latest research on the evidence. In their paper, 'Omega–3 Fatty Acid Docosahexaenoic Acid Is the Precursor of Neuroprotectin D1 in the Nervous System', the authors first review the metabolism of DHA in the nervous system. After ingestion, DHA is processed in the liver and transported by the bloodstream to the central nervous system. Once in the retina and brain, it is incorporated into phospholipids in neuronal and photoreceptor membranes where it promotes proper visual and neural activity. DHA is the precursor to NPD1, a potent neuroprotective lipid-signaling molecule. NPD1 is synthesized in response to oxidative stress, ischemia, and certain neurotrophins. NPD1 has been shown to activate protective anti-apoptotic Bcl-2 proteins including Bcl-2, Bcl-xL, and Bfl-1/A1 while inhibiting pro-apoptotic proteins Bad, Bax, Bid, and Bix. NPD1 also actively inhibits interleukin-1β (IL-1β) induction of cyclooxegenase-2 (COX-2) preventing initiation of the inflammatory cascade. Because of its potent protective activity, NPD1 is a promising candidate to support cell survival/repair in retinal degenerative diseases and reduce damage caused by brain inflammation in conditions such as stroke, Alzheimer disease (AD) and epilepsy.

There is a great interest on the mechanisms by which DHA may have a beneficial effect in patients with AD. Dr. Lukiw in his paper 'Docosahexaenoic Acid and Amyloid-β Peptide Signaling in Alzheimer's Disease' discusses the beneficial actions of free DHA and NPD1. Significant molecular, genetic and epidemiological data support the idea that β-amyloid precursor protein (β-APP)-derived peptide and cytokine-induced oxidative stress, and the generation of reactive oxygen species, play important roles in aging and in the development and progression of neurodegenerative disease. Dr. Lukin discusses the role of β-APP, amyloid-β (Aβ) peptides, oxidative stress and apoptosis in AD. While the degree to which brain inflammation plays a causative role in AD is controversial, there is abundant evidence that pathogenic inflammatory signaling contributes significantly to the maintenance and progression of the AD process. DHA reduces both apoptosis and oxidative stress. Dr. Lukiw points out that DHA suppresses the expression of genes involved in inflammation. DHA through the production of NPD1 and other DHA-derived neuroprotectins, provides additional benefits in patients following trauma or stroke. While the interaction of cholesterol and statins with DHA are just beginning to become understood, DHA supplementation in combination with statin therapy demonstrates a significant enhancement in the reduction of serum cholesterol than is observed with statin treatment alone. The fatty acid composition of neuronal membranes, including DHA and cholesterol content, and cholesterol transporters have direct bearing on whether β-APP is processed into neurotrophic or the more neurotoxic species. Dr. Lukiw concludes: 'The chronic nature of AD suggests that neuroprotective and survival factors are progressively lost, switching from an up-regulation in the expression of anti-apoptotic factors to increases in the expression of pro-apoptotic members of the Bcl-2 gene family. Unlike the actions of excessive cholesterol, the neuroprotective DHA and DHA-derived NPD1 decrease the rate of Aβ peptide generation, aggregation, and it's shifting the balance from the expression of pro-apoptotic factors toward the expression of anti-apoptotic, survival-promoting members of the Bcl-2 gene family.'

Administration of the omega–3 fatty acid DHA to humans or experimental animals can improve cognitive performance; the mechanisms underlying this effect remain uncertain. In general, nutrients or drugs that modify brain function or behavior do so by affecting synaptic transmission, changing the quantities of particular neurotransmitters within synaptic clefts or acting directly on neurotransmitter receptors or downstream signal-transduction molecules.

The next paper, 'Administration of Docosahexaenoic Acid, Uridine and Choline Increases Levels of Synaptic Membranes and Dendritic Spines in Rodent Brain', by Dr. Wurtman et al. presents an extensive review of the biochemistry and metabolism of uridine and choline since DHA's effects on synaptic membrane to a great extent depend on its interactions with brain uridine and choline. The authors found that DHA affects synaptic transmission in mammalian brain: gerbils or rats receiving this fatty acid manifest increased levels of phosphatides and specific pre- or post-synaptic proteins per brain cell, and increased numbers of dendritic spines – a precursor of new synapses – on brain neurons. These actions are markedly enhanced in animals which have also received the other two circulating precursors of phosphatidylcholine – uridine (which gives rise to brain UTP and CTP) and choline (which gives rise to phosphocholine). These findings are reproduced also by eicosapentaenoic acid (EPA), but not by the omega–6 fatty acid AA. Administration of the three compounds (DHA, uridine and choline) also increases neurotransmitter release (acetylcholine; dopamine) and affects animal behavior. Conceivably, this treatment might have some use in patients with synaptic loss, e.g. secondary to neurodegenerative disease, or stroke, or brain injury.

Animal experiments and clinical intervention studies have shown that DHA is essential for learning, behavior and memory. How much DHA is needed for normal growth and development has been estimated from studies with breastfed infants and from clinical intervention studies. Brain development begins shortly after conception. In humans, the brain approaches adult mass within the first 2 years of life during which time the foundation for the neural circuitry of the brain is established. Early access to an adequate supply of substrates for neural development is a key requirement for preventing irreversible cognitive effects.

Hadley et al. in their paper 'An Assessment of Dietary Docosahexaenoic Acid Requirements for Brain Accretion and Turnover during Early Childhood' carried out an extensive review of the data in order to define the DHA requirement during the first 2 years of life by considering data for DHA accretion, concentration and turnover from previously published studies, and prepared a general model for human brain DHA homeostasis. The model is based on physiological demands of the brain rather than on an estimate derived from the caloric contribution of α-linolenic acid (ALA, 18:3n–3). An estimate for the dietary requirement of preformed DHA during early childhood (1–2 years of age) is calculated to be 212 mg/day. This dietary requirement is calculated to be sufficient to support total brain accretion of 3.75 mg/day of DHA.

In the next paper, 'Variation in Lipid-Associated Genes as they Relate to Risk of Advanced Age-Related Macular Degeneration', Dr. SanGiovanni et al. present an extensive review of the functions of both omega–6 and omega–3 long-chain polyunsaturated fatty acids (LCPUFAs), focusing on the role of omega–3 LCPUFAs as factors impacting metabolic processes and environmental exposures implicated in the pathogenesis of AMD. These processes and exposures include neovasucularization, oxidative stress, hemodynamic and hydrodynamic change, and factors affecting cellular survival. Molecules operating with in complex systems to impact AMD pathogenesis include eicosanoids, angiogenic growth factors, matrix metalloproteinases, reactive oxygen species, cyclic nucleotides, neurotransmitters and neuromodulators, pro-inflammatory and immunoregulatory cytokines, and inflammatory phospholipids. The balance and composition of dietary and retinal omega–3 and omega–6 LCPUFAs may affect substrates, availability of biosynthetic enzymes, and gene expression of these molecules; LCPUFAs also act as ligands to a number of transcription factors and serve as precursors to potent cyclooxygenase-, lipoxygenase-, cytochrome P450-derived autocoids that influence vascular sufficiency, cell cycle, and cell survival. In the context of this evidence base, and that on the molecular genetics of AMD, Dr. SanGiovanni and colleagues applied resources from a genome-wide scan to examine the relationship of AMD with polymorphisms in sets of genes encoding enzymes, structural elements, and transcription factors affecting and affected by LCPUFAs and other lipid-based compounds, their precursors, cleavage and biosynthetic enzymes, and metabolites. Their results suggest that variants in genes encoding elements of phosphatidylinositol-based signaling systems are jointly related to a 99-fold increased risk of advanced AMD (odds ratio 99.2, 95% confidence interval 22.3–440.9, $p \leq 1.0 \times 10^{-17}$). This is the first application of joint action models to investigate molecular genetics of AMD related to pathways and gene sets. The pattern of the results suggests that: (1) the phosphatidylinositol signaling system may be acting through pleckstrin homology domains to activate a number of protein kinases, G-protein-based signaling cascades, and phospholipases with potential to impact health and disease of the neural and vascular retina; (2) there is a reasonable basis to investigate the relationship of genetic variants in the inositol pathway and the role of Akt/PI3K and dietary LCPUFAs in calcium homeostasis implicated in retinal disease. Deep sequencing of inositol gene sets in clinical populations and mechanistic studies in model systems may yield useful information on strategies for primary and tertiary prevention of sight-threatening AMD.

This volume on Omega–3 Fatty Acids, the Brain and Retina consists of papers written by the scientists that have contributed immensely to the field on the role of omega–3 fatty acids in maintaining homeostasis and in the prevention and management of neurodegenerative diseases due to the aging process or genetic predisposition. The new studies on the DHA as a precursor of resolvins and protectins is a very exciting area that should continue to advance our knowledge of EPA + DHA in the brain and retina. Therefore, this volume should be of interest to psychologists, physiologists, neuroscientists, psychiatrists, ophthalmologists, geneticists, neurologists, pediatricians, obstetricians, geriatricians, and other physicians, as well as nutritionists, dieticians, and policymakers.

Artemis P. Simopoulos, Washington, D.C.

Simopoulos AP, Bazan NG (eds): Omega-3 Fatty Acids, the Brain and Retina.
World Rev Nutr Diet. Basel, Karger, 2009, vol 99, pp 1–16

Omega−6/Omega−3 Essential Fatty Acids: Biological Effects

Artemis P. Simopoulos

The Center for Genetics, Nutrition and Health, Washington D.C., USA

The interaction of genetics and environment, nature, and nurture is the foundation for all health and disease. In the last two decades, using the techniques of molecular biology, it has been shown that genetic factors determine susceptibility to disease and environmental factors determine which genetically susceptible individuals will be affected [1–6]. Nutrition is an environmental factor of major importance. Using the tools of molecular biology and genetics, research is defining the mechanisms by which genes influence nutrient absorption, metabolism and excretion, taste perception, and degree of satiation, and the mechanisms by which nutrients influence gene expression. Whereas major changes have taken place in our diet over the past 10,000 years since the beginning of the Agricultural Revolution, our genes have not changed. The spontaneous mutation rate for nuclear DNA is estimated at 0.5% per million years. Therefore, over the past 10,000 years there has been time for very little change in our genes, perhaps 0.005%. In fact, our genes today are very similar to the genes of our ancestors during the Paleolithic period 40,000 years ago, at which time our genetic profile was established [7]. Humans today live in a nutritional environment that differs from that for which our genetic constitution was selected. Studies on the evolutionary aspects of diet indicate that major changes have taken place in our diet, particularly in the type and amount of essential fatty acids (EFA) and in the antioxidant content of foods [7–11] (fig. 1).

Today, industrialized societies are characterized by (1) an increase in energy intake and decrease in energy expenditure; (2) an increase in saturated fat, omega−6 fatty acids and *trans* fatty acids, and a decrease in omega−3 fatty acid intake; (3) a decrease in complex carbohydrates and fiber; (4) an increase in cereal grains and a decrease in fruits and vegetables, and (5) a decrease in protein, antioxidants and calcium intake [7, 9, 12–16] (tables 1, 2). The increase in *trans* fatty acids is detrimental to health as shown in table 3 [17]. In addition, *trans* fatty acids interfere with the desaturation and elongation of both omega−6 and omega−3 fatty acids, thus further decreasing the

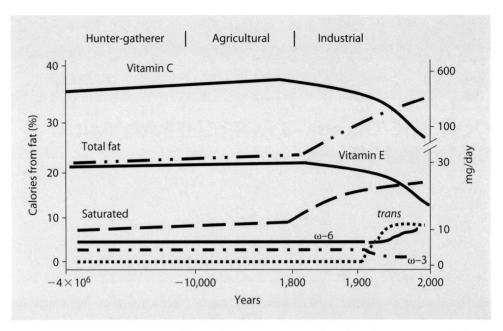

Fig. 1. Hypothetical scheme of fat, fatty acid (ω–6, ω–3, *trans* and total) intake (as percent of calories from fat) and intake of vitamins E and C (mg/day). Data were extrapolated from cross-sectional analyses of contemporary hunter-gatherer populations and from longitudinal observations and their putative changes during the preceding 100 years [9].

amount of arachidonic acid (AA), eicosapentaenoic acid (EPA) and docosahexaenoic acid (DHA) availability for human metabolism [18].

The beneficial health effects of omega–3 fatty acids, EPA and DHA were described first in the Greenland Eskimos who consumed a high seafood diet and had low rates of coronary heart disease, asthma, type 1 diabetes mellitus, and multiple sclerosis. Since that observation, the beneficial health effects of omega–3 fatty acids have been extended to include benefits related to cancer, inflammatory bowel disease, rheumatoid arthritis, and psoriasis [19], as well as depression and other mental illnesses [20–22]. A balanced intake of omega–6 and omega–3 fatty acids is needed for homeostasis and normal development throughout the life cycle.

Imbalance of Omega–6/Omega–3

Food technology and agribusiness provided the economic stimulus that dominated the changes in the food supply [23, 24]. From per capita quantities of foods available for consumption in the US national food supply in 1985, the amount of EPA is reported to be about 50 mg per capita/day and the amount of DHA is 80 mg per capita/day. The two main sources are fish and poultry [25]. It has been estimated that the present Western diet is 'deficient' in omega–3 fatty acids with a ratio of omega–6

Table 1. Estimated omega–3 and omega–6 fatty acid intake in the late Paleolithic period (g/day)[1,2]

Plants	
LA	4.28
ALA	11.40
Animals	
LA	4.56
ALA	1.21
Total	
LA	8.84
ALA	12.60
Animals	
AA (ω–6)	1.81
EPA (ω–3)	0.39
DTA (ω–6)	0.12
DPA (ω–3)	0.42
DHA (ω–3)	0.27
Ratios of ω–6/ω–3	
LA/ALA	0.70
AA+DTA/EPA+DPA+DHA	1.79
Total ω–6/ω–3	0.79[b]

LA = Linoleic acid; ALA = linolenic acid; AA = arachidonic acid; EPA = eicosapentaenoic acid; DTA = docosatetranoic acid; DPA = docosapentaenoic acid; DHA = docosahexaenoic acid.
[1] Data from Eaton et al. [13].
[2] Assuming an energy intake of 35:65 of animal:plant sources.

Table 2. Late Paleolithic and currently recommended nutrient composition for Americans

	Late Paleolithic	Current recommendations
Total dietary energy, %		
Protein	33	12
Carbohydrate	46	58
Fat	21	30
Alcohol	~0	–
P/S ratio	1.41	1.00
Cholesterol, mg	520	300
Fiber, g	100–150	30–60
Sodium, mg	690	1,100–3,300
Calcium, mg	1,500–2,000	800–1,600
Ascorbic acid, mg	440	60

Modified from Eaton et al. [13]. P/S = Polyunsaturated to saturated fat.

Table 3. Adverse effects of *trans* fatty acids [modified from 17]

Decrease or inhibit
Decrease or inhibit incorporation of other fatty acids into cell membranes
Decrease high-density lipoprotein (HDL)
Inhibit Δ–6 desaturase (interfere with elongation and desaturation of essential fatty acids)
Decrease serum testosterone (in male rats)
Cross the placenta and decrease birth weight (in humans)

Increase
Low-density lipoprotein (LDL)
Platelet aggregation
Lipoprotein (a) [Lp(a)]
Body weight
Cholesterol transfer protein (CTP)
Abnormal morphology of sperm (in male rats)

Table 4. Ratios of dietary omega–6:omega–3 fatty acids in the late Paleolithic period and in current Western diets (USA) (g/day)

	Paleolithic	Western
LA:ALA	0.70	18.75
AA+DTA:EPA+DPA+DHA	1.79	3.33
Total	0.79	16.74

LA = Linoleic acid; ALA = linolenic acid; AA = arachidonic acid; EPA = eicosapentaenoic acid; DTA = docosatetranoic acid; DPA = docosapentaenoic acid; DHA = docosahexaenoic acid.
Reprinted with permission from reference 15.

to omega–3 of 15–20/1, instead of 1/1 as is the case with wild animals and presumably human beings [7–11, 13, 26–28] (table 4).

An absolute and relative change of omega–6/omega–3 in the food supply of Western societies has occurred over the last 150 years. A balance existed between omega–6 and omega–3 for millions of years during the long evolutionary history of the genus *Homo*, and genetic changes occurred partly in response to these dietary influences. During evolution, omega–3 fatty acids were found in all foods consumed: meat, wild plants, eggs, fish, nuts and berries [29–38]. Studies by Cordain et al. [39] on wild animals confirm the original observations of Crawford [27] and Sinclair et al. [40]. However, rapid dietary changes over short periods of time as have occurred over the past 100–150 years is a totally new phenomenon in human evolution [13, 15, 41–43] (table 5).

Table 5. Omega–6:omega–3 ratios in various populations

Population	ω–6/ω–3	Ref.
Paleolithic	0.79	13
Greece prior to 1960	1.00–2.00	15
Current Japan	4.00	41
Current India, rural	5–6.1	42
Current UK and Northern Europe	15.00	43
Current USA	16.74	13
Current India, urban	38–50	42

Biological Effects and the Omega–6/Omega–3 Ratio

There are two classes of EFA – omega–6 and omega–3. The distinction between omega–6 and omega–3 fatty acids is based on the location of the first double bond, counting from the methyl end of the fatty acid molecule. In the omega–6 fatty acids, the first double bond is between the 6th and 7th carbon atoms and for the omega–3 fatty acids the first double bond is between the 3rd and 4th carbon atoms. Monounsaturates are represented by oleic acid, an omega–9 fatty acid, which can be synthesized by all mammals including humans. Its double bond is between the 9th and 10th carbon atoms.

Omega–6 and omega–3 fatty acids are essential because humans, like all mammals, cannot make them and must obtain them in their diet. Omega–6 fatty acids are represented by linoleic acid (LA; 18:2ω–6) and omega–3 fatty acids by α-linolenic acid (ALA; 18:3ω–3). LA is plentiful in nature and is found in the seeds of most plants except for coconut, cocoa, and palm. ALA on the other hand is found in the chloroplasts of green leafy vegetables, and in the seeds of flax, rape, chia, perilla and in walnuts. Both EFA are metabolized to longer-chain fatty acids of 20 and 22 carbon atoms. LA is metabolized to AA (20:4ω–6), and LNA to EPA (20:5ω–3) and DHA (22:6ω–3), increasing the chain length and degree of unsaturation by adding extra double bonds to the carboxyl end of the fatty acid molecule (fig. 2).

Humans and other mammals, except for carnivores such as lions, can convert LA to AA and ALA to EPA and DHA, but it is slow [44]. This conversion was shown by using deuterated ALA [45]. There is competition between omega–6 and omega–3 fatty acids for the desaturation enzymes. However, both delta–4 and delta–6 desaturases prefer omega–3 to omega–6 fatty acids [44, 46, 47]. But, a high LA intake interferes with the desaturation and elongation of ALA [45, 48]. *Trans* fatty acids interfere with the desaturation and elongation of both LA and ALA. Delta–6 desaturase is the limiting enzyme and there is some evidence that it decreases with age [44]. Premature infants [49], hypertensive individuals [50], and some diabetics [51] are limited in their ability to make EPA and DHA from ALA. These findings are important and need to

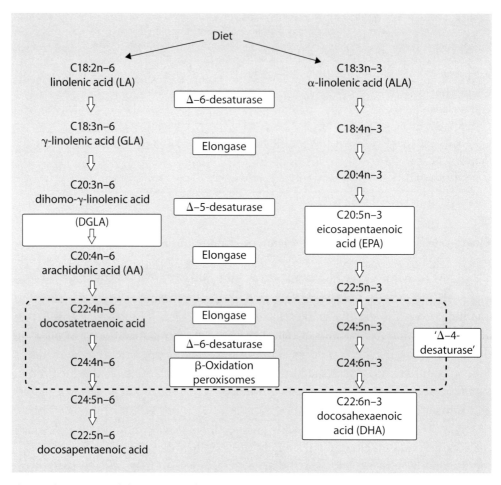

Fig. 2. Elongation and desaturation of omega–6 and omega–3 PUFAs.

be considered when making dietary recommendations. EPA and DHA are found in the oils of fish, particularly fatty fish. AA is found predominantly in the phospholipids of grain-fed animals and eggs.

LA, ALA, and their long-chain derivatives are important components of animal and plant cell membranes. In mammals and birds, the omega-3 fatty acids are distributed selectively among lipid classes. ALA is found in triglycerides, in cholesteryl esters, and in very small amounts in phospholipids. EPA is found in cholesteryl esters, triglycerides, and phospholipids. DHA is found mostly in phospholipids. In mammals, including humans, the cerebral cortex, retina, and testis and sperm are particularly rich in DHA. DHA is one of the most abundant components of the brain's structural lipids. DHA, like EPA, can be derived only from direct ingestion or by synthesis from dietary EPA or ALA.

Mammalian cells cannot convert omega–6 to omega–3 fatty acids because they lack the converting enzyme, delta–3 desaturase. LA, the parent omega–6 fatty acid, and

Table 6. Effects of ingestion of EPA and DHA from fish or fish oil

- Decreased production of prostaglandin E_2 (PGE_2) metabolites
- A decrease in thromboxane A_2, a potent platelet aggregator and vasoconstrictor
- A decrease in leukotriene B_4 formation, an inducer of inflammation, and a powerful inducer of leukocyte chemotaxis and adherence
- An increase in thromboxane A_3, a weak platelet aggregator and weak vasoconstrictor
- An increase in prostacyclin PGI_3, leading to an overall increase in total prostacyclin by increasing PGI3 without a decrease in PGI_2, both PGI_2 and PGI_3 are active vasodilators and inhibitors of platelet aggregation
- An increase in leukotriene B_5, a weak inducer of inflammation and a weak chemotactic agent

ALA, the parent omega–3 fatty acid, and their long-chain derivatives are important components of animal and plant cell membranes (fig. 2). These two classes of EFA are not interconvertible, are metabolically and functionally distinct, and often have important opposing physiological functions. When humans ingest fish or fish oil, the EPA and DHA from the diet partially replace the omega–6 fatty acids, especially AA, in the membranes of probably all cells, but especially in the membranes of platelets, erythrocytes, neutrophils, monocytes, and liver cells [reviewed in 8, 52]. Whereas cellular proteins are genetically determined, the polyunsaturated fatty acid (PUFA) composition of cell membranes is to a great extent dependent on the dietary intake. AA and EPA are the parent compounds for eicosanoid production [8] (tables 6, 7; fig. 3).

Because of the increased amounts of omega–6 fatty acids in the Western diet, the eicosanoid metabolic products from AA, specifically prostaglandins, thromboxanes, leukotrienes, hydroxy fatty acids, and lipoxins, are formed in larger quantities than those formed from omega–3 fatty acids, specifically EPA [8]. The eicosanoids from AA are biologically active in very small quantities and, if they are formed in large amounts, they contribute to the formation of thrombus and atheromas; to allergic and inflammatory disorders, particularly in susceptible people, and to proliferation of cells. Thus, a diet rich in omega–6 fatty acids shifts the physiological state to one that is prothrombotic and proaggregatory, with increases in blood viscosity, vasospasm, and vasoconstriction and decreases in bleeding time. Bleeding time is decreased in groups of patients with hypercholesterolemia, hyperlipoproteinemia, myocardial infarction, other forms of atherosclerotic disease, and diabetes (obesity and hypertriglyceridemia). Bleeding time is longer in women than in men and longer in young than in old people. There are ethnic differences in bleeding time that appear to be related to diet.

Newly Identified Lipid Mediators: Lipoxins, Resolvins and Protectins

Recent studies have shown that additional lipid mediators are produced from AA, EPA and DHA with potent anti-inflammatory properties [53]. Lipoxins are derived

Table 7. Effects of omega–3 fatty acids on factors involved in the pathophysiology of atherosclerosis and inflammation

Factor	Function	Effect of ω–3 fatty acid
Arachidonic acid	Eicosanoid precursor; aggregates platelets; stimulates white blood cells	↓
Thromboxane A_2	Platelet aggregation; vasoconstriction; increase of intracellular Ca^{2+}	↓
Prostacyclin ($PGI_2/_3$)	Prevent platelet aggregation; vasodilation; increase cAMP	↑
Leukotriene (LTB_4)	Neutrophil chemoattractant; increase of intracellular Ca^{2+}	↓
Fibrinogen	A member of the acute phase response and a blood clotting factor	↓
Tissue plasminogen activator	Increase endogenous fibrinolysis	↑
Platelet-activating factor (PAF)	Activates platelets and white blood cells	↓
Platelet-derived growth factor (PDGF)	Chemoattractant and mitogen for smooth muscles and macrophages	↓
Oxygen free radicals	Cellular damage; enhance LDL uptake via scavenger pathway; stimulate arachidonic acid metabolism	↓
Lipid hydroperoxides	Stimulate eicosanoid formation	↓
Interleukin-1 and tumor necrosis factor	Stimulate neutrophil O_2 free radical formation; stimulate lymphocyte proliferation; stimulate PAF; express intercellular adhesion molecule-1 on endothelial cells; inhibit plasminogen activator, thus, procoagulants	↓
Interleukin-6	Stimulates the synthesis of all acute phase proteins involved in the inflammatory response: C-reactive protein; serum amyloid A; fibrinogen; α1-chymotrypsin, and haptoglobin	↓
C-reactive protein (CRP)	An acute phase reactant and an independent risk factor for cardiovascular disease	↓
Endothelial-derived relaxation factor	Reduces arterial vasoconstrictor response	↑
Insulin function		Increases sensitivity to insulin
VLDL	Related to LDL and HDL level	↓
HDL	Decreases the risk for coronary heart disease	↑
Lp(a)	Lipoprotein(a) is a genetically determined protein that has atherogenic and thrombogenic properties	↓
Triglycerides and chylomicrons	Contribute to postprandial lipemia	↓

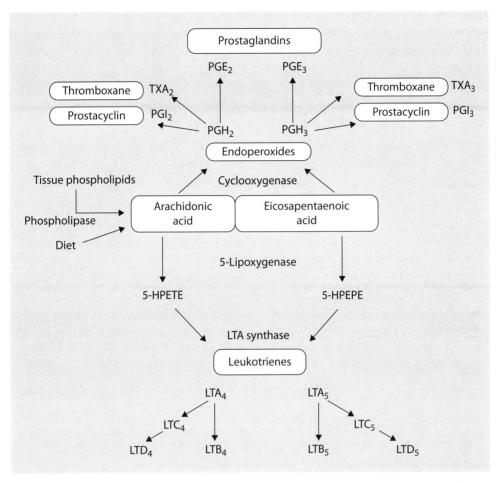

Fig. 3. Oxidative metabolism of AA and EPA by the cyclooxygenase and 5-lipoxygenase pathways. 5-HPETE = 5-Hydroperoxyeicosatetranoic acid, 5-HPEPE = 5-hydroxyeicosapentaenoic acid.

from AA as a result of cell-cell interaction and the sequential transformation by different lipoxygenases. Leukocyte 5-lipoxygenase generates LT4 from AA, which is then transformed to the lipoxin LXA4 in platelets by the oxidase activity of their 12-lipoxygenase. In addition to their anti-inflammatory properties, lipoxins have potent pro-resolution properties, inhibit the formation of inflammatory cytokines, immune cell proliferation and migration. In the presence of aspirin, the acetylation of cyclooxygenase-2 enables it to act as a lipoxygenase forming the lipoxin precursor 15-hydroxyeicosatetraenoic acid from AA, which is then transformed by leukocyte 5-lipoxygenase to 15-epi-LXA4 or 15-epi-LXB4 referred to as aspirin-triggered lipoxins. These aspirin-triggered lipoxins seem to be more potent anti-inflammatory agents than the conventional LX4 [54].

In analogy to the aspirin-triggered lipoxins from AA, bioactive mediators are also produced from EPA + DHA. Serhan and his group [53] used lipidomics and informatics in studies on EPA and DHA metabolites in the resolution of inflammation which are called resolvins. The resolvin from EPA is RvE1. RvE1 inhibits nuclear factor κB by tumor necrosis factor-α (TNF-α). ChemR23 is the receptor for RvE1 and it is a specific G-protein-coupled receptor. Transcription of ChemR23 is found in cardiovascular, gastrointestinal renal, brain, and myeloid tissue. The ChemR23 shares homology with the receptor identified for the AA-derived aspirin-triggered lipoxins but is molecularly distinct.

Resolvins are derived from EPA and DHA with two chemically unique structural forms, the E-series and the D-series respectively. Resolvin E1 is produced in healthy individuals and is increased in the plasma of individuals taking aspirin and or EPA.

DHA is the substrate for two groups of resolvins produced by different biosynthetic routes, referred to as the 17S- and 17RD-series resolvins during the resolution of inflammatory exudates. D-series resolvins have potent anti-inflammatory actions and are particularly interesting because the brain, synapses and retina are highly enriched in DHA. The D-series resolvins are of interest in the control of inflammation resolution in host defense and in neural tissues.

Another class of lipid mediators produced from DHA are the 10,17S-docosatriene, now known as protectins. When produced by neural tissues is termed neuroprotectin D1 because of its biosynthetic origin. Protectin D1 blocks T-cell migration in vivo, reduces TNF and interferon-γ (IFN-γ) secretion and promotes T-cell apoptosis.

Resolvin E1 and protectin D1 derived from EPA + DHA respectively are potent resolution agonists that activate cell type, neutrophils, macrophages, and epithelial cells to accelerate resolution.

Lipoxins, resolvins and protectins have potent multilevel mechanisms of action in disease models and promote resolution in animal models of oral, lung, ocular, kidney, skin and gastrointestinal inflammation, as well as in ischemia-reperfusion injury and angiogenesis.

Lipoxins, resolvin E1 and protectins act on T cells, dendritic cells and phagocytic cells, therefore they represent a link between the innate and the immune system. Considering that lipoxins, resolvin E1, and protectins are produced from AA, EPA + DHA, it follows that these fatty acids represent a molecular link between the two systems.

Inflammation is at the base of many chronic diseases such as cardiovascular disease, obesity, diabetes, arthritis, mental illnesses and cancer, as well as many autoimmune diseases. These diseases are characterized by increased amounts of IL-1 and IL-6. Increased dietary intake of omega–6 fatty acids is associated with higher levels of TXA_2 and LTB_4. LTB_4 is a proinflammatory AA metabolite that along with IL-1 and IL-6 contributes to inflammation. The discovery of the newly identified mediators lipoxins, resolvins, protectins and neuroprotectins form AA (lipoxins) EPA (resolvins) and DHA (protectins and neuroprotectins) indicate that the resolution of inflammation is not just a passive termination of inflammation, but rather an active biochemical and metabolic process. These families of endogenous pro-resolution molecules are not immunosuppressive but instead function in the resolution of inflammation by activating specific mechanisms to promote homeostasis [54].

The Balance of Omega–6/Omega–3 Fatty Acids Is Important for Health: Evidence from Gene Transfer Studies

Further support for the need to balance the omega–6/omega–3 EFA comes from the studies of Kang et al. [55, 56], which clearly show the ability of both normal rat cardiomyocytes and human breast cancer cells in culture to form all the omega–3s from omega–6 fatty acids when fed the cDNA encoding omega–3 fatty acid desaturase obtained from the roundworm *Caenorhabditis elegans*. The omega–3 desaturase efficiently and quickly converted the omega–6 fatty acids that were fed to the cardiomyocytes in culture to the corresponding omega–3 fatty acids. Thus, omega–6 LA was converted to omega–3 ALA and AA was converted to EPA, so that at equilibrium, the ratio of omega–6 to omega–3 PUFA was close to 1/1. Further studies demonstrated that the cancer cells expressing the omega–3 desaturase underwent apoptotic death whereas the control cancer cells with a high omega–6/omega–3 ratio continued to proliferate [57]. More recently, Kang et al. [58–60] showed that transgenic mice and pigs expressing the *C. elegans fat-1* gene encoding an omega–3 fatty acid desaturase are capable of producing omega–3 from omega–6 fatty acids, leading to enrichment of omega–3 fatty acids with reduced levels of omega–6 fatty acids in almost all organs and tissues, including muscles and milk, with no need of dietary omega–3 fatty acid supply. This discovery provides a unique tool and new opportunities for omega–3 research, and raises the potential of production of *fat-1* transgenic livestock as a new and ideal source of omega–3 fatty acids to meet the human nutritional needs. Furthermore, the transgenic mouse model is being used widely by scientists for the study of chronic diseases and for the study of mechanisms of the beneficial effects of omega–3 fatty acids [61]. The fat-1 transgenic mice produce and store higher levels of EPA + DHA in their tissues than wild-type mice, and as a result generate increased levels of resolvins and protectins.

Omega–3 Fatty Acids and Gene Expression

Previous studies have shown that fatty acids released from membrane phospholipids by cellular phospholipases, or made available to the cell from the diet or other aspects of the extracellular environment, are important cell signaling molecules. They can act as second messengers or substitute for the classical second messengers of the inositide phospholipid and the cyclic AMP signal transduction pathways. They can also act as modulator molecules mediating responses of the cell to extracellular signals. Recently it has been shown that fatty acids rapidly and directly alter the transcription of specific genes [62]. In the case of genes involved in inflammation, such as IL-1β, EPA and DHA suppress IL-1β mRNA whereas AA does not, and the same effect appears in studies on growth-related early response gene expression and growth factor [62]. In the case of vascular cell adhesion molecule (VCAM), AA has a modest suppressing effect relative to DHA. The latter situation may explain the protective effect of fish oil toward colonic carcinogenesis, since EPA and DHA did not stimulate protein kinase C. PUFA regulation of gene expression extends beyond the liver and includes genes such as adipocyte glucose transporter-4, lymphocyte stearoyl-CoA desaturase-2 in the brain, peripheral monocytes (IL-1β and VCAM-1) and platelets [platelet-derived growth factor (PDGF)]. Whereas some of the transcriptional effects of PUFA appear to be mediated by eicosanoids, the PUFA suppression of lipogenic and glycolytic genes is independent of eicosanoid synthesis, and appears to involve a nuclear mechanism directly modified by PUFA.

Mental Health and Eye Disease

Psychologic stress in humans induces the production of proinflammatory cytokines such as IFN-γ, TNF-α, IL-6 and IL-1. An imbalance of omega–6 and omega–3 PUFA in the peripheral blood causes an overproduction of proinflammatory cytokines. There is evidence that changes in fatty acid composition are involved in the pathophysiology of major depression [63]. Changes in serotonin (5-HT) receptor number and function caused by changes in PUFA provide the theoretical rationale connecting fatty acids with the current receptor and neurotransmitter theories of depression [64–68]. The increased C20:4ω–6/C20:5ω–3 ratio and the imbalance in the omega–6/ omega–3 PUFA ratio in major depression may be related to the increased production of proinflammatory cytokines and eicosanoids in that illness [66]. There are a number of studies evaluating the therapeutic effect of EPA and DHA in major depression. Stoll and colleagues [69, 70] have shown that EPA and DHA prolong remission, that is, reduce the risk of relapse in patients with bipolar disorder.

Kiecolt-Glaser et al. [71] studied depressive symptoms, omega–6/omega–3 fatty acid ratio and inflammation in older adults. As the dietary ratio of omega–6/omega–3 increased, the depressive symptoms, TNF-α, IL-6, and IL-6 soluble receptor (sIL-6r) increased. The authors concluded that diets with a high omega–6/omega–3 ratio may enhance the risk for both depression and inflammatory diseases.

Dry eye syndrome (DES) is one of the most prevalent conditions. Inflammation of the lacrimal gland, the meibomian gland, and the ocular surface plays a significant role in DES [72, 73]. An increased concentration of inflammatory cytokines, such as IL-1, IL-6, and TNF-α, has been found in tear film in patients with DES [74]. Miljanovic et al. [75] investigated the relation of dietary intake of omega–3 fatty acids and the ratio of omega–6 to omega–3 with DES incidence in a large population of women participating in the Women's Health Study. A higher ratio of omega–6/

omega–3 consumption was associated with a significantly increased risk of DES (OR 2.51; 95% CI 1.13, 5.58) for >15:1 vs. <4.1 (p for trend = 0.01). These results suggest that a higher dietary intake of omega–3 fatty acids is associated with a decreased incidence of DES in women and a high omega–6/omega–3 ratio is associated with a greater risk.

Age-related macular degeneration (AMD) is the leading cause of vision loss among people 65 and older. Both AMD and cardiovascular disease share similar modifiable factors [76–80]. Fish intake has been reported to have protective properties in lowering the risk of AMD [81, 85], especially when LA intake was low [81, 82]. In a study involving twins, Seddon et al. [86] showed that fish consumption and omega–3 fatty acid intake reduce the risk of AMD whereas cigarette smoking increases the risk for AMD.

Conclusions and Recommendations

Western diets are characterized by high omega–6 and low omega–3 fatty acid intake, whereas during the Paleolithic period when human's genetic profile was established, there was a balance between omega–6 and omega–3 fatty acids. Therefore, humans today live in a nutritional environment that differs from that for which our genetic constitution was selected.

Both omega–6 and omega–3 fatty acids influence gene expression. The balance of omega–6/omega–3 fatty acids is an important determinant in maintaining homeostasis, normal development, and mental health throughout the life cycle.

The new lipid mediators from AA, EPA + DHA such as lipoxins, resolvins, and protectins are potent pro-resolution and anti-inflammatory agents and appear to be the molecular link between the innate and adaptive immune systems, indicating the importance of nutrition in maintaining homeostasis and the need to decrease omega–6 fatty acid intake while increasing omega–3 fatty acid intake.

References

1 Simopoulos AP, Childs B (eds): Genetic Variation and Nutrition. World Rev Nutr Diet. Basel, Karger, 1990, vol 63.

2 Simopoulos AP, Robinson J: The Omega Diet. The Lifesaving Nutritional Program Based on the Diet of the Island of Crete. New York, HarperCollins, 1999.

3 Simopoulos AP, Nestel PJ (eds): Genetic Variation and Dietary Response. World Rev Nutr Diet. Basel, Karger, 1997, vol 80.

4 Simopoulos AP, Pavlou KN (eds): Nutrition and Fitness 1: Diet, Genes, Physical Activity and Health. World Rev Nutr Diet. Basel, Karger, 2001, vol 89.

5 Simopoulos AP: Genetic variation and dietary response: Nutrigenetics/nutrigenomics. Asia Pacific J Clin Nutr 2002;11(suppl 6):S117–S128.

6 Simopoulos AP, Ordovas JM (eds): Nutrigenetics and Nutrigenomics. World Rev Nutr Diet. Basel, Karger, 2004, vol 93.

7 Eaton SB, Konner M: Paleolithic nutrition. A consideration of its nature and current implications. N Engl J Med 1985;312:283–289.

8 Simopoulos AP: Omega–3 fatty acids in health and disease and in growth and development. Am J Clin Nutr 1991;54:438–463.

9 Simopoulos AP: Genetic variation and evolutionary aspects of diet; in Papas A (ed): Antioxidants in Nutrition and Health. Boca Raton, CRC Press, 1999, pp 65–88.

10 Simopoulos AP: Evolutionary aspects of omega–3 fatty acids in the food supply. Prostaglandins Leukotr Essent Fatty Acids 1999;60:421–429.

11 Simopoulos AP: New products from the agri-food industry: the return of n–3 fatty acids into the food supply. Lipids 1999;34(suppl):S297–S301.

12 Eaton SB, Konner M, Shostak M: Stone agers in the fast lane: chronic degenerative diseases in evolutionary perspective. Am J Med 1988;84:739–749.

13 Eaton SB, Eaton SB III, Sinclair AJ, Cordain L, Mann NJ: Dietary intake of long-chain polyunsaturated fatty acids during the Paleolithic. World Rev Nutr Diet. Basel, Karger, 1998, vol 83, pp 12–23.

14 Leaf A, Weber PC: A new era for science in nutrition. Am J Clin Nutr 1987;45:1048–1053.

15 Simopoulos AP: Overview of evolutionary aspects of ω–3 fatty acids in the diet. World Rev Nutr Diet. Basel, Karger, 1998, vol 83, pp 1–11.

16 Weber PC: Are we what we eat? Fatty acids in nutrition and in cell membranes: cell functions and disorders induced by dietary conditions. Svanoybukt/Norway, Svanoy Foundation, 1989, Report No 4, pp 9–18.

17 Simopoulos AP: Evolutionary aspects of diet: fatty acids, insulin resistance and obesity; in VanItallie TB, Simopoulos AP (eds). Obesity: New Directions in Assessment and Management. Philadelphia, Charles Press, 1995, pp 241–261.

18 Simopoulos AP: Trans fatty acids; in Spiller GA (ed): Handbook of Lipids in Human Nutrition. Boca Raton, CRC Press, 1995, pp 91–99.

19 Simopoulos AP: Omega–3 fatty acids in inflammation an autoimmune diseases. J Am Coll Nutr 2002; 21:495–505.

20 Freeman MP, Hibbeln JR, Wisner KL, Davis JM, Mischoulon D, Peet M, Keck PE Jr, Marangell LB, Richardson AJ, Lake J, Stoll AL: Omega–3 fatty acids: evidence basis for treatment and future research in psychiatry. J Clin Psychiatry 2006; 67:1954–1967.

21 Lin PY, Su KP: A meta-analytic review of double-blind, placebo-controlled trials of antidepressant efficacy of omega–3 fatty acids. J Clin Psychiatry 2007;68:1056–1061.

22 Bourre JM: Dietary omega–3 fatty acids and psychiatry: mood, behavior, stress, depression, dementia and aging. J Nutr Health Aging 2005;9:31–38.

23 Hunter JE: Omega–3 fatty acids from vegetable oils; in Galli C, Simopoulos AP (eds): Biological Effects and Nutritional Essentiality. Series A: Life Sciences. New York, Plenum Press, 1989, vol 171, pp 43–55.

24 Litin L, Sacks F: Trans-fatty-acid content of common foods. N Engl J Med 1993;329:1969–1970.

25 Raper NR, Cronin FJ, Exler J: Omega–3 fatty acid content of the US food supply. J Am College Nutr 1992;11:304.

26 Ledger HP: Body composition as a basis for a comparative study of some East African animals. Symp Zool Soc Lond 1968;21:289–310.

27 Crawford MA: Fatty acid ratios in free-living and domestic animals. Lancet 1968;i:1329–1333.

28 Crawford MA, Gale MM, Woodford MH: Linoleic acid and linolenic acid elongation products in muscle tissue of Syncerus caffer and other ruminant species. Biochem J 1969;115:25–27.

29 Simopoulos AP, Norman HA, Gillaspy JE, Duke JA: Common purslane: a source of omega–3 fatty acids and antioxidants. J Am College Nutr 1992;11:374–382.

30 Simopoulos AP, Norman HA, Gillaspy JE: Purslane in human nutrition and its potential for world agriculture. World Rev Nutr Diet. Basel, Karger, 1995, vol 77, pp 47–74.

31 Simopoulos AP, Salem N Jr: Purslane: a terrestrial source of omega–3 fatty acids. N Engl J Med 1986; 315:833.

32 Simopoulos AP, Gopalan C (eds): Plants in Human Health and Nutrition Policy. World Rev Nutr Diet. Basel, Karger, 2003, vol 91.

33 Zeghichi S, Kallithrka S, Simopoulos AP, Kypriotakis Z: Nutritional composition of selected wild plants in the diet of Crete. 2003, vol 91, pp 22–40.

34 Simopoulos AP: Omega–3 fatty acids in wild plants, seeds and nuts. Asian Pacific J Clin Nutr 2002; 11(suppl 6):S163–S173.

35 Simopoulos AP: Omega–3 fatty acids and antioxidants in edible wild plants. Biol Res 2004;37:263–277.

36 Simopoulos AP, Salem N Jr: n–3 fatty acids in eggs from range-fed Greek chickens. N Engl J Med 1989; 321:1412.

37 Simopoulos AP, Salem N Jr: Egg yolk as a source of long-chain polyunsaturated fatty acids in infant feeding. Am J Clin Nutr 1992;55:411–414.

38 Van Vliet T, Katan MB: Lower ratio of n–3 to n–6 fatty acids in cultured than in wild fish. Am J Clin Nutr 1990:51:1–2.

39 Cordain L, Martin C, Florant G, Watkins BA: The fatty acid composition of muscle, brain, marrow and adipose tissue in elk: evolutionary implications for human dietary requirements. World Rev Nutr Diet. Basel, Karger, 1998, vol 83, p 225.

40 Sinclair AJ, Slattery WJ, O'Dea K: The analysis of polyunsaturated fatty acids in meat by capillary gas-liquid chromotography. J Food Sci Agric 1982;33: 771–776.

41 Sugano M, Hirahara F: Polyunsaturated fatty acids in the food chain in Japan. Am J Clin Nutr 2000; 71(suppl):189S–196S.

42 Pella D, Dubnov G, Singh RB, Sharma R: Effects of an Indo-Mediterranean diet on the omega–6/omega–3 ratio in patients at high risk of coronary artery disease: the Indian paradox. World Rev Nutr Diet. Basel, Karger, 2003, vol 92, pp 74–80.

43 Sanders TAB: Polyunsaturated fatty acids in the food chain in Europe. Am J Clin Nutr 2000; 71(suppl):S176–S178.

44 De Gòmez Dumm IN, Brenner RR: Oxidative desaturation of α-linolenic, linoleic, and stearic acids by human liver microsomes. Lipids 1975;10: 315–317.

45 Emken EA, Adlof RO, Rakoff H, Rohwedder WK: Metabolism of deuterium-labeled linolenic, linoleic, oleic, stearic and palmitic acid in human subjects; in Baillie TA, Jones JR (eds): Synthesis and Application of Isotopically Labeled Compounds 1988. Amsterdam, Elsevier Science, 1989, pp 713–716.

46 Hague TA, Christoffersen BO: Effect of dietary fats on arachidonic acid and eicosapentaenoic acid biosynthesis and conversion to C22 fatty acids in isolated liver cells. Biochim Biophys Acta 1984;796: 205–217.

47 Hague TA, Christoffersen BO: Evidence for peroxisomal retroconversion of adrenic acid (22:4n–6) and docosahexaenoic acid (22:6n–3) in isolated liver cells. Biochim Biophys Acta 1986;875:165–173.

48 Indu M, Ghafoorunissa G: n–3 fatty acids in Indian diets – comparison of the effects of precursor (α-linolenic acid) vs. product (long chain n–3 polyunsaturated fatty acids). Nutr Res 1992;12:569–582.

49 Carlson SE, Rhodes PG, Ferguson MG: Docosahexaenoic acid status of preterm infants at birth and following feeding with human milk or formula. Am J Clin Nutr 1986;44:798–804.

50 Singer P, Jaeger W, Voigt S, Theil H: Defective desaturation and elongation of n–6 and n–3 fatty acids in hypertensive patients. Prostaglandins Leukot Med 1984;15:159–165.

51 Honigmann G, Schimke E, Beitz J, Mest HJ, Schliack V: Influence of a diet rich in linolenic acid on lipids, thrombocyte aggregation and prostaglandins in type I (insulin-dependent) diabetes (abstract). Diabetologia 1982;23:175.

52 Simopoulos AP: Essential fatty acids in health and chronic disease. Am J Clin Nutr 1999;70(suppl):560S–569S.

53 Serhan CN, Chiang N, Van Dyke TE: Resolving inflammation: dual anti-inflammatory and pro-resolution lipid mediators. Nat Rev Immunol 2008;8:349–361.

54 McMahon B, Godson C: Lipoxins: endogenous regulators of inflammation. Am J Physiol Renal Physiol 2004;286:F189–F201.

55 Kang ZB, Ge Y, Chen Z, Brown J, Lapasota M, Leaf A, Kang JX: Adenoviral transfer of Caenorhabditis elegans n–3 fatty acid desaturase optimizes fatty acid composition in mammalian heart cells. Proc Natl Acad Sci USA 2001;98:4050–4054.

56 Ge Y-L, Chen Z, Kang ZB, Cluette-Brown J, Laposata M, Kang JX: Effects of adenoviral transfer of Caenorhabditis elegans n–3 fatty acid desaturase on the lipid profile and growth of human breast cancer cells. Anticancer Res 2002;22:537–544.

57 Kang JX: The importance of omega–6/omega–3 fatty acid ratio in cell function. The gene transfer of omega–3 fatty acid desaturase. World Rev Nutr Diet. Basel, Karger, 2003, vol 92, pp 23–36.

58 Kang JX, Wang J, Wu L, Kang ZB: Fat-1 mice convert n–6 to n–3 fatty acids. Nature 2004;427:504.

59 Kang JX: Balance of omega–6/omega–3 fatty acids is important for health: the evidence from gene transfer studies. World Rev Nutr Diet. Basel, Karger, 2004, vol 95, pp 93–102.

60 Lai L, Kang JX, Li R, Wang J, Witt WT, Yong HY, Hao Y, Was DM, Murphy CN, Rieke A, Samuel M, Linville ML, Korte SW, Evans RW, Starzl TE, Prather RS, Dai Y: Generation of cloned transgenic pigs rich in omega–3 fatty acids. Nat Biotechnol 2006;4:435–436.

61 Kang JX: Fat-1 transgenic mice: a new model for omega–3 research. Prostaglandins Leukot Essent Fatty Acids 2007;77:263–267.

62 Simopoulos AP: The role of fatty acids in gene expression: health implications. Ann Nutr Metab 1996;40:303–311.

63 Hibbeln JR, Salem N Jr: Dietary polyunsaturated fatty acids and depression: when cholesterol does not satisfy. Am J Clin Nutr 1995;62:1–9.

64 Hibbeln JR, Umhau JC, Linnoila M George DT, Ragan PW, Shoaf SE, Vaughan MR, Rawlings R, Salem N Jr: A replication study of violent and nonviolent subjects: cerebrospinal fluid metabolites of serotonin and dopamine are predicted by plasma essential fatty acids. Biol Psychiatry 1998;44:243–249.

65 Hibbeln JR, Linnoila M, Umhau JC, Rawlings R, George DT, Salem N Jr: Essential fatty acids predict metabolites of serotonin and dopamine in cerebrospinal fluid among healthy control subjects, and early- and late-onset alcoholics. Biol Psychiatry 1998;44:235–242.

66 Maes M, Smith R, Christophe A, Cosyns P, Desnyder R, Meltzer H: Fatty acid composition in major depression: decreased ω-3 fractions in cholesteryl esters and increased C20:4ω–6/C20:5ω–3 ratio in cholesteryl esters and phospholipids. J Affect Disord 1996;38:35–46.

67 Maes M, Smith R, Christophe A, Vandoolaeghe E, Van Gastel A, Neels H, Demedts P, Wauters A, Meltzer HY: Lower serum high-density lipoprotein cholesterol in major depression and in depressed men with serious suicidal attempts: relationship with immune inflammatory markers. Acta Psychiatr Scand 1997;95:212–221.

68 Peet M, Murphy B, Shay J, Horrobin D: Depletion of omega–3 fatty acid levels in red blood cell membranes of depressive patients. Biol Psychiatry 1998; 43:315–319.

69 Locke CA, Stoll AL: Omega–3 fatty acids in major depression. World Rev Nutr Diet. Basel, Karger, 2001, vol 89, pp 173–185.

70 Stoll AL, Severus WE, Freeman MP, Rueter S, Zboyan HA, Diamond E, Cress KK, Marangell LB: Omega–3 fatty acids in bipolar disorder: a preliminary double-blind, placebo-controlled trial. Arch Gen Psychiatry 1999;56:407–412.

71 Kiecolt-Glaser JK, Belury MA, Porter K, Beversdorf DQ, Lemeshow S, Glaser R: Depressive symptoms, omega–6:omega–3 fatty acids, and inflammation in older adults. Psychosom Med 2007;69:217–224.

72 Kunert KS, Tisdale AS, Stern ME, Smith JA, Gipson IK: Analysis of topical cyclosporine treatment of patients with dry eye syndrome: effect of conjunctival lymphocytes. Arch Ophthalmol 2000;118:1489–1496.

73 Marsh P, Pflugfelder SC: Topical nonpreserved methylprednisolone therapy for keratoconjuntivitis sicca in Sjögren syndrome. Ophthalmology 1999; 106:811–816.

74 Solomon A, Dursun D, Liu Z, Xie Y, Macri A, Pflugfelder SC: Pro- and anti-inflammatory forms of interleukin-1 in the tear fluid and conjunctiva of patients with dry-eye disease. Invest Opthalmol Vis Sci 2001;42:2283–2292.

75 Miljanovic B, Trivedi KA, Dana MR, Gilbard JP, Buring JE, Schaumberg DA: Relation between dietary n–3 and n–6 fatty acids and clinically diagnosed dry eye syndrome in women. Am J Clin Nutr 2005;82:887–893.

76 Snow KK, Seddon JM: Do age-related macular degeneration and cardiovascular disease share common antecedents? Ophthalmic Epidemiol 1999;6: 125–143.

77 Seddon JM, Chen CA: Epidemiology of age-related macular degeneration; in Ryan SJ (ed): Retina, ed 4, vol 2: Medical Retina. St Louis, Mosby, 2005.

78 Seddon JM, Hankinson S, Speizer F, Willett WC: A prospective study of cigarette smoking and age-related macular degeneration in women. JAMA 1996;276:1141–1146.

79 Tomany SC, Wang JJ, van Leeuwen R, Klein R, Mitchell P, Vingerling JR, Klein BE, Smith W, De Jong PT: Risk factors for incident age-related macular degeneration: pooled findings from three continents. Ophthalmology 2004;11:1280–1287.

80 Report of the Surgeon General, 2005: The Health Consequences of Smoking. http://www.cdc.gov/ tobacco/data_statistics/sgr/sgr_2004/index.htm (accessed April 18, 2007).

81 Seddon JM, Rosner B, Sperduto RD, Yannuzzi L, Haller JA, Blair NP, Willett W: Dietary fat and risk for advanced age-related macular degeneration. Arch Ophthalmol 2001;119:1191–1199.

82 Seddon JM, Cote J, Rosner B: Progression of age-related macular degeneration: association with dietary fat, transunsaturated fat, nuts, and fish intake. Arch Ophthalmol 2003;121:1728–1737.

83 Cho E, Hung S, Willett W, Rimm EB, Seddon JM, Colditz GA, Hankinson SE: Prospective study of dietary fat and the risk of age-related macular degeneration. Am J Clin Nutr 2001;73:209–218.

84 Smith W, Mitchell P, Leeder SR: Dietary fat and fish intake and age-related maculopathy. Arch Ophthalmol 2000;118:401–404.

85 Seddon J, Ajani U, Sperduto R: Dietary fat intake and age-related macular degeneration (ARVO abstract). Invest Ophthalmol Vis Sci 1994;35:2003.

86 Seddon JM, George S, Rosner B: Cigarette smoking, fish consumption, omega–3 fatty acid intake, and associations with age-related macular degeneration. The US Twin Study of Age-Related Macular Degeneration. Arch Ophthalmol 2006;124:995–1001.

Artemis P. Simopoulos, MD, President
The Center for Genetics, Nutrition and Health
2001 S Street, NW, Suite 530, Washington, DC 20009 (USA)
Tel. +1 202 462 5062, Fax +1 202 462 5241, E-Mail cgnh@bellatlantic.net

Simopoulos AP, Bazan NG (eds): Omega-3 Fatty Acids, the Brain and Retina.
World Rev Nutr Diet. Basel, Karger, 2009, vol 99, pp 17–30

Depression, Suicide and Deficiencies of Omega–3 Essential Fatty Acids in Modern Diets

Joseph R. Hibbeln

National Institutes Alcohol Abuse and Alcoholism, NIH, Bethesda, Md., USA

Background

Optimal brain function requires the ready availability of brain critical nutrients, especially during periods of extreme stress. Deficiencies of brain-specific nutrients, in addition to inadequate calories, may not only substantially contribute to suboptimal cognition and alertness, but may manifest as severe psychiatric disorders including adjustment disorders, major depression, impulsive violence and suicide. The mammalian brain is primarily composed of fats and lipids, usually 60% wet weight. Approximately 30% of fatty acid pool cannot be made de novo and must be obtained through the diet and are thus termed essential fatty acids. Seafood, fish oils and fortified foods are rich sources of the long-chain ω–3 fatty acids (ω–3 LCFAs: eicosapentaenoic (EPA), docosapentaenoic (DPAω–3), and docosahexaenoic acids (DHA)). DHA is selectively concentrated in neuronal membranes comprising 14% of total fatty acids. Plausible biological mechanisms linking dietary deficiencies of ω–3 LCFAs with psychiatric illness include: depletion of serotonin and dopamine levels by 50% in animal models [1], impaired neuronal migration, connectivity, timed apoptosis, and dendritic arborization, such that there is an irreversible disruption in the neuronal pathways that regulate behavior [2] neuroinflammatory processes and dysregulation of the hypothalamic pituitary adrenal axis [3].

This work does not represent any policy or position of the National Institutes of Health and is solely the scientific opinion of the author.

Defining Deficiency

The absence of signs of deficiency related to critical target tissues has been considered in formulation of required dietary intakes. DHA is selectively concentrated in synaptic neuronal membranes and, comprises nearly 14% of all brain fatty acids and is necessary for optimal neurological function [4]. Thus, deficit intakes of DHA or ω–3 LCFAs supporting DHA are likely to manifest as signs or symptoms of neural dysfunction including neurodevelopmental and neuropsychiatric impairments. Neurodevelopmental impairments are identified as signs and symptoms of deficiency in setting the dietary reference intakes (DRIs) [5] for biotin, folate, iodine and iron. Psychiatric and neurocognitive impairments are also identified as signs and symptoms of deficiency in setting the DRIs [5] for vitamin B_6; depression and confusion, vitamin B_{12}; mood changes, confusion, insomnia and cognitive impairments, biotin; depression, lethargy and hallucinations, folate; irritability and difficulty concentrating, niacin; depression and apathy, pantothenic acid; irritability, restlessness, apathy and malaise, thiamin; apathy, irritability, confusion decreased short-term memory, iodine; hypothyroidism and learning impairments and iron; impaired cognition and decreased work capacity. Severe symptoms of major depression may be used as a categorical diagnosis and can potentially be used to calculate an estimated average requirement. Major depression is commonly a chronic degenerative disease. Neurodevelopmental and neuropsychiatric impairments are clearly identified by the Food and Nutrition Board as signs and symptoms of deficiencies for several nutrients [5], thus setting a precedent potentially applicable to ω–3 LCFA's deficiencies in similar outcome parameters.

The viewpoints of Sir Austin Bradford Hill [6] are routinely evaluated in assessing the strength of the body of epidemiological and other evidence for possible relationships to causality. We posit that DHA and ω–3 LCFA deficiencies are causally related to an increase risk of psychiatric disorders, specifically major depression. Evidence linking deficiencies in ω–3 LCFAs in psychiatric disorders has recently been reviewed in a UK Parliamentary Inquiry Report on Nutrients and Mental Health [7] and by the American Psychiatric Association in the treatment recommendations issued for ω–3 LCFAs in psychiatric patients [8]. Both find consistent data across ecological cross-national studies, epidemiological studies, case-control comparisons of blood and brain tissues, in double-blind randomized placebo-controlled trials and meta-analyses of these trials, that low fish consumption or low ω–3 body compositional status increases risk of depression and other affective illnesses. Here we assess in detail ecological, epidemiological dietary intake data, blood and tissue composition data and randomized clinical intervention trials for evidence of causal links between low intakes of ω–3 fatty acid and risk of significant depressive symptoms. Data linking low intakes of ω–3 LCFAs to risk of suicide or suicidal ideation is beginning to emerge and shows great promise.

Hill 'Criteria'

Strength
The ecological and epidemiological associations between low seafood and ω–3 LCFA intake are strong. Ecological studies indicate that in comparison to countries with the highest consumption, low seafood consumption is associated with a 65-fold higher risk for lifetime prevalence of major depression (r = –0.84, p < 0.0001) [9], a 50-fold higher risk for postnatal depression (r = –0.81, p < 0.0001) [10], a 30-fold higher risk for bipolar spectrum disorder (r = –0.80, p < 0.0003) [11], and a 10-fold higher risk of death from homicide mortality (r = –0.63, p < 0.0006) [12]. Correlation coefficients in these ranges are considered to be strong.

Consistency
'Consistent findings observed by different persons in different places with different samples strengthen the likelihood of an effect' [6]. We find a relationship of low ω–3 LCFA status and greater risk of affective illnesses to be consistent across ecological studies, epidemiological studies, case-control studies and biological tissue sample studies. In particular, epidemiological studies have reported strong associations between low seafood intake and greater risk of depression with a high degree of consistency. Among 1,767 subjects in Northern Finland, Tanskanen et al. [13] found that both the risk of being depressed (odds ratio (OR) 0.63; 95% confidence interval (CI) 0.43–0.94; p = 0.02) and the risk of having suicidal ideation (OR 0.57; 95% CI 0.35–0.95; p = 0.03) were significantly lower among frequent lake-fish consumers compared with more infrequent consumers. In a birth cohort of 5,689 Finnish subjects, the risk of depression was 2.6-fold (95% CI 1.4–5.1) greater and risk of suicidal thinking was 1.5-fold (95% CI 1.0–3.0) greater comparing females with rare fish consumption to regular consumers [14]. Finnish fishermen (n = 6,410) consume twice as much fish but have a lower risk of mortality from alcohol-related diseases (OR 0.59; 95% CI 0.41–0.82) and suicides (OR 0.61; 95% CI 0.39–0.91) compared to the general population, after adjustment [15]. In contrast, Hakkarainen et al. [16] found no associations between the dietary intake of ω–3 fatty acids or fish consumption and self-report of depressed mood, hospitalization for a major depressive episode, or suicide among 29,133 Finnish men. However, there was a high covariance with fish and ω–6 linoleate consumption, which was 20-fold higher than ω–3 LCFA from fish [17]. Thus, it is difficult to determine which factor was specifically associated with an increased risk of depression. Among 21,835 Norwegians, users of cod liver oil were significantly less likely to have depressive symptoms than non-users after adjusting for multiple possible confounding factors (OR 0.71; 95% CI 0.52–0.97) [18]. In a longitudinal follow-up study of 13,017 French subjects, subjects consuming fatty fish, or having an ω–3 LCFA intake >1 en%, had significantly reduced risk of single or recurrent depressive episodes [19]. In the Zutphen Study of the Elderly, high intakes of ω–3 LCFAs (mean 407 mg/day) were associated with lower risk of

depressive symptoms (OR 0.46; 95% CI 0.22–0.95) compared with low intakes (21 mg/day) [20]. Among 7,903 Spanish subjects, moderate consumption of fish had a relative risk reduction of >30% [21]. Among 10,602 men from Northern Ireland and France, the greater depressed mood is associated with lower fish intake in a non-linear relationship [22]. A similar non-linear relationship between greater depression and lower fish intake was described among a UK population (n = 2,982) [23]. Jacka et al. [24] also found no association between fish consumption and depression defined by DSM-III criteria in a New Zealand population (n = 755). Murakami et al. [25] found no association between fish intake and lower risk of depressive symptoms among 618 adults. However, the mean ω–3 LCFA intake was approximately 0.37 en% far above the putative estimated average requirements and recommended dietary allowances presented here, thus the majority of the population may have adequate intakes. We conclude that epidemiological studies based on reports of dietary intakes have found an association between low ω–3 LCFA intake and significant depressive symptoms with good consistency.

Specificity

Tissue compositional studies have fairly consistently reported a lower ω–3 LCFA status and/or a higher ω–6 LCFA status among depressed subjects. The most specific evidence of tissue compositional deficits is the finding that DHA was 22% lower in the postmortem orbitofrontal cortex of patients with a major depressive disorder [26]. A similar deficit of DHA was found in the orbitofrontal cortex of patients with a bipolar disorder [27]. The pathophysiology of depressive disorders is thought to involve deficits in orbitofrontal cortex function [34]. These specific deficits in brain composition, combined with the epidemiologically based tissue compositional studies, indicate that deficits of ω–3 LCFA, in particular EPA and DHA, are associated with depressive illnesses. Adams et al. [28] found a significant positive correlation between the severity of depression and both the erythrocyte phospholipid arachidonic acid (AA) and EPA ratio and erythrocyte EPA alone. Maes et al. [29] found lower ω–3 LCFAs in serum phospholipids and cholesteryl esters of depressed patients compared to controls. Edwards et al. [30] reported lower EPA and DHA concentrations in the erythrocytes of depressed compared to control subjects. They also noted a biological gradient in which lower erythrocyte DHA correlated with greater severity of symptoms (r = 0.80, p < 0.01). Peet et al. [31] also reported a nearly 50% reduction in DHA in the erythrocytes of depressed subjects. Among a community sample of the elderly in Bordeaux, plasma EPA alone was inversely associated with severity of depressive symptoms [32]. Among adolescents in Crete (n = 90), depressive symptoms were negatively associated with EPA and positively associated with the ω–6 fatty acid dihomo-γ-linolenic acid in adipose tissue [33]. Among 247 healthy males in Crete, mildly depressed subjects had significantly reduced (–34.6%) adipose tissue DHA levels compared to non-depressed subjects. Multiple linear regression analysis indicated that depression related negatively to adipose tissue DHA levels [34]. Among 3,884 elderly subjects in Rotterdam, ω–3 LCFAs were significantly lower (5.2 vs. 5.9%, p = 0.02) and ratios of ω–6 to ω–3 LCFAs were higher (7.2 vs. 6.6, p = 0.01) comparing subjects with depressive disorders to controls [35]. Among a US community sample (n = 207), higher plasma AA and lower EPA concentrations were associated with greater depression and neuroticism [36] and erythrocyte ω–3 LCFAs are decreased in patients with social anxiety disorder [37]. EPA levels in erythrocytes were significantly lower in suicide attempters than those of the control subjects [38]. When the highest and lowest quartiles of EPA in RBCs were compared, the ORs of suicide attempt was 0.12 in the highest quartile (95% CI 0.04–0.36, p for trend = 0.0001) after adjustment for possible confounding factors [38]. A bias against publications failing to find tissue compositional differences may exist, however most published studies indicate a lower ω–3 LCFA body composition status among depressed subjects.

Depression Associated with Other Medical Disorders

Compared to controls, depressed patients with acute coronary syndromes had significantly lower concentrations of total ω–3 and DHA, and higher ratios of AA/DHA and AA/EPA [39]. A second study of patients with acute coronary syndromes reported higher depression severity scores which were significantly associated with lower DHA levels, with similar but non-significant trends observed for EPA and total ω–3 LCFA levels [40]. Consistent with these reports, Schins et al. [41] found higher plasma AA/EPA ratios comparing depressed to non-depressed subjects among 50 postmyocardial infarction patients. Kobayakawa et al. [42] found no differences comparing depressed and non-depressed lung cancer patients, but used a very low cut point to define depression. No differences in ω–3 LCFA compositions were found comparing depressed and non-depressed patients with multiple sclerosis [43].

Temporality
Deficits in ω–3 LCFA tissue status can be caused by either low intakes of ω–3 LCFA and/or excessive intakes of competing ω–6 fatty acids, for example greater dietary intakes of ω–6 linoleic acid, ranging from 1 to 8 en%, results in 10-fold lower tissue concentrations of ω–3 LCFA [44]. Strong temporal relationships have been reported between increasing intakes of the ω–6 fatty acid, linoleic acid and greater prevalence rates of major depression [45] and homicide mortality in five different countries between 1960 and 2000 (20-fold higher risk, r = 0.94, p < 0.0001) [46].

Biological Gradient
A biological gradient in the reduction of risk of depression is evident in ecological studies and epidemiological studies. Progressively greater exposure to ω–3 LCFA from fish consumption generally leads to a progressively lower incidence of

psychiatric symptoms and illness as reviewed above. Direct compositional analyses of tissue composition usually report a similar biological gradient, as reviewed above. In ecological and epidemiological studies, negative exponential equations consistently best describe the biological gradient relationships [44].

Plausibility

DHA is a nutrient required for neurological development and cannot be substituted by any other molecule [4, 47]. Studies of the multiple interacting mechanisms linking ω–3 LCFA and depressive symptoms have recently been reviewed [2, 48]. Plausible biological mechanisms linking dietary deficiencies of ω–3 LCFAs with psychiatric illness include: depletion of serotonin and dopamine levels by 50% in animal models, impaired neuronal migration, connectivity, timed apoptosis, and dendritic arborization, such that there is an irreversible disruption in the neuronal pathways that regulate behavior [2], neuroinflammatory processes [29, 49] and dysregulation of the hypothalamic pituitary adrenal axis [3]. ω–3 LCFAs may prevent vascular contributions to depression [50]. Inadequate serotonergic and dopaminergic function has long been recognized in the pathophysiology of depression and is the target of most pharmaceutical treatments. Concentrations of serotonin and dopamine were nearly doubled in the frontal cortex of piglets among piglets fed infant formula supplemented with DHA and AA for 18 days [1]. Unconditioned mild stress induced a significant decrease in the tissue levels of serotonin in the frontal cortex, striatum and hippocampus in the range of 40–65%. Interestingly, the ω–3 LCFA supplementation reversed this stress-induced reduction in 5-HT levels and decreased aggressive behavior [51]. One generation of ω–3 LCFA deficiency markedly increased depressive and aggressive behaviors in rats [52]. Consistent with these animal studies, Hibbeln et al. [53] found the lower plasma DHA concentrations were correlated with lower concentrations of the metabolites of both serotonin and dopamine in cerebrospinal fluid among healthy controls. Low cerebrospinal fluid concentrations of these metabolites have been repeatedly reported among suicidal and impulsive patients. Chronic alcohol use, in the context of a low ω–3 diet, depleted DHA levels by 50% in rhesus frontal cortex (from 14 to 7%), suggesting that depression and impulsive behaviors associated with alcohol may be attributable, in part, to depletion of ω–3 LCFAs [54]. Alcohol-induced depletion of neural tissues may contribute to the high rates of violence and depression among alcoholics [45]. We conclude that many known biological mechanisms plausibly link ω–3 LCFA deficiencies to depressive and aggressive pathologies.

Coherence

'Coherence between epidemiological and laboratory findings increases the likelihood of an effect' [6]. One example of the coherence is the role of ω–3 LCFA in relationship to depressive symptoms in pregnancy. We posited that since maternal DHA is selectively transported to the fetus, mothers without sufficient dietary intakes may become depleted, leaving them more vulnerable to depression symptoms during or after

pregnancy [10]. A cross-national ecological study supported this proposition linking both low maternal milk DHA composition and low seafood consumption with higher rates of postnatal depression [10]. In a series of animal experiments, Levant et al. [55–57] have demonstrated depletion of regionally specific brain DHA in a single reproductive cycle, with multiple parity and alterations of dopamine and dopamine-related behaviors. Decreased brain DHA was associated with decreased hippocampal brain-derived neurotrophic factor, increased corticosterone responses to stress and increased immobility on the forced swim test [58]. Otto et al. [59] found that post-partum depression symptoms were associated with a slower recovery of DHA plasma status. A recent randomized controlled trial among pregnant women reported significantly lower depression scores and higher rates of clinical response (62%) to 3.5 g/day of ω–3 fatty acids compared to placebo (27%) [60]. Another randomized controlled trial reported a trend towards efficacy, but was described by the authors as under-powered [61]. Recent non-blinded trials of EPA and DHA supplementation have also reported a reduction of depressive symptoms related to pregnancy of 50% [62, 63]. Two prior epidemiological studies (from New Zealand and Japan) reported no association between seafood consumption and pregnancy-related depressive symptoms. The New Zealand study included only 80 women [64] and consequently did not have sufficient power. Although the Japanese study had much larger numbers (n = 865) it used a cut point of 9+ (rather than 13+) on the Edinburgh Postnatal Depression Scale and almost all the subjects had a relatively high intake of oily fish with very few subjects consuming zero ω–3 from seafood [65]. In contrast, Sontrop and Campbell [66] found low intakes of ω–3 LCFAs from seafood among smoking and single women associated depressive symptoms in pregnancy when more clinically significant cut points were used. In summary, the status of studies in pregnancy-related depression is coherent and promising: animal studies, adequately powered intervention and epidemiological studies do support the proposition that ω–3 LCFAs may have therapeutic benefit.

Experiment

The specificity and efficacy of ω–3 LCFAs in reducing significant depressive symptoms has been assessed in the meta-analyses of randomized placebo-controlled trials. Three recent meta-analyses of up to 11 randomized placebo-controlled trials of ω–3 fatty acids have each reported large treatment effect sizes of ω–3 LCFA in reducing significant depressive symptoms [63, 67, 68]. In 2006 the accumulation of data was sufficient enough for the American Psychiatric Association to issue treatment recommendation for ω–3 LCFAs [63]. Since that time, several confirmatory studies have also been published. Jazayeri et al. [69] reported similar response rates (defined as a 50% reduction in depressive symptoms) comparing patients receiving 1 g of EPA alone (50%) to fluoxetine (56%) but significantly better rates (81%) when patients received both EPA and fluoxetine in combination. Antypa et al. [70] found a reduction of depression-related cognitive symptoms even among healthy controls. Mischoulon et al. [71] reported anti-depressant efficacy of DHA 1 g/day, but not at higher doses. Dinan et al. [72] reported that ω–3 LCFA levels and ratios of EPA to AA predicted clinical responses to anti-depressants. Freund-Levi et al. [73] found that reduction of aggressive and depressive symptoms in Alzheimer's patients to ω–3 LCFAs appeared to depend upon their APOEω4 genotype. Some randomized controlled trials have failed to find treatment effects [74–77]. However, Elkin et al. [78] have established that if clinical trials include subjects without a sufficiently high initial severity of depression, antidepressants were unlikely to demonstrate treatment effects because of inadequate power and floor effects inherent in the clinical study of depression [78]. A common feature of the clinical trials that have failed to find antidepressive effects of ω–3 LCFAs has been the enrollment of patients below the cut points of depressive symptom severity established by Elkin et al. [78] with one exception [75]. Thus, insufficiently powered trials should not be considered as definitively negative trials. The demonstration of efficacy in randomized trials appears to depend upon adequate symptom severity, baseline ω–3 LCFA status, perhaps the relative amounts of EPA and DHA, and perhaps allelic variance. The evidence from the currently published placebo-controlled randomized trials and meta-analyses of these trials indicate that ω–3 LCFAs are effective in treating severe depression.

Analogy

Nutritional deficiencies in vitamin B_6, vitamin B_{12}, niacin, folate, pantothenic acid iodine and iron results in reversible neuropsychiatric symptoms. Deficiency symptoms for these nutrients are rarely confined to one organ system. Deficiencies in ω–3 LCFAs may similarly increase risk of several chronic diseases. We have previously proposed that an increased risk of cardiovascular disease and an increased risk of affective disorders are two different manifestations of a common deficiency of ω–3 LCFAs [45].

Suicide Risk, Prevention and Treatment

Epidemiologic data indicate that low fish consumption is a risk factor, but certainly not a sole determinant for suicide mortality. In a 17-year follow-up of 256,118 Japanese subjects [79], those who ate fish daily had a lower risk of death from suicide (OR 0.81; 95% CI 0.27–0.91) compared to subjects eating fish less than daily, but that result was not adjusted for confounding variables. We examined 1,767 subjects in northern Finland and reported that frequent fish consumption (twice per week or more) significantly reduced the risk of reporting depressive symptoms (OR 0.63, $p < 0.03$) and of reporting suicidal thinking (OR 0.57, $p < 0.04$) after adjustment for confounding variables [80]. De Vriese et al. [81] reported that the seasonal variation in ω–3 plasma status closely correlated with the seasonal variation in suicide rates in Belgium.

These epidemiological observations are consistent with the assessment of ω–3 LCFA body compositions directly among patients. Among suicide attempters without depression as a primary diagnosis, low concentrations of plasma EPA alone were robustly correlated with greater psychopathology on rating scales of impulsivity, guilt, future suicide risk, and most subscales of the Comprehensive Psychopathological Rating Scale [82]. In a case-control study of 200 subjects in Dalian, China, Huan et al. [38] found 30% lower RBC concentrations of EPA among suicide attempters and a dose response association of low EPA status and greater risk. Low DHA status predicted greater risk of a new suicide attempt in a follow-up study of more than 800 days, 5% of subjects above the median split had new attempts compared to 50% having new attempts among those below the median split [83]. These subjects also had resting PET scans quantifying regional glucose uptake. Future suicide attempters had greater activity in the anterior cingulate and limbic forebrain, consistent with the suspected pathophysiology of severe depression and posttraumatic stress disorder (PTSD). Low DHA in plasma phospholipid robustly predicted this regional hyperactivity ($r = -0.86$, $p < 0.0001$) indicating that low DHA status may increase limbic system-mediated anxiety [83]. In a randomized blinded placebo-controlled trial, we have reported a 45% reduction in suicidal thinking and a 30% reduction in depression among patients with recurrent self-harm recruited from an emergency room 84]. This intervention used 2 g/day of ω–3 LCFAs in a 12-week trial of 49 subjects. Subjects also reported a reduced perception of daily stresses and anxiety which is likely relevant to reduction of risk of the development of PTSD. While substantial work needs to be conducted in the study of ω–3 deficiencies and increased suicide risk, current data suggest an apparent beneficial effect.

Cost Savings to Healthcare Systems

Because of the well-established benefits to cardiovascular health, cost-efficacy analyses have been conducted for use of ω–3 LCFAs for secondary prevention for cardiovascular disease. The Lewin Group (2006) [89] determined that supplementation with 1,800 mg/day of ω–3 long-chain fatty acids was estimated to prevent 384,303,000 hospitalizations due to cardiovascular disease and save USD 3.1 billion over 5 years in the USA, using Congressional Budget office methodology. Similar reductions in misery and economic costs could be expected for the reduction in burden of neuropsychiatric illnesses. For example, depressive disorders appear to respond to ω–3 LCFAs more rapidly (within 2–4 weeks) and have a larger treatment effect size, in comparison to the well-documented effects in the reduction in cardiovascular risk [44]. The use of ω–3 LCFAs in primary prevention is likely to be much more cost-effective than providing treatment of established neuropsychaitric illness. A RAND study indicated that evidence-based care using psychotherapy techniques, for PTSD and major depression, could save as much as USD 1.7 billion, or USD 1,063 per returning veteran; the savings come from increases in productivity, as well as from reductions in the expected number of suicides [85]. The use of ω–3 LCFAs in primary prevention of cardiovascular disease and psychiatric illness could potentially result in much greater savings in cost and human misery.

Cultural Symbolism

It may not be too broad a leap to begin to question if our societal happiness or sense of collective meaning be impaired by deficiencies in ω–3 fatty acids? One approach to examining that question has been an evaluation of the meaning of fish as a cultural symbol [86]. The data from randomized studies in major depression, suicide and aggression indicate that fish is a food with psychotropic properties because it is rich in long-chain ω–3 fatty acids that improve mental wellbeing, i.e. change emotional states. Central to the neuroscience of the assignment of meaning to a visual object is the pairing of that object to an emotional state. Symbols of foods or other substances with psychotropic properties may become paired to the emotional states the substances induce. We posited that traditional cultural medical practices and religious symbolism reflect the ability of long-chain ω–3 fatty acids in fish and seafood to reduce depressive or dysphoric states [86]. Symbols of fish may have become consciously and unconsciously associated with the healing of mental illness and the optimization of emotional wellbeing sacred to both religion and healing. Throughout time, religious and spiritual practitioners have altered their dietary practices, observed their altered internal states, and linked dietary practices to spiritual beliefs using religious and cultural symbols. In traditional Chinese medicine, seafood is used to calm excessive aggression. In Hinduism, Buddhism, Shinto, Islam, ancient Middle Eastern religions, Judaism, and Christianity, fish is symbolically associated with central tenets of faith and healing. For at least six millennia among independent cultures, fish has nearly universally been symbolically associated with sacred symbols of peace and religion. A recent study of a religious group that strictly adheres to the Christian Orthodox Church is remarkably consistent with this proposition [87]. As proscribed by the Church, adherents followed dietary laws for abstinence from meat, eggs, and dairy products for most Wednesdays, Fridays and other periods such as 40 days before Christmas and 40 days before Easter, as well as August 1–15 and other shorter periods, adding up to about 180 days per year [88]. Seafood is not only allowed but is also expected to be eaten and resulted in higher levels of adipose DHA in comparison to controls [87]. These higher adipose DHA levels were also correlated with lower levels of depressive symptoms. Thus, the culturally encoded dietary laws which affirm their religious identity also changed their body compositions of DHA and improved mental wellbeing. The treatment recommendations of the American Heart Association and American Psychiatric Association to consume seafood 2–3 times per week are remarkably similar to the dietary practices of the Christian Orthodox Church.

Acknowledgement

This research was supported in part by the Intramural Research Program of the NIAAA, NIH.

References

1 De la Presa Owens S, Innis SM: Docosahexaenoic and arachidonic acid prevent a decrease in dopaminergic and serotoninergic neurotransmitters in frontal cortex caused by a linoleic and α-linolenic acid deficient diet in formula-fed piglets. J Nutr 1999; 129:2088–2093.

2 Sinclair AJ, Begg D, Mathai M, Weisinger RS: Omega–3 fatty acids and the brain: review of studies in depression. Asia Pac J Clin Nutr 2007;16(suppl 1): 391–397.

3 Hibbeln JR, Bissette G, Umhau JC, George DT: Omega–3 status and cerebrospinal fluid corticotrophin-releasing hormone in perpetrators of domestic violence. Biol Psychiatry 2004;56:895–897.

4 Salem N Jr, Litman B, Kim HY, Gawrisch K: Mechanisms of action of docosahexaenoic acid in the nervous system. Lipids 2001;36:945–959.

5 Hellwig JP, Meyers LD: Dietary reference intakes: the essential guide to nutrient requirements. Washington, National Academy of Sciences Press, 2006.

6 Hill AB: The environment and disease: association or causation? Proc R Soc Med 1965;58:295–300.

7 The Associate Parliamentary Food and Health Forum: The Links between Diet and Behaviour. The Influence of Nutrition on Mental Health. London, Parliament of the United Kingdom, 2008.

8 Freeman MP, Hibbeln JR, Wisner KL, et al: Omega–3 fatty acids: evidence basis for treatment and future research in psychiatry. J Clin Psychiatry 2006;67:1954–1967.

9 Hibbeln JR: Fish consumption and major depression. Lancet 1998;351:1213.

10 Hibbeln JR: Seafood consumption, the DHA content of mothers' milk and prevalence rates of post-partum depression: a cross-national, ecological analysis. J Affect Disord 2002;69:15–29.

11 Noaghiul S, Hibbeln JR: Cross-national comparisons of seafood consumption and rates of bipolar disorders. Am J Psychiatry 2003;160:2222–2227.

12 Hibbeln JR: Seafood consumption and homicide mortality. World Rev Nutr Diet. Basel, Karger, 2001, vol 85, pp 41–46.

13 Tanskanen A, Hibbeln JR, Hintikka J, Haatainen K, Honkalampi K, Viinamäki H: Fish consumption, depression, and suicidality in a general population. Arch Gen Psychiatry 2001;58:512–513.

14 Timonen M, Horrobin D, Jokelainen J, Laitinen J, Herva A, Rasanen P: Fish consumption and depression: the Northern Finland 1966 birth cohort study. J Affect Disord 2004;82:447–452.

15 Turunen AW, Verkasalo PK, Kiviranta H, et al: Mortality in a cohort with high fish consumption. Int J Epidemiol 2008.

16 Hakkarainen R, Partonen T, Haukka J, Virtamo J, Albanes D, Lonnqvist J: Is low dietary intake of omega–3 fatty acids associated with depression? Am J Psychiatry 2004;161:567–569.

17 Hakkarainen R, Partonen T, Haukka J, Virtamo J, Albanes D, Lonnqvist J: Food and nutrient intake in relation to mental wellbeing. Nutr J 2004;3:14.

18 Raeder MB, Steen VM, Vollset SE, Bjelland I: Associations between cod liver oil use and symptoms of depression: the Hordaland Health Study. J Affect Disord 2007;101:245–249.

19 Astorg P, Couthouis A, Bertrais S, et al: Association of fish and long-chain n–3 polyunsaturated fatty acid intakes with the occurrence of depressive episodes in middle-aged French men and women. Prostaglandins Leukot Essent Fatty Acids 2008;78:171–182.

20 Kamphuis MH, Geerlings MI, Tijhuis MA, Kalmijn S, Grobbee DE, Kromhout D: Depression and cardiovascular mortality: a role for n–3 fatty acids? Am J Clin Nutr 2006;84:1513–1517.

21 Sanchez-Villegas A, Henriquez P, Figueiras A, Ortuno F, Lahortiga F, Martinez-Gonzalez MA: Long chain omega–3 fatty acids intake, fish consumption and mental disorders in the SUN cohort study. Eur J Nutr 2007;46:337–346.

22 Appleton KM, Woodside JV, Yarnell JW, et al: Depressed mood and dietary fish intake: direct relationship or indirect relationship as a result of diet and lifestyle? J Affect Disord 2007;104:217–223.

23 Appleton KM, Peters TJ, Hayward RC, et al: Depressed mood and n–3 polyunsaturated fatty acid intake from fish: non-linear or confounded association? Soc Psychiatry Psychiatr Epidemiol 2007;42:100–104.

24 Jacka FN, Pasco JA, Henry MJ, Kotowicz MA, Nicholson GC, Berk M: Dietary omega–3 fatty acids and depression in a community sample. Nutr Neurosci 2004;7:101–106.

25 Murakami K, Mizoue T, Sasaki S, et al: Dietary intake of folate, other B vitamins, and omega–3 polyunsaturated fatty acids in relation to depressive symptoms in Japanese adults. Nutrition 2008;24:140–147.

26 McNamara RK, Hahn CG, Jandacek R, et al: Selective deficits in the omega–3 fatty acid docosahexaenoic acid in the postmortem orbitofrontal cortex of patients with major depressive disorder. Biol Psychiatry 2007;62:17–24.

27 McNamara RK, Jandacek R, Rider T, et al: Deficits in docosahexaenoic acid and associated elevations in the metabolism of arachidonic acid and saturated fatty acids in the postmortem orbitofrontal cortex of patients with bipolar disorder. Psychiatry Res 2008;160:285–299.

28 Adams PB, Lawson S, Sanigorski A, Sinclair AJ: Arachidonic acid to eicosapentaenoic acid ratio in blood correlates positively with clinical symptoms of depression. Lipids 1996;31(suppl):S157–S161.

29 Maes M, Christophe A, Delanghe J, Altamura C, Neels H, Meltzer HY: Lowered omega–3 polyunsaturated fatty acids in serum phospholipids and cholesteryl esters of depressed patients. Psychiatry Res 1999;85:275–291.

30 Edwards R, Peet M, Shay J, Horrobin D: Omega–3 polyunsaturated fatty acid levels in the diet and in red blood cell membranes of depressed patients. J Affect Disord 1998;48:149–155.

31 Peet M, Murphy B, Edwards R, Shay J, Horrobin D: Depletion of docosahexaenoic acid in erythrocyte membranes of depressed patients. Biol Psychiatry 1998;43:315–319.

32 Feart C, Peuchant E, Letenneur L, et al: Plasma eicosapentaenoic acid is inversely associated with severity of depressive symptomatology in the elderly: data from the Bordeaux sample of the Three-City Study. Am J Clin Nutr 2008;87:1156–1162.

33 Mamalakis G, Jansen E, Cremers H, Kiriakakis M, Tsibinos G, Kafatos A: Depression and adipose and serum cholesteryl ester polyunsaturated fatty acids in the survivors of the seven countries study population of Crete. Eur J Clin Nutr 2006;60:1016–1023.

34 Mamalakis G, Tornaritis M, Kafatos A: Depression and adipose essential polyunsaturated fatty acids. Prostaglandins Leukot Essent Fatty Acids 2002;67: 311–318.

35 Tiemeier H, van Tuijl HR, Hofman A, Kiliaan AJ, Breteler MM: Plasma fatty acid composition and depression are associated in the elderly: the Rotterdam Study. Am J Clin Nutr 2003;78:40–46.

36 Conklin SM, Manuck SB, Yao JK, Flory JD, Hibbeln JR, Muldoon MF: High omega–6 and low omega–3 fatty acids are associated with depressive symptoms and neuroticism. Psychosom Med 2007;69:932–934.

37 Green P, Hermesh H, Monselise A, Marom S, Presburger G, Weizman A: Red cell membrane omega–3 fatty acids are decreased in nondepressed patients with social anxiety disorder. Eur Neuropsychopharmacol 2006;16:107–113.

38 Huan M, Hamazaki K, Sun Y, et al: Suicide attempt and n–3 fatty acid levels in red blood cells: a case-control study in China. Biol Psychiatry 2004;56:490–496.

39 Frasure-Smith N, Lesperance F, Julien P: Major depression is associated with lower omega–3 fatty acid levels in patients with recent acute coronary syndromes. Biol Psychiatry 2004;55:891–896.

40 Parker GB, Heruc GA, Hilton TM, et al: Low levels of docosahexaenoic acid identified in acute coronary syndrome patients with depression. Psychiatry Res 2006;141:279–286.

41 Schins A, Crijns HJ, Brummer RJ, et al: Altered omega–3 polyunsaturated fatty acid status in depressed post-myocardial infarction patients. Acta Psychiatr Scand 2007;115:35–40.

42 Kobayakawa M, Yamawaki S, Hamazaki K, Akechi T, Inagaki M, Uchitomi Y: Levels of omega–3 fatty acid in serum phospholipids and depression in patients with lung cancer. Br J Cancer 2005;93:1329–1333.

43 Aupperle RL, Denney DR, Lynch SG, Carlson SE, Sullivan DK: Omega–3 fatty acids and multiple sclerosis: relationship to depression. J Behav Med 2008;31:127–135.

44 Hibbeln JR, Nieminen LR, Blasbalg TL, Riggs JA, Lands WE: Healthy intakes of n–3 and n–6 fatty acids: estimations considering worldwide diversity. Am J Clin Nutr 2006;83:1483S–1493S.

45 Hibbeln JR, Salem N Jr: Dietary polyunsaturated fatty acids and depression: when cholesterol does not satisfy. Am J Clin Nutr 1995;62:1–9.

46 Hibbeln JR, Nieminen LR, Lands WE: Increasing homicide rates and linoleic acid consumption among five Western countries, 1961–2000. Lipids 2004;39:1207–1213.

47 Salem N Jr, Niebylski CD: The nervous system has an absolute molecular species requirement for proper function. Mol Membr Biol 1995;12:131–134.

48 McNamara RK, Carlson SE: Role of omega–3 fatty acids in brain development and function: potential implications for the pathogenesis and prevention of psychopathology. Prostaglandins Leukot Essent Fatty Acids 2006;75:329–349.

49 Smith RS: The macrophage theory of depression. Med Hypotheses 1991;35:298–306.

50 Teper E, O'Brien JT: Vascular factors and depression. Int J Geriatr Psychiatry 2008.

51 Vancassel S, Leman S, Hanonick L, et al: n–3 polyunsaturated fatty acid supplementation reverses stress-induced modifications on brain monoamine levels in mice. J Lipid Res 2008;49:340–348.

52 DeMar JC Jr, Ma K, Bell JM, Igarashi M, Greenstein D, Rapoport SI: One generation of n–3 polyunsaturated fatty acid deprivation increases depression and aggression test scores in rats. J Lipid Res 2006; 47:172–180.

53 Hibbeln JR, Linnoila M, Umhau JC, Rawlings R, George DT, Salem N Jr: Essential fatty acids predict metabolites of serotonin and dopamine in cerebrospinal fluid among healthy control subjects, and early- and late-onset alcoholics. Biol Psychiatry 1998;44:235–242.

54 Pawlosky RJ, Bacher J, Salem N Jr: Ethanol consumption alters electroretinograms and depletes neural tissues of docosahexaenoic acid in rhesus monkeys: nutritional consequences of a low n–3 fatty acid diet. Alcohol Clin Exp Res 2001;25:1758–1765.

55 Levant B, Ozias MK, Carlson SE: Diet (n–3) poly-unsaturated fatty acid content and parity interact to alter maternal rat brain phospholipid fatty acid composition. J Nutr 2006;136:2236–2242.

56 Levant B, Ozias MK, Carlson SE: Specific brain regions of female rats are differentially depleted of docosahexaenoic acid by reproductive activity and an (n–3) fatty acid-deficient diet. J Nutr 2007;137: 130–134.

57 Levant B, Radel JD, Carlson SE: Decreased brain docosahexaenoic acid during development alters dopamine-related behaviors in adult rats that are differentially affected by dietary remediation. Behav Brain Res 2004;152:49–57.

58 Levant B, Ozias MK, Davis PF, et al: Decreased brain docosahexaenoic acid content produces neurobiological effects associated with depression: interactions with reproductive status in female rats. Psychoneuroendocrinology 2008;33:1279–1292.

59 Otto SJ, de Groot RH, Hornstra G: Increased risk of postpartum depressive symptoms is associated with slower normalization after pregnancy of the functional docosahexaenoic acid status. Prostaglandins Leukot Essent Fatty Acids 2003;69:237–243.

60 Su KP, Huang SY, Chiu TH, et al: Omega–3 fatty acids for major depressive disorder during pregnancy: results from a randomized, double-blind, placebo-controlled trial. J Clin Psychiatry 2008; 69:644–651.

61 Rees AM, Austin MP, Parker GB: Omega–3 fatty acids as a treatment for perinatal depression: randomized double-blind placebo-controlled trial. Aust NZ J Psychiatry 2008;42:199–205.

62 Freeman MP, Davis M, Sinha P, Wisner KL, Hibbeln JR, Gelenberg AJ: Omega–3 fatty acids and supportive psychotherapy for perinatal depression: a randomized placebo-controlled study. J Affect Disord 2008;110:142–148.

63 Freeman MP, Hibbeln JR, Wisner KL, Brumbach BH, Watchman M, Gelenberg AJ: Randomized dose-ranging pilot trial of omega–3 fatty acids for postpartum depression. Acta Psychiatr Scand 2006; 113:31–35.

64 Browne JC, Scott KM, Silvers KM: Fish consumption in pregnancy and omega–3 status after birth are not associated with postnatal depression. J Affect Disord 2006;90:131–139.

65 Miyake Y, Sasaki S, Yokoyama T, et al: Risk of postpartum depression in relation to dietary fish and fat intake in Japan: the Osaka Maternal and Child Health Study. Psychol Med 2006;36:1727–1735.

66 Sontrop J, Campbell MK: Omega–3 polyunsaturated fatty acids and depression: a review of the evidence and a methodological critique. Prev Med 2006;42:4–13.

67 Appleton KM, Hayward RC, Gunnell D, et al: Effects of n–3 long-chain polyunsaturated fatty acids on depressed mood: systematic review of published trials. Am J Clin Nutr 2006;84:1308–1316.

68 Lin PY, Su KP: A meta-analytic review of double-blind, placebo-controlled trials of antidepressant efficacy of omega–3 fatty acids. J Clin Psychiatry 2007;68:1056–1061.

69 Jazayeri S, Tehrani-Doost M, Keshavarz SA, et al: Comparison of therapeutic effects of omega–3 fatty acid eicosapentaenoic acid and fluoxetine, separately and in combination, in major depressive disorder. Aust NZ J Psychiatry 2008;42:192–198.

70 Antypa N, Van der Does AJ, Smelt AH, Rogers RD: Omega–3 fatty acids (fish-oil) and depression-related cognition in healthy volunteers. J Psychopharmacol 2008.

71 Mischoulon D, Best-Popescu C, Laposata M, et al: A double-blind dose-finding pilot study of docosahexaenoic acid for major depressive disorder. Eur Neuropsychopharmacol 2008;18:639–645.

72 Dinan T, Siggins L, Scully P, O'Brien S, Ross P, Stanton C: Investigating the inflammatory phenotype of major depression: focus on cytokines and polyunsaturated fatty acids. J Psychiatr Res 2008.

73 Freund-Levi Y, Basun H, Cederholm T, Faxén-Irving G, Garlind A, Grut M, Vedin I, Palmblad J, Wahlund LO, Eriksdotter-Jönhagen M: Omega–3 supplementation in mild to moderate Alzheimer's disease: effects on neuropsychiatric symptoms. Int J Geriatr Psychiatry 2008;23:161–169.

74 Grenyer BF, Crowe T, Meyer B, et al: Fish oil supplementation in the treatment of major depression: a randomised double-blind placebo-controlled trial. Prog Neuropsychopharmacol Biol Psychiatry 2007; 31:1393–1396.

75 Marangell LB, Martinez JM, Zboyan HA, Kertz B, Kim HF, Puryear LJ: A double-blind, placebo-controlled study of the omega–3 fatty acid docosahexaenoic acid in the treatment of major depression. Am J Psychiatry 2003;160:996–998.

76 Silvers KM, Woolley CC, Hamilton FC, Watts PM, Watson RA: Randomised double-blind placebo-controlled trial of fish oil in the treatment of depression. Prostaglandins Leukot Essent Fatty Acids 2005;72:211–218.

77 Rogers PJ, Appleton KM, Kessler D, et al: No effect of n–3 long-chain polyunsaturated fatty acid (EPA and DHA) supplementation on depressed mood and cognitive function: a randomised controlled trial. Br J Nutr 2008;99:421–431.

78 Elkin I, Gibbons RD, Shea MT, et al: Initial severity and differential treatment outcome in the National Institute of Mental Health Treatment of Depression Collaborative Research Program. J Consult Clin Psychol 1995;63:841–847.

79 Hirayama T: Lifestyle and Mortality. A Large-Scale Census-Based Cohort Study in Japan. New York, Karger, 1990.

80 Tanskanen A, Hibbeln JR, Tuomilehto J, et al: Fish consumption and depressive symptoms in the general population in Finland. Psychiatr Serv 2001; 52:529–531.

81 De Vriese SR, Christophe AB, Maes M: In humans, the seasonal variation in poly-unsaturated fatty acids is related to the seasonal variation in violent suicide and serotonergic markers of violent suicide. Prostaglandins Leukot Essent Fatty Acids 2004;71: 13–18.

82 Hibbeln JR, Enstrom G, Majchrzak S, Salem N Jr, Traskman-Benz L: Suicide attempters and PUFAs: lower plasma eicosapentaenoic acid alone predicts greater psychopathology. 4th Congress of the International Society for the Study of Fatty Acids and Lipids, Tsukuba 2000, p 104.

83 Sublette ME, Hibbeln JR, Galfalvy H, Oquendo MA, Mann JJ: Omega–3 polyunsaturated essential fatty acid status as a predictor of future suicide risk. Am J Psychiatry 2006;163:1100–1102.

84 Hallahan B, Hibbeln JR, Davis JM, Garland MR: Omega–3 fatty acid supplementation in patients with recurrent self-harm. Single-centre double-blind randomised controlled trial. Br J Psychiatry 2007;190:118–122.

85 Tanielian T, Jaycox LH (eds): Invisible wounds of war. Psychological and Cognitive Injuries, Their Consequences, and Services to Assist Recovery 2008; The Rand Corporation, Santa Monica, CA.

86 Reis LC, Hibbeln JR: Cultural symbolism of fish and the psychotropic properties of omega–3 fatty acids. Prostaglandins Leukot Essent Fatty Acids 2006;75: 227–236.

87 Sarri KO, Linardakis M, Tzanakis N, Kafatos AG: Adipose DHA inversely associated with depression as measured by the Beck Depression Inventory. Prostaglandins Leukot Essent Fatty Acids 2008;78: 117–122.

88 Simopoulos AP: What Is So Special about the Diet of Greece: The Scientific Evidence. World Rev Nutr Diet. Basel, Karger, 2005, vol 95, pp 80–92.

89 DaVanzo JE, Dobson A, Tannamor M, Dollard J: An Evidence Based Study of the Role of Dietary Supplements in Helping Seniors Maintain their Independence Lewin Group Inc., Prepared for: Dietary Supplement Education Alliance. http://www.supplementinfo.org/anm/templates/?a=_&z=

Capt. Joseph R. Hibbeln, MD
LMBB, NIAAA, NIH
5625 Fishers Lane, Rm 3N-07, MSC 9410
Bethesda, MD 20892 (USA)
Tel. +1 301 594 3034, Fax +1 301 594 0035, E-Mail jhibbeln@mail.nih.gov

Simopoulos AP, Bazan NG (eds): Omega-3 Fatty Acids, the Brain and Retina.
World Rev Nutr Diet. Basel, Karger, 2009, vol 99, pp 31–45

Serial Structural MRI Analysis and Proton and ^{31}PMR Spectroscopy in the Investigation of Cerebral Fatty Acids in Major Depressive Disorder, Huntington's Disease, Myalgic Encephalomyelitis and in Forensic Schizophrenic Patients

Basant K. Puri · Sofia Tsaluchidu · Ian H. Treasaden

MRI Unit, Imaging Sciences Department, MRC Clinical Sciences Centre, Imperial College London, Hammersmith Hospital, London, UK

Magnetic Resonance Scanning

Spectroscopy revolutionized the study of organic chemistry and biochemistry during the last century. While X-ray crystallography, mass spectrometry and infrared spectroscopy cannot be used non-invasively in the study of fatty acid metabolism in adult human brains, fortunately nuclear magnetic resonance spectroscopy can be so used. In the context of human in vivo studies, nuclear magnetic resonance spectroscopy is more commonly referred to as magnetic resonance spectroscopy, partly to avoid the potentially pejorative and upsetting word 'nuclear' when talking to human volunteers and patients, and partly because the technique involves the use of the same magnetic resonance imaging (MRI) scanners as are employed to carry out structural MRI.

The technique requires a strong magnetic field, preferably at least 1.5 T when applied to the adult human brain. Certain atomic nuclei in the brain interact with this strong static magnetic field. These include protons and the 13-carbon and 31-phosphorus isotopes. In lay terms, each of these nuclei can be considered to possess more than one possible energy level in the magnetic field. Upon exposure of the brain to a short pulse of radiofrequency energy in a magnetic resonance scanner, some of these nuclei absorb the radiofrequency energy and enter a higher quantum energy state. Recovery of the previous, lower, quantum energy state is associated with the reverse process of the release of energy. The latter is measured as an amplified signal by the head coil receiver.

With all such measurements, there is the phenomenon of 'noise'. For example, when a normal radio receiver is not tuned correctly to a radio station, then one hears a lot of static – noise. (Actually, some of this noise may derive from electromagnetic radiation which had its origin in the big bang.) Then, as one tunes in to a correct station frequency (a resonance frequency), the signal-to-noise ratio becomes high enough to allow the station to be heard clearly. The individual nuclei also have particular resonance frequencies. In order to improve the signal-to-noise ratio, multiple readings are taken. Since the noise is assumed to be random, successive additions of the readings lead to relative enhancement of the true signals against a diminishing background of noise signals which tend to cancel each other out. Furthermore, in a given molecule, all the protons do not usually resonate at the same frequency, and all the 31-phosphorus nuclei do not usually resonate at another single frequency (different from that for the protons). This is because the resonance frequencies for given nuclei are partly determined by the electron structure of the molecule. (In classical electromagnetic physics, one can consider that the motion of these charged electrons in a magnetic field gives rise to an electric current which in turn gives rise to an associated and opposing magnetic field, in accordance with Maxwell's equations; this causes varying levels of shielding of the nuclei from the applied external magnetic field.) The difference between the resonance frequencies of a given nucleus and of a reference nucleus is calculated and the chemical shift of the given nucleus is then defined in terms of the ratio of this difference to the resonance frequency of the reference nucleus. The chemical shift is usually expressed in parts per million (ppm). The signals from the brain are plotted as peaks against the chemical shift, the latter constituting the abscissa of the graph. The area under each peak is directly proportional to the concentration of the corresponding nucleus in the sample (for instance, a brain voxel) under study. Moreover, the shape of the peak(s) yields information about the electrochemical environment of the nucleus in the molecule. Further details of this technique are beyond the scope of this article but may be found in the paper by Cox and Puri [1].

Magnetic resonance scanning also offers a non-invasive method of studying brain structure which, as with magnetic resonance spectroscopy, does not involve the use of ionizing radiation. Serially acquired high-resolution structural MRI scans of the brain can now be registered, that is to say, they can be positionally matched, with great accuracy. Upon successful anatomical registration, the scan first acquired chronologically may be electronically subtracted from the second scan. The resulting subtraction image highlights any regions of anatomical change in the brain, to the resolution of the technique used.

The registration technique used by our group in studying cerebral structural changes in relation to fatty acids, as described in this article, is a rigid-body sub-voxel technique whose development was pioneered by Hajnal and Bydder [2]. In this technique, the brain is considered to be a rigid body whose spatial coordinates have changed between scans, in respect to the scanner, owing to spatial and rotational transformations. In mathematical terms, the technique assumes 6 rigid-body degrees of freedom: 3 spatial and 3 rotational. The data matrix corresponding to the second (and subsequent) scan is spatially transformed in each of three mutually orthogonal directions and rotated about three mutually orthogonal axes and the resulting matrix compared with the matrix corresponding to the first, baseline, scan. The differences between the two matrices are then evaluated, and a chi-squared statistical index of goodness-of-fit is calculated. Based on these results, the whole process is repeated, in order to try to minimize the overall difference between the two sets of data. By means of such an iterative process, an optimum positional match between the two datasets is achieved. It turns out that this method can detect differences in position which are far smaller than the dimensions of a voxel; that is, the procedure can detect subvoxel shifts [3]. Such subvoxel shifts are particularly detectable at steep signal intensity boundaries, such as those which occur between cerebral tissue and cerebrospinal fluid, such as the boundary of the lateral ventricles. In a further development of this technique, Nadeem Saeed and Basant Puri developed a semi-automated method for the quantification of ventricular volumes. Further mathematical details of both techniques are beyond the scope of this article but may be found in a paper by Puri [4].

Depression

While working with ultra-pure eicosapentaenoic acid in patients with schizophrenia, schizoaffective disorder, and dyslexia, including a large double-blind, placebo-controlled trial in schizophrenia, the first author became convinced that eicosapentaenoic acid appeared to have antidepressant properties. This hypothesis found support from epidemiological and biochemical evidence, which are now briefly outlined.

In his epidemiological study of the annual prevalence of major depression versus apparent fish consumption (fish catch plus fish imports minus fish exports) in nine countries, Hibbeln [5] found a significant negative correlation between these two variables.

Maes et al. [6] reported a seasonal variation in the severity of depression in 104 consecutively admitted depressed patients between November 1983 and April 1985, with peaks in Zung Self-Rating Depression Scale scores being found in April-May, with lows occurring in August-September. They also reported a significant seasonality for suicide but not homicide from an analysis of the data on suicide, violent suicide, non-violent suicide, and homicide (categorized according to ICD-9) for all of Belgium for the period 1979–1987 [7]. Seasonality was present in violent but not in non-violent suicide. The number of violent suicides increased with age and was more prominent in men. The violent suicide spectral chronograms of younger and elderly persons were distinct in the occurrence of peaks in March-April and August, and lows in December-January. There was no significant relationship between violent suicide and homicide. The same group subsequently took monthly blood samples from 23 healthy volunteers from Belgium, during the period from December 1991 to December 1992, to test for polyunsaturated fatty acid (PUFA) composition in serum phospholipids. Significant annual rhythms were detected in the long-chain PUFAs arachidonic acid (C20:4n–6), eicosapentaenoic acid (C20:5n–3), and docosahexaenoic acid (C22:6n–3) [8]. Comparing these data with their previous seasonal findings, the group found a significant correlation between, on the one hand, the changes over the previous 2 weeks in arachidonic acid and eicosapentaenoic acid, and, on the other hand, the mean weekly number of violent, but not non-violent, suicide deaths in Belgium. (There was also a significant correlation between the PUFAs arachidonic acid and docosahexaenoic acid, and the B_{max} [^{3}H]-paroxetine binding to platelets.)

This Belgian group also studied serum phospholipids in post-fasting samples in 36 patients with DSM-III-R major depression, 14 patients with DSM-III-R adjustment disorder with depressed mood and dysthymia, and 24 normal controls [9]. Compared with the normal controls, the major depression group showed a higher ratio of arachidonic acid to eicosapentaenoic acid, and lower eicosapentaenoic acid levels in the serum cholesteryl fraction and in phospholipids.

Adams et al. [10] from Australia published an important study of 20 moderately to severely depressed patients, diagnosed using research diagnostic criteria and excluding known bipolar mood disorder and reactive depression, in which they investigated relationships between severity of depression and levels and ratios of n–3 and n–6 PUFA in plasma and erythrocyte phospholipids. Severity of depression was measured using the 21-item Hamilton Depression Rating Scale and a second linear rating scale of severity of depressive symptoms that omitted anxiety symptoms. They reported a significant correlation between the ratio of erythrocyte phospholipid arachidonic acid to eicosapentaenoic acid and severity of depression as rated by both scales. A significant negative correlation was also found between erythrocyte eicosapentaenoic acid and the linear rating scale of severity of depressive symptoms. The arachidonic acid to eicosapentaenoic acid ratio in plasma phospholipids and the ratio of erythrocyte long-chain (C20 and C22 carbon) n–6 to long-chain n–3 PUFAs were also significantly correlated with this linear rating scale. The authors commented that their findings did not appear to be simply explained by differences in dietary intake of eicosapentaenoic acid. They further suggested that their findings provided a basis for studying the effect in depressed patients of nutritional supplementation aimed at reducing the ratio of arachidonic acid to eicosapentaenoic acid in tissues on the severity of depression. (Clearly this could be achieved by increasing the intake of eicosapentaenoic acid.)

Similar findings were reported in the British study by Edwards et al. [11] in which erythrocyte membrane fatty acid levels, dietary PUFA intake, and the level of depressive symptomatology (assessed using Beck Depression Inventory) were measured in 10 depressed patients and 14 matched healthy control subjects. They reported a significant depletion of erythrocyte membrane n–3 PUFAs in the depressed patients which was not the result of reduced omega–3 fatty acid intake. Furthermore, the severity of depression was found to correlate negatively with erythrocyte membrane levels and with dietary intake of n–3 PUFAs. In line with the paper by Adams et al., in this paper the authors suggested that their findings raised the possibility that depressive symptoms may be alleviated by n–3 PUFA supplementation.

Based on the above evidence, our group became the first actively to treat major depression with eicosapentaenoic acid. The first published case of a patient with depression to be treated with eicosapentaenoic acid underwent cerebral 31-phosphorus magnetic resonance spectroscopy at baseline and at 79-month follow-up [12]. The patient was a 21-year-old male student with a 7-year history of unremitting depressive symptoms. In this severe case of treatment-resistant depression, no conventional antidepressant treatment or combination of conventional treatment (for example, a selective serotonin re-uptake inhibitor with a lithium salt) has proved effective. However, the addition of ultra-pure eicosapentaenoic acid, in the form of its ethyl ester, was followed by clinical improvement. This included the cessation within 1 month of previously unremitting severe suicidal ideation, and also a marked improvement in previously troubling social phobia symptomatology. The improvement continued and by 9 months the patient's depressive symptoms had disappeared altogether, without any apparent adverse side effects from taking the nutritional supplementation of pure eicosapentaenoic acid. During this 9-month period, the relative phosphomonoester peak value, expressed as a ratio to the total 31-phosphorus signal, increased markedly from 9.23 to 14.11%, representing a 52.9% increase. This 31-phosphorus spectroscopy peak contains contributions from freely mobile phosphomonoesters, including phosphocholine and phosphoethanolamine, and small contributions from inositol phosphate, glycerophosphate, phosphothreonine, and L-phosphoserine. It also contains contributions from phosphomonoester-containing molecules which are less mobile, including some phosphorylated proteins, and from neuronal cytoskeletal protein components. Therefore the area under this peak indexes the level of membrane phospholipid anabolism. In contrast, over the same 9-month period the relative phosphodiester peak value, again expressed as a ratio to the total 31-phosphorus signal, decreased from 46.60 to 41.99%, representing a 9.8% increase in value. This 31-phosphorus phosphodiester spectroscopy peak contains contributions from freely mobile phosphodiesters, including glycerophosphocholine and glycerophosphoethanolamine, as well as contributions from less mobile phosphodiester-containing molecules including some involved in cell membrane structure, the latter including not just the outer cell membrane but also intracellular organelle membranes. Therefore, the area under this phosphodiester peak indexes the level of membrane phospholipid catabolism. Taken together, these neurospectroscopy results were consistent with the hypothesis that nutritional supplementation with pure eicosapentaenoic acid was associated with a reduction in neuronal phospholipid turnover, with increased cerebral membrane phospholipid biosynthesis and decreased cerebral membrane phospholipid breakdown. They were also in line with the finding that the volumetric niacin response, which indexes arachidonic acid-related signal transduction [13], showed an increase of 30% over the same 9-month period.

High-resolution structural MRI scanning was also carried out at the same time as the 31-phosphorus neurospectroscopy. The structural data obtained underwent subvoxel registration using a sinc interpolation function. The sinc function is defined as:

$$\operatorname{sinc} z = (\sin z)/z, \text{ where } z \in \mathbb{C}$$

This is used as it is the appropriate in-plane point spread function for magnetic resonance image data acquired in the Fourier domain over a bounded region of k-space, with band-limited frequency content [14]. The right-hand side of the above equation may worry some readers as, clearly, z may need to take the value $0 \in \mathbb{C}$, and this may lead to the concern that a singularity is being produced through the division of sin 0 (which equals zero) by zero. However, since the numerator may be expressed as a Taylor series, as $z - z^3/3! + \ldots$, it follows that sinc z is given by:

$$\operatorname{sinc} z = 1 - z^2/3! + \ldots \ (z \in \mathbb{C})$$

and hence sinc 0 is unity and so the domain of the function is the whole of $\mathbb{C}$, including zero. Following subtraction of the subvoxel-registered images (follow-up minus baseline), detailed analysis revealed definite structural changes in the brain. In particular, during the 9-month initial period of nutritional supplementation with the ultra-pure eicosapentaenoic acid, not only had the patient's previous treatment-resistant depressive symptomatology markedly improved, but his lateral ventricles had actually shrunk in size [12, 15], again consistent with the 31-phosphorus neurospectroscopy changes described above.

Subsequent randomized, double-blind, placebo-controlled supplementation trials in depression with either ultra-pure eicosapentaenoic acid or a mixture of eicosapentaenoic acid and docosahexaenoic acid have generally been associated with clinically positive results [16].

Huntington's Disease

Huntington's disease, also known as Huntington's chorea, is a progressive inherited neurodegenerative disease which is associated with abnormal involuntary movements, psychiatric disturbance, and cognitive deterioration with progression to dementia and death over 10–20 years. The movement disorder typically includes choreiform movements in head, face, and arms, and a wide-spaced gait with sudden lurching. The psychiatric disturbance is variable but common. Initial insight may lead to depression, while prodromal personality changes, antisocial behavior with substance misuse, affective or schizophreniform disorders may occur. The initial insight may give way to mild euphoria, explosive outbursts, irritability, and rage. Unfortunately there is no effective treatment for Huntington's disease, although tetrabenazine, a benzoquinolizine derivative initially developed in the 1950s as an antipsychotic medication, may help with the movement disorder [17]. Huntington's disease is inherited as an autosomal dominant disorder, with complete penetrance, caused by an expansion in the number of CAG repeats in the gene for huntingtin on chromosome 4p16.3, coding for polyglutamine [18]. Huntingtin interacts with many other proteins, including calmodulin (a Ca^{2+}-binding regulatory protein), CREB-binding protein (a transcriptional coactivator), mSin3a (a transcriptional co-repressor), cystathionine B-synthase (a metabolic enzyme), GAPDH (a glycolytic enzyme and translational regulator), HAP-1 (involved with membrane trafficking), HAP-40 (unknown function), HIP-1 (a pro-apoptotic protein involved in actin organization and endocytosis), HIP-2 (ubiquitin-conjugating enzyme), HYP-A (a WW-domain protein involved in mRNA splicing), HYP-B (a WW-domain protein which acts as a transcription factor), HYP-C (a WW-domain protein involved in mRNA splicing), MLK2 (JNK activator), N-CoR (nuclear receptor co-repressor), p53 (a transcription factor), SH3GL3 (involved with clathrin-mediated endocytosis and the recycling of synaptic vesicles), Shc (a signaling protein), and EGF receptor (a signaling protein).

Several converging lines of evidence lent support to the suggestion by the first author of this article that ultra-pure eicosapentaenoic acid might be therapeutic in Huntington's disease. These included two single-case studies, findings relating to membrane phospholipid metabolism from a post-mortem study, impaired phospho-lipid-related signal transduction, a study of the effects of fatty acids on a transgenic mouse model of the disease, and the cerebral effects of eicosapentaenoic acid in other neuropsychiatric disorders. We shall now outline each of these in turn.

The two single-case studies in Huntington's disease were published by Vaddadi [19]. These 2 Australian patients showed improvement in some of their symptomatology following supplementation with fatty acids, mainly from evening primrose oil, and therefore mainly containing linoleic acid and γ-linolenic acid.

Ellison et al. [20] carried out measurements of both phosphoethanolamine and ethanolamine in post-mortem brain samples from patients with Huntington's disease using high-performance liquid chromatography with electrochemical detection. The concentrations of phosphoethanolamine were significantly reduced by 76% in the caudate, 53% in the putamen and 48% in the nucleus accumbens, while ethanolamine concentrations showed similar but smaller reductions. Since both phosphoethanolamine and ethanolamine are involved in phospholipid metabolism, these findings suggested that phospholipid metabolism might be impaired in Huntington's disease.

The first author of this paper carried out a study of the volumetric niacin response, which indexes phospholipid-related signal transduction [13], in patients with advanced (stage III) Huntington's disease. Compared with age- and sex-matched control subjects, who had a mean volumetric niacin response of 28.3 mol s l^{-1}, the

Huntington's disease patients were found to have a reduced mean volumetric niacin response of 16.3 mol s l^{-1} [21].

Clifford et al. [22] described the systematic effects of treatment with fatty acids or placebo, given throughout life, on the emergence and progression of phenotype in the R6/1 transgenic mouse model of Huntington's disease using assessment techniques which included a novel, ethologically based, approach to dissect neurological impairment into topographical domains of function at a naturalistic level. Transgenic R6/1 mice incorporate a human genomic fragment containing promoter elements exon 1 and a portion of intron 2 of the huntingtin gene and they develop late-onset neurological deficits, as occurs with the motor abnormalities of Huntington's disease. In this study, R6/1 and normal mice were randomized to receive a mixture of fatty acids, containing linoleic acid, γ-linolenic acid, eicosapentaenoic acid, and docosahexaenoic acid, or placebo on alternate days throughout life. Over mid-adulthood, topographical assessment of behavior revealed the R6/1 transgenic mice to evidence progressive shortening of stride length, with progressive reductions in locomotion, elements of rearing, sniffing, sifting and chewing, and an increase in grooming, deficits which were either not evident or markedly diminished in the R6/1 transgenic mice receiving the fatty acids. The latter also showed reductions in body mass and in brain dopamine D_1-like and D_2-like quantitative receptor autoradiography which were unaltered by the fatty acid supplementation. The authors concluded that these findings indicated that early and sustained treatment with fatty acids were able to protect against motor deficits in R6/1 transgenic mice expressing exon 1 and a portion of intron 2 of the huntingtin gene, and they suggested that fatty acids may have therapeutic potential in (human) Huntington's disease.

The final strand of evidence related to the cerebral effects of eicosapentaenoic acid in neuropsychiatric disorders other than Huntington's disease. These effects in relation to depression have been described above. Similar benefits were also found in schizophrenia, with clear evidence of a reversal of the previously increasing ventricle-to-brain ratio accompanying clinical benefits in the first patient with schizophrenia to be treated solely with ultra-pure eicosapentaenoic acid (in the absence of any other medication, including antipsychotics) [23, 24].

Based on the above evidence, we carried out the first pilot study of ultra-pure eicosapentaenoic acid in Huntington's disease. This consisted of a 6-month randomized, placebo-controlled study of the ethyl ester of eicosapentaenoic acid in 7 inpatients with advanced (stage III) Huntington's disease (3 on eicosapentaenoic acid, 4 on placebo; no significant difference in age or sex between the groups) [25]. At 6-month follow-up all the patients treated with eicosapentaenoic acid were found to have improved on the orofacial component of the Unified Huntington's Disease Rating Scale while all the patients on placebo deteriorated on this scale (p < 0.03). Following subvoxel registration of follow-up 3D MRI brain scans with baseline scans, subtraction images showed that while the placebo was associated with progressive cerebral atrophy, the eicosapentaenoic acid supplementation was associated with a reverse process. From this pilot study we concluded that treatment with eicosapentaenoic acid appeared to be associated with beneficial motor and MRI changes.

As a result of this pilot study, a larger, phase III, multicenter, double-blind, placebo-controlled trial was carried out by us [26]. A total of 135 patients with either stage I (a decline in functional capacity to work with impaired motor function and emotional control, including irritability and depression, but fully able to maintain his or her own activities of daily living) or stage II (unable to work or drive a car, reliant on family or other carers for activities of daily living but with assistance can remain at home, increasing dysarthria, dysphasia, loss of motor control and cognitive function) Huntington's disease entered into the study to receive either ultra-pure eicosapentaenoic acid (as the ethyl ester) or placebo daily. All the patients had symptomatic, genetically confirmed Huntington's disease or had a family history of Huntington's disease. The inclusion criteria also included having a score from 50 (24-hour supervision appropriate: assistance required for bathing, eating, toileting) to 90 (no physical care needed if difficult tasks are avoided) on the Independence Scale component of the Unified Huntington's Disease Rating Scale. Pharmacotherapy with depot antipsychotics was not allowed. The primary efficacy variable was the Total Motor Score 4 subscale of the Unified Huntington's Disease Rating Scale. The items of this motor subscale are: maximal dystonia (five locations); maximal chorea (seven locations); ocular pursuit (two tests); tongue protrusion; retropulsion pull test; finger tapping (right and left); pronation and supination of the hands (right and left); rigidity (right and left), and tandem walking. A total of 121 patients completed 12 months, and 83 did so without protocol violations (the per protocol cohort). Intent-to-treat analysis revealed no significant difference between eicosapentaenoic acid and placebo on the Total Motor Score 4 subscale. In the per protocol cohort, however, eicosapentaenoic acid proved significantly better than placebo on this Total Motor Score 4 subscale. Exploration of moderators of the efficacy of eicosapentaenoic acid on the motor signs of the Total Motor Score 4 subscale showed a significant interaction between treatment and a factor defining patients with high versus low CAG repeat number at 4p16.3. Reported adverse events were distributed equally between treatment arms.

Two potential mechanisms of action of eicosapentaenoic acid in Huntington's disease have recently been proposed [27, 28]. They are based on two pathways which might be of pathophysiologic significance in this disease. In the first pathway, interleukin-1β (IL-1β), lipopolysaccharide, and glutamate may induce nuclear factor-κB (NF-κB), a transcription factor which is a critical regulator of neuronal survival, via an IKK complex, p65, IκBα, and p50, while in the second pathway huntingtin, lipopolysaccharide, and radiation may activate c-jun N-terminal kinases (JNK), which may mediate neuronal degeneration via JNK-AP-1. Eicosapentaenoic acid appears to inhibit both NF-κB and JNK-AP-1, and this may therefore help explain its efficacy in Huntington's disease. Our finding that the clinical efficacy of eicosapentaenoic acid in Huntington's disease varied according to the CAG repeat number is more difficult to explain at present, but a partial explanation may lie in the fact that the CAG repeat length determines the extent of mitochondrial sensitivity towards (metabolic) challenges; further research is clearly indicated.

Myalgic Encephalomyelitis

Myalgic encephalomyelitis, also known as chronic fatigue syndrome, is a devastating disease which, according to the Revised CDC (Centers for Disease Control and Prevention) Criteria, include the following symptoms and signs in addition to chronic fatigue: impaired memory or concentration; sore throat; tender cervical or axillary lymph nodes; myalgia; multi-joint pains; new headaches; unrefreshing sleep, and post-exertion malaise [29]. The etiology of myalgic encephalomyelitis is currently unknown. However, there is evidence that LC-PUFAs may have an important role to play [30]. A key part of the evidence for this came from proton neurospectroscopy studies.

The first such systematic proton neurospectroscopy study was carried out by our group, in which 8 patients with myalgic encephalomyelitis (chronic fatigue syndrome), diagnosed according to the Revised CDC Criteria, were compared with 8 matched control subjects [31]. The key finding was an increased level of cerebral choline (the area of the peak associated with free choline-containing compounds) in the myalgic encephalomyelitis patients. The second systematic proton neurospectroscopy study was carried out by Chaudhuri et al. [32] in Scotland, using the same number of patients and controls as we had in our study. Again, this group reported a significant increase in the area of the peak associated with free choline-containing compounds in the myalgic encephalomyelitis patients compared with the matched control subjects. A series of 3 cases of juvenile myalgic encephalomyelitis was reported by Tomoda et al. [33] from Japan, and again included the finding of a raised level of the choline peak on proton neurospectroscopy.

We have hypothesized that the raised level of choline-containing compounds in the brain in myalgic encephalomyelitis may be the result of reduced incorporation of the choline polar head group in phospholipid molecules (at the Sn3 position) in both outer cell membranes and intracellular organelle membranes in neurons and glial cells [30]. In turn, this might be the result of impaired biosynthesis of membrane phospholipid molecules in the brain, caused by reduced biosynthesis of long-chain PUFAs (at the Sn2 position of phospholipids) by putative viral infectious inhibition of the first LC-PUFA biosynthetic step catalyzed by Δ6-desaturase.

Intriguingly, there exist other lines of evidence pointing to a possible viral etiology for myalgic encephalomyelitis [30]. One is that many clinical features of epidemics of myalgic encephalomyelitis-like illnesses, such as the Los Angeles County Hospital epidemic of 1934 and the Royal Free Hospital (in London, UK) epidemic of 1955, are consistent with viral infections. Another is that the general pattern of immune system changes in myalgic encephalomyelitis is consistent with a pre-existing long-term viral infection. Again, direct analysis of blood fatty acids has shown decreased levels of certain long-chain PUFAs in myalgic encephalomyelitis patients compared with matched control subjects.

The recent report by Kerr's group [34] of up-regulation of the mitochondrial translation initiation factor EIF4G1 transcript variant 5 in myalgic encephalomyelitis is consistent with a persistent virus infection. Virus infections, through their inhibition of Δ6-desaturase, might then cause a deficiency of long-chain PUFAs.

Two placebo-controlled, double-blind trials of the use of fatty acids in chronic fatigue patients have been published. The first, by Behan et al. [35], showed a significant benefit, while the second, by Peet's group [36], proved negative. In the first neuroimaging study of fatty acid supplementation in a patient with myalgic encephalomyelitis, our group carried out high-resolution MRI brain scanning at baseline and after just 16 weeks in a female patient in her mid-20s who had a 6-year history of unremitting symptoms of this illness [37]. The fatty acid supplementation was associated with both clinical improvement and, upon subvoxel registration of the structural MRI scans, a reduction in the ventricle-to-brain ratio, with the baseline lateral ventricular volume of 28,940 mm^3 decreasing to just 23,660 mm^3 at 16-week follow-up. This is clearly an area that requires further research.

Forensic Patients with Schizophrenia

We have already mentioned the first case report of the successful use of ultra-pure eicosapentaenoic acid (in the absence of any other form of pharmacotherapy) in the treatment of a patient with a long history of positive and negative symptoms of schizophrenia; the rapid clinical improvement was accompanied by improvements in indices of cerebral structure, including a reduction in the lateral ventricular volume and in the associated ventricle-to-brain ratio [23, 24]. These results were consistent with the membrane hypothesis of schizophrenia, formulated largely by the late David Horrobin.

However, schizophrenia is a heterogeneous disorder. While the majority of structural brain-scanning studies of schizophrenia have indicated that the disorder is associated with ventricular enlargement, a study of first-episode schizophrenia, carried out by our group, that utilized the monomodal rigid-body subvoxel registration technique outlined earlier, showed that lateral ventricular volumes can alter in either direction early on in the course of the illness [38]. Moreover, the direction of change may relate to schizophrenia syndromes. Compared with the control subjects, the schizophrenia patients categorized as suffering from the withdrawn syndrome showed progressive ventricular enlargement, with an increase in ventricle-to-brain volume ratio, whereas the schizophrenia patients suffering from the active syndrome showed a reduction in ventricle-to-brain volume ratio, with a change opposite in sign and smaller in magnitude [39]. The active syndrome consists of raised activity levels, accelerated cognition, positive thought disorder, positive labile affect, and affective delusions, and has been said to be associated with a greater left than right functional activation, while the opposite pattern of functional hemispheric imbalance has been said to be associated with the withdrawn syndrome, which comprises the essential negative features of schizophrenia [40]. In studying schizophrenia, therefore, it is helpful to select a group which is relatively well circumscribed clinically. We have chosen to do so by studying those patients with schizophrenia who have seriously and violently offended while psychotic; we were interested to ascertain whether the subgroup of patients with schizophrenia who are violent offenders may suffer from abnormal membrane phospholipid metabolism.

Accordingly, we carried out 31-phosporus neurospectroscopy on 15 male patients with DSM-IV schizophrenia who were all inpatients in the largest European Medium Secure Unit and on a comparison group of 13 healthy normal age-matched male controls with no known medical or psychiatric disorder [41]. Expert psychiatric opinion, accepted in court, was that all the patients had violently offended directly as a result of schizophrenia prior to admission. These offences consisted of homicide, attempted murder, or wounding with intent to cause grievous bodily harm. Interestingly, we found no direct neurospectroscopic evidence of a membrane phospholipid abnormality in the brain in this cohort of patients, which underlines the heterogeneous nature of the illness. However, the level of β-nucleotide triphosphate (β-NTP) was found to be lower, and the level of γ-nucleotide triphosphate (γ-NTP) higher, in the forensic schizophrenia patient group compared with the control group. While β-NTP indexes ATP (adenosine triphosphate), the majority of ADP (adenosine diphosphate) is nuclear magnetic resonance-invisible, although the γ-NTP signal overlaps with signals from β-ADP, although the signal of γ-NTP is much stronger. Therefore, our results were consistent with increased cerebral energy metabolism taking place in this particular group of schizophrenia patients.

We then decided to examine the association of arachidonic acid-related signal transduction, as quantified using the volumetric niacin response [13], with cerebral metabolism, measured using 31-phosphorus neurospectroscopy, in this group of schizophrenia patients [42]. There was a strong, and negative, correlation between the volumetric niacin response and the cerebral metabolite concentration of inorganic phosphate expressed as a ratio of the total 31-phosphorus signal. There was also a trend towards a negative correlation between the volumetric niacin response and the metabolite concentration of α-NTP expressed as a ratio of the total 31-phosphorus signal. This suggests that reduced phospholipid signal transduction may be related to higher cerebral energy metabolism in this group of schizophrenia patients. However, since the volumetric niacin response is reduced in patients with schizophrenia compared with normal controls, this suggests that a lower response is likely to be associated with increased severity of illness. Hence, these results lead to the possibility that patients with schizophrenia who have violently offended and have poor phospholipid-related signal transduction may have higher levels of cerebral energy metabolism.

Discussion and Conclusions

In this paper we have demonstrated the utility of applying serial structural MRI analysis and proton and 31-phosphorus magnetic resonance spectroscopy to the investigation of cerebral fatty acids in neurologic and psychiatric disorders. While most of these applications have thus far been mainly related to advancing our understanding of the basic scientific foundations of the relationship of lipids to the pathophysiology of the disorders described, it seems probable that they will increasingly contribute to the study of the effects of dietary supplementation in these disorders.

References

1 Cox IJ, Puri BK: In vivo MR spectroscopy in diagnosis and research of neuropsychiatric disorders. Prostaglandins Leukot Essent Fatty Acids 2004;70: 357–360.

2 Hajnal JV, Saeed N, Soar EJ, Oatridge A, Young IR, Bydder GM: A registration and interpolation procedure for subvoxel matching of serially acquired MR images. J Comput Assist Tomogr 1995;19:289–296.

3 Bydder GM, Hajnal JV: Registration and subtraction of serial magnetic resonance images. Part 2. Image interpretation; in Bradley WG, Bydder GM (eds): Advanced MR Imaging Techniques. London, Dunitz, 1997, pp 239–257.

4 Puri BK: High-resolution magnetic resonance imaging sinc-interpolation-based subvoxel registration and semi-automated quantitative lateral ventricular morphology employing threshold computation and binary image creation in the study of fatty acid interventions in schizophrenia, depression, chronic fatigue syndrome and Huntington's disease. Int Rev Psychiatry 2006;18:149–154.

5 Hibbeln JR: Fish consumption and major depression. Lancet 1998;351:1213.

6 Maes M, Meltzer HY, Suy E, De Meyer F: Seasonality in severity of depression: relationships to suicide and homicide occurrence. Acta Psychiatr Scand 1993;88:156–161.

7 Maes M, Cosyns P, Meltzer HY, De Meyer F, Peeters D: Seasonality in violent suicide but not in nonviolent suicide or homicide. Am J Psychiatry 1993;150: 1380–1385.

8 De Vriese SR, Christophe AB, Maes M: In humans, the seasonal variation in poly-unsaturated fatty acids is related to the seasonal variation in violent suicide and serotonergic markers of violent suicide. Prostaglandins Leukot Essent Fatty Acids 2004;71: 13–18.

9 Maes M, Smith R, Christophe AB, Cosyns P, Desnyder R, Meltzer H: Fatty acid composition in major depression: decreased omega–3 fractions in cholesteryl esters and increased C20:4ω–6/C20: 5ω–3 ratio in cholesteryl esters and phospholipids. J Affect Disord 1996;38:35–46.

10 Adams PB, Lawson S, Sanigorski A, Sinclair AJ: Arachidonic acid to eicosapentaenoic acid ratio in blood correlates positively with clinical symptoms of depression. Lipids 1996;31(suppl):S157–S161.

11 Edwards R, Peet M, Shay J, Horrobin D: Omega–3 polyunsaturated fatty acid levels in the diet and in red blood cell membranes of depressed patients. J Affect Disord 1998;48:149–155.

12 Puri BK, Counsell SJ, Hamilton G, Richardson AJ, Horrobin DF: Eicosapentaenoic acid treatment in treatment-resistant depression associated with symptom remission, structural brain changes and reduced neuronal phospholipid turnover. Int J Clin Pract 2001;55:560–563.

13 Puri BK, Hirsch SR, Easton T, Richardson AJ: A volumetric biochemical niacin flush-based index that noninvasively detects fatty acid deficiency in schizophrenia. Prog Neuropsychopharmacol Biol Psychiatry 2002;26:49–52.

14 Jain AK: Fundamentals of Digital Image Processing. Englewood Cliffs, Prentice Hall, 1989.

15 Puri BK, Counsell SJ, Richardson AJ, Horrobin DF: Eicosapentaenoic acid in treatment-resistant depression. Arch Gen Psychiatry 2002;59:91–92.

16 Ross BM, Seguin J, Sieswerda LE: Omega–3 fatty acids as treatments for mental illness: which disorder and which fatty acid? Lipids Health Dis 2007;6: 21.

17 Kenney C, Jankovic J: Tetrabenazine in the treatment of hyperkinetic movement disorders. Expert Rev Neurother 2006;6:7–17.

18   Huntington's Disease Collaborative Research Group: A novel gene containing a trinucleotide repeat that is expanded and unstable on Huntington's disease chromosomes. Cell 1993;72:971–983.

19   Vaddadi K: Dyskinesias and their treatment with essential fatty acids: a review. Prostaglandins Leukot Essent Fatty Acids 1996;55:89–94.

20   Ellison DW, Beal MF, Martin JB: Phosphoethanolamine and ethanolamine are decreased in Alzheimer's disease and Huntington's disease. Brain Res 1987;417:389–392.

21   Puri BK: Impaired phospholipid-related signal transduction in advanced Huntington's disease. Exp Physiol 2001;86:683–685.

22   Clifford JJ, Drago J, Natoli AL, Wong JY, Kinsella A, Waddington JL, Vaddadi KS: Essential fatty acids given from conception prevent topographies of motor deficit in a transgenic model of Huntington's disease. Neuroscience 2002;109:81–88.

23   Puri BK, Richardson AJ: Sustained remission of positive and negative symptoms of schizophrenia following treatment with eicosapentaenoic acid. Arch Gen Psychiatry 1998;55:188–189.

24   Puri BK, Richardson AJ, Horrobin DF, Easton T, Saeed N, Oatridge A, Hajnal JV, Bydder GM: Eicosapentaenoic acid treatment in schizophrenia associated with symptom remission, normalisation of blood fatty acids, reduced neuronal membrane phospholipid turnover and structural brain changes. Int J Clin Pract 2000;54:57–63.

25   Puri BK, Bydder GM, Counsell SJ, Corridan BJ, Richardson AJ, Hajnal JV, Appel C, Mckee HM, Vaddadi KS, Horrobin DF: MRI and neuropsychological improvement in Huntington disease following ethyl-EPA treatment. Neuroreport 2002;13:123–126.

26   Puri BK, Leavitt BR, Hayden MR, Ross CA, Rosenblatt A, Greenamyre JT, Hersch S, Vaddadi KS, Sword A, Horrobin DF, Manku M, Murck H: Ethyl-EPA in Huntington disease: a double-blind, randomized, placebo-controlled trial. Neurology 2005;65:286–292.

27   Delerive P, Fruchart J-C, Staels B: Peroxisome proliferator-activated receptors in inflammation control. J Endocrinol 2001;169:453–459.

28   Murck H, Manku M: Ethyl-EPA in Huntington disease: potentially relevant mechanism of action. Brain Res Bull 2007;72:159–164.

29   Fukuda K, Straus SE, Hickie I, Sharpe MC, Dobbins JG, Komaroff A: The chronic fatigue syndrome: a comprehensive approach to its definition and study. International Chronic Fatigue Syndrome Study Group. Ann Intern Med 1994;121:953–959.

30   Puri BK: Long-chain polyunsaturated fatty acids and the pathophysiology of myalgic encephalomyelitis (chronic fatigue syndrome). J Clin Pathol 2007;60:122–124.

31   Puri BK, Counsell SJ, Zaman R, Main J, Collins AG, Hajnal JV, Davey NJ: Relative increase in choline in the occipital cortex in chronic fatigue syndrome. Acta Psychiatr Scand 2002;106:224–226.

32   Chaudhuri A, Condon BR, Gow JW, Brennan D, Hadley DM: Proton magnetic resonance spectroscopy of basal ganglia in chronic fatigue syndrome. Neuroreport 2003;14:225–228.

33   Tomoda A, Miike T, Yamada E, Honda H, Moroi T, Ogawa M, Ohtani Y, Morishita S: Chronic fatigue syndrome in childhood. Brain Dev 2000;22:60–64.

34   Kaushik N, Fear D, Richards SC, McDermott CR, Nuwaysir EF, Kellam P, Harrison TJ, Wilkinson RJ, Tyrrell DA, Holgate ST, Kerr JR: Gene expression in peripheral blood mononuclear cells from patients with chronic fatigue syndrome. J Clin Pathol 2005;58:826–832.

35   Behan PO, Behan WM, Horrobin D: Effect of high doses of essential fatty acids on the postviral fatigue syndrome. Acta Neurol Scand 1990;82:209–216.

36   Warren G, McKendrick M, Peet M: The role of essential fatty acids (EFA) in chronic fatigue syndrome. A case-controlled study of red-cell membrane EFA and a placebo-controlled treatment study with high dose of EFA. Acta Neurol Scand 1999;99:112–116.

37   Puri BK, Holmes J, Hamilton G: Eicosapentaenoic acid-rich essential fatty acid supplementation in chronic fatigue syndrome associated with symptom remission and structural brain changes. Int J Clin Pract 2004;58:297–299.

38   Puri BK, Hutton SB, Saeed N, Oatridge A, Hajnal JV, Duncan L, Chapman MJ, Barnes TR, Bydder GM, Joyce EM: A serial longitudinal quantitative MRI study of cerebral changes in first-episode schizophrenia using image segmentation and subvoxel registration. Psychiatry Res 2001;106:141–150.

39   Puri BK, Saeed N, Richardson AJ, Oatridge A, Hajnal JV, Bydder GM: Schizophrenia syndromes associated with changes in ventricle-to-brain ratios: a serial high-resolution three-dimensional magnetic resonance imaging study in first-episode schizophrenia patients using subvoxel registration and semiautomated quantification. Int J Clin Pract 2005;59:399–402.

40   Gruzelier JH: The factorial structure of schizotypy. Part I. Affinities with syndromes of schizophrenia. Schizophr Bull 1996;22:611–620.

41 Puri BK, Counsell SJ, Hamilton G, Bustos MG, Horrobin DF, Richardson AJ, Treasaden IH: Cerebral metabolism in male patients with schizophrenia who have seriously and dangerously violently offended: a ^{31}P magnetic resonance spectroscopy study. Prostaglandins Leukot Essent Fatty Acids 2004;70: 409–411.

42 Puri BK, Richardson AJ, Counsell SJ, Ward PE, Bustos MG, Hamilton G, Bhakoo KK, Treasaden IH: Negative correlation between cerebral inorganic phosphate and the volumetric niacin response in male patients with schizophrenia who have seriously and dangerously violently offended: a ^{31}P magnetic resonance spectroscopy study. Prostaglandins Leukot Essent Fatty Acids 2007;77: 97–99.

Basant K. Puri
MRI Unit, Hammersmith Hospital
Du Cane Road, London W12 0HS (UK)
Tel. +44 0208 383 2412, Fax +44 0208 383 3038, E-Mail basant.puri@csc.mrc.ac.uk

Simopoulos AP, Bazan NG (eds): Omega-3 Fatty Acids, the Brain and Retina.
World Rev Nutr Diet. Basel, Karger, 2009, vol 99, pp 46–54

Omega–3 Fatty Acid Docosahexaenoic Acid Is the Precursor of Neuroprotectin D1 in the Nervous System

Tiffany D. Niemoller · David T. Stark · Nicolas G. Bazan

Neuroscience Center of Excellence and Department of Ophthalmology, Louisiana State University Health Sciences Center, School of Medicine, New Orleans, La., USA

Omega–3 fatty acids cannot be made de novo in the human body. They are derived from linolenic acid (18:3,n–3) and are an essential part of the human diet. A substantial body of research exists indicating the beneficial effects of increased dietary intake of essential omega–3 fatty acids on cardiovascular and brain health. They are required to maintain membrane integrity and necessary for optimal cellular function [1].

Docosahexaenoic acid (DHA, 22:6,n–3) is an essential omega–3 fatty acid obtained from the diet mostly in the form of fish oil and marine algae. It is highly concentrated in membrane phospholipids of the retina and brain [2]. Lipids comprise 22% of the cerebral cortex and DHA is the most abundant omega–3 fatty acid in the phospholipid bilayer of neurons. DHA has been shown to be essential for proper maturation and maintenance of the visual cortex and retina [3]. Free DHA has been shown to limit oxidative-stress induced apoptosis via the production of neuroprotectin D1 (NPD1), a transient, yet powerful, signaling molecule.

As the name suggests, NPD1 is a potent anti-inflammatory, anti-apoptotic agent with great neuroprotective utility in multiple disease processes. D1 indicates that NPD1 is the first of presumably several neuroprotective signaling molecules derived from DHA in circumstances of oxidative stress and cellular damage (fig. 1). Enhancing our understanding of and influence on DHA's endogenous anti-inflammatory signaling potential, including the synthesis of NPD1, will provide a means for developing therapeutic strategies aimed at decreasing the morbidity and mortality of many devastating diseases, including retinal degenerative diseases, stroke, Alzheimer's disease (AD), and epilepsy.

T.D.N· and D.T.S. contributed equally to this work.

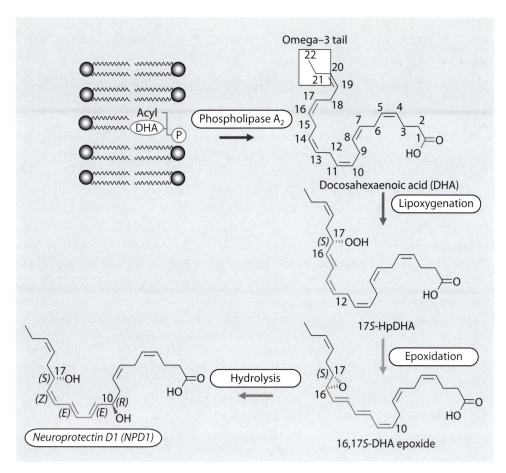

Fig. 1. Biosynthesis of NPD1. Phospholipase A_2 hydrolyzes membrane phospholipids releasing free DHA. Lipoxygenation is then followed by epoxidation and hydrolysis to generate NPD1 (reprinted from Bazan [46] with permission of The Association for Research in Vision and Ophthalmology).

Adequate Stores of DHA Are Required for Proper CNS Function

The consumption of large amounts of DHA has been associated with multiple health benefits. DHA has been shown to be involved with brain and retinal development, aging, memory formation, synaptic membrane function, photoreceptor biogenesis and function, and neuroprotection [2, 4]. DHA-supplemented infant formula enhances maturation of retinal function, visual acuity, and mental performance in preterm and term infants [2]. In age-related macular degeneration, there is an inverse relationship between diets high in DHA and risk for the disease [5]. Finally, epidemiologic studies indicate that diets enriched with DHA are associated with reduced risk of cognitive impairment and slow the progression of dementia and AD [6].

Certain individuals with low dietary intake of DHA, such as vegans, vegetarians, and the elderly, have been shown to have less brain DHA [7]. The fatty acid composition of brain lipids can be modified by diet. While lack of DHA in the diet will eventually result in loss of DHA content from brain and retina, both the brain and retina actively conserve DHA pools displaying a striking ability to retain DHA even after prolonged dietary deficiencies [8]. In cases of prolonged essential omega–3 fatty acid deficiency, decreased amounts of DHA in neuronal membranes alter membrane fluidity and signaling properties [6].

Depleted stores of DHA are associated with several health risks. It has been suggested that a lack of specific dietary nutrients, such as essential omega–3 fatty acids, may significantly contribute to cognitive decline and increased risk and severity of brain injury. When rats are fed low-DHA diets for one or more generations, clear deficits in cognition are observed [6]. Blood DHA levels are decreased in various forms of retinitis pigmentosa, in Usher's syndrome, and in animal models of inherited retinal degeneration [2].

Aging is associated with decreased levels of DHA in both rat and human brains, especially the frontal cortex [6]. In addition to decreased dietary intake and reduced liver fatty acid desaturase capacity, age-related defects in antioxidant systems result in an increase in lipid peroxidation that further reduces DHA levels [6]. Therefore, the elderly population is specifically at risk for the cognitive and cellular impairments associated with depleted DHA levels.

DHA Is Delivered to the CNS via the Bloodstream

DHA is concentrated in the brain and retina. DHA and its lipid precursor, linolenic acid (18:3,n–3), are provided by the diet. Linolenic acid is elongated and desaturated in liver hepatocytes to form DHA. Hepatic stores of DHA are then activated (22:6-CoA) and acylated into phospholipids and released as lipoproteins from the liver into the bloodstream for distribution to the central nervous system (CNS) [9].

Once processed in the liver and released into the blood, retinal pigment epithelial (RPE) cells take up newly elongated DHA via the choriocapillaris [2]. Intraperitoneal injection of [^{3}H]DHA demonstrates that DHA first accumulates in RPE cells prior to being incorporated into the inner segments of photoreceptors [10, 11]. Under in vitro conditions, the retina has been shown to incorporate approximately 60–90% of physiologically meaningful administrations of [^{3}H]DHA (i.e., nanomolar range) into the retina in the form of esterified phospholipids within 4 h [12].

Phospholipids Containing DHA Are Incorporated into Photoreceptors

RPE cells are derived from the neuroectoderm and are closely associated with photoreceptors. In humans, approximately 23 photoreceptors interact with each RPE cell. They are specialized to maintain optimal photoreceptor health by providing nutrition, protection, synthesis/secretion of neurotrophic growth factors, and phagocytosing/ processing of aged photoreceptor outer segment tips [13]. After RPE cells absorb DHA from the choriocapillaries, they release DHA into the interphotoreceptor matrix, where it is preferentially taken up by the myoid region of the photoreceptor inner segment and activated by coenzyme A. DHA is then esterified into both the SN-1 and SN-2 position of phosphatidic acid and triacylglycerol, ultimately producing multiple DHA-containing membrane phospholipids including phosphatidylethanolamine, phosphatidylinositol, phosphatidylserine, and phosphatidylcholine [14–17].

Previous research has indicated that photoreceptors are rich in a supraenoic form of the phospholipid phosphatidylcholine. This phospholipid incorporates a DHA in position SN-2 and a 24-6-36:6 elongation product of DHA in position SN-1 that tightly bind rhodopsin [18]. The SN-1 tail functions to 'curl' and restrict rhodopsin motion [19]. This interaction between DHA and rhodopsin is required for photoreceptor function and vision. In healthy individuals, DHA must be provided in adequate quantities for successful photoreceptor formation during prenatal and perinatal development; DHA must be provided over the lifetime of the individual in order to carry out photoreceptor repair and membrane turnover.

Photoreceptors have outer segments composed of stacks of photosensitive disks that respond to light exposure. These photosensitive membrane disks are continuously formed in the basal portion of the photoreceptor outer segment with a proportional amount shed from the outer segment tips. As more and more membrane disks are assembled and accumulate in the basal region, older disks are advanced toward the photoreceptor tip where they are ultimately shed and phagocytosed by closely associated RPE cells. The rate of membrane shedding and the rate of membrane biogenesis is identical, resulting in successful outer segment renewal/turnover with no modification in outer segment length [10].

Electron microscopic autoradiography, using labeled [³H]DHA, tracks disk labeling and progression. [³H]DHA is not observed at the tips of the photoreceptors prior to labeled disk migration into the tip region. In addition, the density of [³H]DHA incorporated into each disk membrane in the basal region of the photoreceptor outer segment remains stable throughout the life of the disk membrane [10]. Thus, there is no further redistribution of DHA once it is loaded onto a disk membrane at the basal region of the outer segment [10]. Rather, photoreceptors incorporate DHA into disks at the base of the outer segment where DHA molecules will remain until eventual outer segment shedding and phagocytosis by the RPE cells [10].

The body actively conserves DHA stores in order to prevent DHA depletion. This is especially true in the retina. After RPE cells phagocytize shed photoreceptor outer segment tips during routine photoreceptor maintenance, DHA, like vitamin A, is recycled back to the inner segments of the photoreceptor via the interphotoreceptor matrix. In one experiment, frogs were injected with [³H]DHA until the entire photoreceptor outer segment was heavily labeled (~30 days after injection). During subsequent shedding of photoreceptor tips and the uptake of those phagosomes into the RPE cells, a pulse of labeled

[^{3}H]DHA was observed entering the RPE cell. Once inside the RPE cell, the transient oil droplets containing [^{3}H]DHA-labeled phospholipids immediately underwent degradation and dissipated. It was observed that during the experiment, 12% of the labeled [^{3}H]DHA was phagocytized into the RPE cell, while total retinal [^{3}H]DHA remained unchanged [10]. The stable [^{3}H] signal in photoreceptors indicates that [^{3}H]DHA is not lost during outer segment shedding. Rather, RPE cells must successfully recycle [^{3}H]DHA back to the photoreceptor inner segment for subsequent use in new membrane disks [10]. Although this efficient recycling of DHA back and forth from the RPE cells to the photoreceptors via the interphotoreceptor matrix (IPM) has been observed, it is still poorly characterized regarding the mechanisms of DHA uptake into the photoreceptor inner segment as well as a detailed description of the specific form of DHA transported across the IPM.

DHA in Neurodegenerative Disease

DHA has been implicated as a risk modifier for several CNS pathologies. Some prospective and case-control epidemiological studies have suggested that increased dietary intake of DHA lowers the long-term risk for developing AD and that a low concentration of DHA in the blood is an AD risk factor [20]. Post-mortem studies have shown that DHA is reduced in the hippocampi of AD patients [21]. Additionally, animal models of AD are more vulnerable to DHA depletion than controls, and DHA reduces several pathological hallmarks of AD (e.g., synaptic dropout, τ protein hyper-phosphorylation, and Aβ peptide aggregation) [20].

In AD, abnormal accumulation of the Aβ peptides results in cell death associated with Ca^+ excitotoxicity and a general oxidative stress response. We have recently shown that DHA downregulates Aβ peptide secretion from aging human neural (HN) cell cultures [21]. This response is associated with a concomitant increase in NPD1 synthesis. The soluble amyloid precursor protein-α (sAPPα) is a product of β-amyloid precursor protein (β-APP) cleavage by the α-secretase pathway and is known to reduce Aβ peptide secretion. Application of sAPPα to HN cells also significantly increases NPD1 synthesis, and application of a small concentration (50 nM) of exogenous NPD1 protects HN cells from Aβ42 peptide-induced apoptosis. Exogenous NPD1 exerts this effect by activation of a neuroprotective program that counteracts oxidative stress by upregulation of anti-apoptotic Bcl-2 family proteins (Bcl-2; Bcl-xl; Bfl-1/A1), down-regulation of pro-apoptotic Bcl-2 family proteins (Bad; Bax; Bid; Bik), and inhibition of pro-inflammatory gene expression (COX-2 [prostaglandin synthase-2, cyclooxygenase-2]; CEX-1 [chemokine exodus protein-1]; B-94 [TNF-α-inducible pro-inflammatory element]). Moreover, in the same study, both unesterified DHA and NPD1 were found to be significantly reduced in the hippocampi from AD patients as compared to age-matched controls. These data suggest that DHA acts to induce an anti-apoptotic, neuroprotective gene-expression program that counteracts Aβ42-induced inflammation by serving as a precursor to the potently bioactive oxygenation product NPD1.

DHA in Epilepsy, Epileptogenesis, and Synaptic Plasticity

Alterations in fatty acid metabolism have been proposed to contribute to the efficacy of the ketogenic diet used to treat refractory epilepsy in children [22–24]. Ketogenic diets have been shown to increase plasma DHA in rats and humans [25, 26], and rats consuming a ketogenic diet showed a 15% increase in brain DHA as compared to controls [22]. Multiple mechanisms have been proposed for DHA's role in modulation of seizure activity and pathological sequelae, including attenuation of neuronal membrane excitability via direct interaction with ion channels, regulation of expression and activity of mitochondrial uncoupling proteins, and regulation of genes linked to energy metabolism [24]. However, strong evidence for reduced seizure activity in patients fed DHA-enriched diets has remained elusive [27, 28].

DHA added to hippocampal slices may elicit anti-epileptogenic activity, modulate ion channels and neurotransmitter receptors, and in turn regulate synaptic plasticity. There are conflicting observations on the effects of DHA using extracellular and intracellular recordings of hippocampal slices. DHA facilitates N-methyl-D-aspartate (NMDA) responses [29], and it blocks delayed-rectifier K^+ channels [30, 31]. Thus a consequence of these DHA actions would be enhancement of neuronal excitability and worsening of seizure activity. In contrast, DHA added to hippocampal slices significantly reduced the frequency of evoked action potentials in CA1 neurons, hyperpolarized the resting membrane potential, and raised the stimulatory threshold for action potential generation [32]. At lower stimulation frequencies than in the studies described in previous reports [30, 31], it was found that DHA does not exert actions on multiple spikes induced by bicuculline or in Mg^{2+}-free medium, indicating that DHA does not directly interact with NMDA or non-NMDA receptors [33]. However, DHA may attenuate synaptic transmission and epileptiform activity in rat hippocampis by frequency-dependent Na^+ channel blockade [33]. Most of these electrophysiologic studies have used added DHA at relatively high concentrations (e.g., 50 μM). In contrast, we reported that 50 nM of added NPD1 exerts potent bioactivity [21, 34–36]. We now propose a new approach to define the significance of DHA in epilepsy: that is the finding that very small amounts of systemically infused DHA elicit profound down-regulation of kindling-induced epileptogenesis [unpubl. observations] due to the fact that DHA is used as a precursor for NPD1. Brain DHA is the substrate for the synthesis of NPD1 in the hippocampus during kindling, and this offers a different explanation for the involvement of DHA in epileptogenesis.

COX-2 regulates neuronal excitability and activity-dependent induction of long-term potentiation in the hippocampus via synthesis of prostaglandin E_2 (PGE_2), which is derived from arachidonic acid (AA) (20:4,n–6), the major omega–6 fatty acid in CNS cellular membranes. PGE_2 increases neuronal excitability by modulating K^+ channels, hyperpolarization-activated cation channels, and tetrodotoxin-resistant Na^+ channels [37–39], and it facilitates back-propagation of axonal action potentials required for long-term potentiation [40]. COX-2 and phospholipase A_2, which cleaves

AA (and DHA) from membrane phospholipids, become activated during kindling epileptogenesis, and the resulting prostaglandin synthesis is believed to mediate the development of aberrant neuronal connectivity [41].

Interestingly, in hippocampal synaptosomal fractions, bicuculline-induced status epilepticus promotes the accumulation of free (unesterified) DHA, which is also cleaved from membrane phospholipids by PLA_2 [40]. In turn, seizures elicit the synthesis of NPD1, indicating activation of an auto-neuroprotective signaling after seizures that counteracts seizure-induced increases in COX-2 expression [unpubl. observations].

DHA in Ischemia-Reperfusion Injury

In ischemia-reperfusion injury, pathological events stemming from energy depletion lead to non-specific glutamate release and glutamate reuptake inhibition, intracellular Ca^{2+} overload, mitochondrial dysfunction, and generation of reactive oxygen species. Increases in unesterified DHA are triggered by ischemia-reperfusion injury [41–43]. Under these circumstances, DHA can contribute to cellular injury through its non-enzymatic conversion to lipid peroxides. However, we showed, using a mouse model of ischemia-reperfusion injury, that DHA is also converted to NPD1 upon its release from membrane phospholipids [44]. In the presence of aspirin, DHA was converted into a series of 17R-hydroxy-containing DHA oxygenation products (D series resolvins), which possess pro-resolution bioactivity in inflammatory processes [45]. After infusing exogenous NPD1 into the third ventricle of mice undergoing ischemia-reperfusion injury, we found a dramatic decrease in polymorphonuclear leukocyte infiltration into infarcted areas, and the volume of infarction was greatly reduced as compared to vehicle-treated controls. These changes were associated with NPD1 attenuation of ischemia-induced up-regulation of COX-2 expression. In the same study [44], NPD1 was shown to inhibit IL-1β-mediated COX-2 expression. These findings have important implications for potential new experimental therapeutics for stroke, as well as other neurologic diseases sharing cytokine-mediated inflammatory processes.

Future Directions

In spite of all that has been discovered, many questions remain concerning DHA and its product NPD1. First, during situations of cellular stress, how do the retina and brain signal for the release of lipoproteins containing DHA from the liver? It is known that the liver is capable of releasing DHA when the CNS is threatened, but how does the CNS communicate that message to the liver (perhaps a plasma messenger)? Second, it is known that certain neurotrophins induce the synthesis of NPD1 (such as PEDF), but which receptor do they bind and how does that receptor signal for the release of free DHA and synthesis of NPD1? Finally, once synthesized, how does NPD1 traverse the nuclear membrane in order to modulate gene expression? Also, what is the nature of the signal that 'turns off' this gene expression? In time, we hope to discover the answers to these and many more questions in order to harness NPD1's extraordinary neuroprotective potential and find beneficial therapies in the treatment of retinal disorders and neurologic diseases.

References

1 Simopoulos AP: Essential fatty acids in health and chronic disease. Am J Clin Nutr 1999;70:560S–569S.
2 Bazan NG: Cell survival matters: docosahexaenoic acid signaling, neuroprotection and photoreceptors. Trends Neurosci 2006;29:263–271.
3 Uauy RD, Birch DG, Birch EE, Tyson JE, Hoffman DR: Effect of dietary omega–3 fatty acids on retinal function of very-low-birth-weight neonates. Pediatr Res 1990;28:485–492.
4 Bazan NG: Synaptic lipid signaling: significance of polyunsaturated fatty acids and platelet-activating factor: J Lipid Res 2003;44:2221–2233.
5 Bazan NG: Neuroprotectin D1: a DHA-derived mediator that protects brain and retina against cell injury-induced oxidative stress. Brain Pathol 2005;15:159–166.
6 Uauy R, Dangour AD: Nutrition in brain development and aging: role of essential fatty acids. Nutr Rev 2006;64:S24–S33.
7 Muskiet FA, Fokkema MR, Schaafsma A, Boersma ER, Crawford MA: Is docosahexaenoic acid (DHA) essential? Lessons from DHA status regulation, our ancient diet, epidemiology and randomized controlled trials. J Nutr 2004;134:183–186.
8 Neuringer M, Connor WE, Lin DS, Barstad L, Luck S: Biochemical and functional effects of prenatal and postnatal omega–3 fatty acid deficiency on retina and brain in rhesus monkeys. Proc Natl Acad Sci USA 1986;83:4021–4025.
9 Scott BL, Bazan NG: Membrane docosahexaenoate is supplied to the developing brain and retina by the liver. Proc Natl Acad Sci USA 1989;86:2903–2907.
10 Gordon WC, Rodriguez de Turco EB, Bazan NG: Retinal pigment epithelial cells play a central role in the conservation of docosahexaenoic acid by photoreceptor cells after shedding and phagocytosis. Curr Eye Res 1992;11:73–83.
11 Gordon WC, Bazan NG: Visualization of [³H]docosahexaenoic acid trafficking through photoreceptors and retinal pigment epithelium by electron microscopic autoradiography. Invest Ophthalmol Vis Sci 1993;34:2402–2411.
12 Bazan NG, Rodriguez de Turco EB, Gordon WC: Pathways for the uptake and conservation of docosahexaenoic acid in photoreceptors and synapses: biochemical and autoradiographic studies. Can J Physiol Pharmacol 1993;71:690–698.
13 Young RW: Shedding of discs from rod outer segments in the rhesus monkey. J Ultrastruct Res 1971;34:190–203.
14 Reddy TS, Bazan NG: Activation of polyunsaturated fatty acids by rat tissues in vitro. Lipids 1984;19:987–989.
15 Reddy TS, Bazan NG: Synthesis of arachidonoyl coenzyme A and docosahexaenoyl coenzyme A in retina. Curr Eye Res 1984;3:1225–1232.
16 Reddy TS, Bazan NG: Synthesis of arachidonoyl coenzyme A and docosahexaenoyl coenzyme A in synaptic plasma membranes of cerebrum and microsomes of cerebrum, cerebellum, and brain stem of rat brain. J Neurosci Res 1985;13:381–390.
17 Reddy TS, Bazan NG: Synthesis of docosahexaenoyl-, arachidonoyl- and palmitoyl-coenzyme A in ocular tissues. Exp Eye Res 1985;41:87–95.
18 Aveldano MI: Phospholipid species containing long and very long polyenoic fatty acids remain with rhodopsin after hexane extraction of photoreceptor membranes. Biochemistry 1988;27:1229–1239.
19 Aveldano MI, Bazan NG: Molecular species of phosphatidylcholine, -ethanolamine, -serine, and -inositol in microsomal and photoreceptor membranes of bovine retina. J Lipid Res 1983;24:620–627.
20 Calon F, Cole G: Neuroprotective action of omega–3 polyunsaturated fatty acids against neurodegenerative diseases: evidence from animal studies. Prostaglandins Leukot Essent Fatty Acids 2007;77:287–293.
21 Lukiw WJ, Cui JG, Marcheselli VL, Bodker M, Botkjaer A, Gotlinger K, Serhan CN, Bazan NG: A role for docosahexaenoic acid-derived neuroprotectin D1 in neural cell survival and Alzheimer disease. J Clin Invest 2005;115:2774–2783.
22 Taha AY, Ryan MA, Cunnane SC: Despite transient ketosis, the classic high-fat ketogenic diet induces marked changes in fatty acid metabolism in rats. Metabolism 2005;54:1127–1132.

23 Dahlin M, Hjelte L, Nilsson S, Amark P: Plasma phospholipid fatty acids are influenced by a ketogenic diet enriched with n–3 fatty acids in children with epilepsy. Epilepsy Res 2007;73:199–207.

24 Bough KJ, Rho JM: Anticonvulsant mechanisms of the ketogenic diet. Epilepsia 2007;48:43–58.

25 Cunnane SC, Musa K, Ryan MA, Whiting S, Fraser DD: Potential role of polyunsaturates in seizure protection achieved with the ketogenic diet. Prostaglandins Leukot Essent Fatty Acids 2002;67:131–135.

26 Fraser DD, Whiting S, Andrew RD, Macdonald EA, Musa-Veloso K, Cunnane SC: Elevated polyunsaturated fatty acids in blood serum obtained from children on the ketogenic diet. Neurology 2003;60:1026–1029.

27 Yuen AW, Sander JW, Fluegel D, Patsalos PN, Bell GS, Johnson T, Koepp MJ: Omega–3 fatty acid supplementation in patients with chronic epilepsy: a randomized trial. Epilepsy Behav 2005;7:253–258.

28 Bromfield E, Dworetzky B, Hurwitz S, Eluri Z, Lane L, Replansky S, Mostofsky D: A randomized trial of polyunsaturated fatty acids for refractory epilepsy. Epilepsy Behav 2008;12:187–190.

29 Nishikawa M, Kimura S, Akaike N: Facilitatory effect of docosahexaenoic acid on N-methyl-D-aspartate response in pyramidal neurones of rat cerebral cortex. J Physiol 1994;475:83–93.

30 Poling JS, Karanian JW, Salem N Jr, Vicini S: Time- and voltage-dependent block of delayed rectifier potassium channels by docosahexaenoic acid. Mol Pharmacol 1995;47:381–390.

31 Poling JS, Vicini S, Rogawski MA, Salem N Jr: Docosahexaenoic acid block of neuronal voltage-gated K$^+$ channels: subunit selective antagonism by zinc. Neuropharmacology 1996;35:969–982.

32 Xiao Y, Li X: Polyunsaturated fatty acids modify mouse hippocampal neuronal excitability during excitotoxic or convulsant stimulation. Brain Res 1999;846:112–121.

33 Young C, Gean PW, Chiou LC, Shen YZ: Docosahexaenoic acid inhibits synaptic transmission and epileptiform activity in the rat hippocampus. Synapse 2000;37:90–94.

34 Mukherjee PK, Marcheselli VL, Serhan CN, Bazan NG: Neuroprotectin D1: a docosahexaenoic acid-derived docosatriene protects human retinal pigment epithelial cells from oxidative stress. Proc Natl Acad Sci USA 2004;101:8491–8496.

35 Gold MS, Levine JD, Correa AM: Modulation of TTX-R INa by PKC and PKA and their role in PGE$_2$-induced sensitization of rat sensory neurons in vitro. J Neurosci 1998;18:10345–10355.

36 Ingram SL, Williams JT: Modulation of the hyperpolarization-activated current (Ih) by cyclic nucleotides in guinea-pig primary afferent neurons. J Physiol 1996;492:97–106.

37 Nicol GD, Vasko MR, Evans AR: Prostaglandins suppress an outward potassium current in embryonic rat sensory neurons. J Neurophysiol 1997;77:167–176.

38 Chen C, Magee JC, Bazan NG: Cyclooxygenase-2 regulates prostaglandin E$_2$ signaling in hippocampal long-term synaptic plasticity. J Neurophysiol 2002;87:2851–2857.

39 Tu B, Bazan NG: Hippocampal kindling epileptogenesis upregulates neuronal cyclooxygenase-2 expression in neocortex. Exp Neurol 2003;179:167–175.

40 Birkle DL, Bazan NG: Effect of bicuculline-induced status epilepticus on prostaglandins and hydroxyeicosatetraenoic acids in rat brain subcellular fractions. J Neurochem 1987;48:1768–1778.

41 Bazan NG Jr: Effects of ischemia and electroconvulsive shock on free fatty acid pool in the brain. Biochim Biophys Acta 1970;218:1–10.

42 Aveldano MI, Bazan NG: Differential lipid deacylation during brain ischemia in a homeotherm and a poikilotherm. Content and composition of free fatty acids and triacylglycerols. Brain Res 1975;100:99–110.

43 Yoshida S, Harik SI, Busto R, Santiso M, Martinez E, Ginsberg MD: Free fatty acids and energy metabolites in ischemic cerebral cortex with noradrenaline depletion. J Neurochem 1984;42:711–717.

44 Marcheselli VL, Hong S, Lukiw WJ, Tian XH, Gronert K, Musto A, Hardy M, Gimenez JM, Chiang N, Serhan CN, Bazan NG: Novel docosanoids inhibit brain ischemia-reperfusion-mediated leukocyte infiltration and pro-inflammatory gene expression. J Biol Chem 2003;278:43807–43817.

45 Serhan CN: Resolution phase of inflammation: novel endogenous anti-inflammatory and proresolving lipid mediators and pathways. Annu Rev Immunol 2007;25:101–137.

46 Bazan N: Homeostatic regulation of photoreceptor cell integrity: significance of the potent mediator neuroprotectin D1 biosynthesized from docosahexaenoic acid. The Proctor Lecture. Invest Ophthalmol Vis Sci 2007;48:4866–4881.

N.G. Bazan
Neuroscience Center of Excellence and Department of Ophthalmology
Louisiana State University Health Sciences Center, School of Medicine
2020 Gravier St. Ste. D, New Orleans, LA 70112 (USA)
Tel. +1 504 599 0831, Fax +1 504 568 5801, E-Mail nbazan@lsuhsc.edu

Simopoulos AP, Bazan NG (eds): Omega-3 Fatty Acids, the Brain and Retina.
World Rev Nutr Diet. Basel, Karger, 2009, vol 99, pp 55–70

Docosahexaenoic acid and Amyloid-β Peptide Signaling in Alzheimer's Disease

Walter J. Lukiw

LSU Neuroscience Center of Excellence and Department of Ophthalmology, Louisiana State University Health Sciences Center, New Orleans, La., USA

Docosahexaenoic acid (22:6,n–3, DHA), an essential marine-derived omega–3 poly-unsaturated fatty acid, is selectively concentrated in neuronal, synaptic and retinal membranes. 60% of fatty acids esterified in neocortical neuronal cell membrane phospholipid stores consist of DHA, so brain cells have a convenient and readily accessible reserve of DHA, that through phospholipase activities, liberate membrane-bound DHA into unesterified (free) DHA that serves in neural signaling, survival, and cell fate pathways.

Stereospecific oxygenated derivatives of DHA created through lipoxygenase action on free DHA further generate neuroprotectin D1 (NPD1) that elicits potent cyto- and neuroprotective effects. The neurophysiological actions of esterified DHA occur in part through the maintenance of neuronal plasma membrane integrity and lipid bilayer biophysics. The beneficial actions of free DHA and NPD1 occur (a) through the repression of the induction of inflammatory signaling mediators such as the inducible cyclooxygenase-2 (COX-2) enzyme, (b) through the recruitment of anti-apoptotic members of the Bcl-2 gene family, and (c) through the repression of pro-inflammatory and pro-apoptotic signaling genes and their translation products. DHA is essential for prenatal brain development and normal, homeostatic brain function. Dietary deficiencies in DHA are associated with retinal and neurological dysfunction and visual and cognitive decline. Deficits in DHA and NPD1 abundance are associated with the neurodegenerative mechanisms that characterize Alzheimer's disease (AD), the leading cause of neurodegeneration and cognitive impairment in our society. AD exhibits a progressive deposition of ragged amyloid-β (Aβ) peptides derived from the β-γ secretase pathway that processes β-amyloid precursor protein (βAPP) into the more toxic forms of βAPP-derived fragments. Aβ peptides themselves, and downstream consequences of Aβ peptide signaling, are pro-oxidative, neurotoxic, pro-inflammatory and pro-apoptotic. The enzymatic generation, speciation and trafficking of βAPP and Aβ peptides in AD and in experimental AD models are impacted by DHA abundance, the bioavailability of unesterified (free) DHA, and by derivatives of DHA such as NPD1.

This paper will review the interplay of DHA, NPD1, βAPP and Aβ peptide-related oxidative mechanisms in homeostatic brain function and in the development and progression of AD, currently the most prevalent neurological dysfunction in aging Western and Asian populations.

β-Amyloid Precursor Protein, Amyloid-β Peptides, Oxidative Stress and Apoptosis in Alzheimer's Disease

Significant molecular, genetic and epidemiological data support the idea that βAPP-derived peptide- and cytokine-induced oxidative stress, and the generation of reactive oxygen species (ROS), play important roles in aging and in the development and progression of neurodegenerative disease [1–20]. These pathogenic processes exhibit two key features: (a) they act in an accumulative fashion over the lifespan of the organism and (b) once begun, their deleterious effects on brain cell structure and function exhibit positive feedback, often perpetuating until the substrate is consumed or until the oxidative reactions are quenched or terminated. Mitochondrial dysfunction and focused oxidative damage, including primary peroxidation of cell components by ROS, appears to be among the earliest events in pathological aging and in the onset, development and progression of AD [14–22]. Free radical oxidative damage to brain plasma membrane lipids, which contain a high proportion of DHA, is thought to be one of the early critical and determining events involved in initiating brain cell membrane instability, dysfunction and degeneration. A related hallmark event in AD is the evolution from βAPP of soluble Aβ peptides into dense, fibrous insoluble deposits of extracellular congophilic, agyrophilic, neuropathological lesions called neuritic plaques. Neuritic plaques accumulate in the extracellular space and around the endothelial cell walls of cerebral blood vessels and especially in brain microvasculature [5, 6, 9, 21, 23–27]. Importantly, the generation of Aβ peptide oligomers, thought to be a 'priming' event in the pathogenesis of AD, appears to precede the formation of τ-positive paired helical filaments in neurofibrillary tangles [23, 24, 28, 29]. The βAPP holoprotein, comprising the substrate of the 'γ-secretase complex' that consists of presenilin 1 and/or 2 (PS1/PS2; essential components of γ-secretase) and nicastrin, gives rise to neurotoxic Aβ peptides 37–43 amino acids in length (Aβ37–Aβ43). The 'γ-secretase complex' thereby contains both peripheral and trans-membrane domains intimately associated with the lipid bilayers of neuronal lysosomal, Golgi, endoplasmic reticular and plasma membranes. The interaction of DHA with specific components of the 'γ-secretase complex' is not well understood, however, DHA-induced alterations in synaptic plasma membrane fluidity may contribute to learning-related memory retention in Aβ-peptide infused rats (see below) [23, 24, 30]. Both Aβ peptides and mature neuritic plaques support oxidative stress, partly through an incompletely understood direct action through metal-ion induced Fenton chemistries, and indirectly through a brain-specific glial-mediated inflammatory response [4–17]. Aβ peptide accumulation in the cerebral vasculature disturbs homeostatic functions of the blood-brain barrier, alters blood vessel neurophysiology, obstructs regional cerebral blood flow, and generates directly or further facilitates the production of ROS and oxidative stresses that progressively contribute to neuronal dysfunction and cognitive decline [5, 8–10, 31, 32]. Peripheral sources of Aβ peptides and inflammatory lipids, either by transversing a damaged or leaky blood-brain barrier, may further contribute to Aβ peptide deposition in the AD brain [4, 19, 25, 26]. The presence of neuritic plaques triggers an immune attack by brain microglia, resulting in a robust release of microglia-derived cytokines such as interleukin-1β (IL-1β) and tumor necrosis factor-α (TNF-α), and excessive local production of ROS, actions which may in part be catalyzed by trace amounts of neurotoxic metal ions [1, 4, 6, 15, 17, 33, 34]. The state of aggregation and compactness of Aβ peptides and maturation stage of neuritic plaques are associated with their potential for ROS generation and their ability to induce oxidative stress and to promote apoptotic signaling [5, 17, 20, 35, 36]. Apoptosis in turn is in part regulated by pro-apoptotic or anti-apoptotic proteins of a growing 20+ member Bcl-2 gene family [37–40]. Pro-apoptotic members such as Bad, Bax and Bik trigger apoptosis via their translocation into the mitochondrial membrane while promoting loss of calcium homeostasis and cytochrome c release. In response to apoptotic stimuli, mitochondria can also release caspase-independent cell death effectors such as apoptosis inducing factor (AIF), a flavoprotein induced by noxious stimuli, neurotoxic metals and by the redox state of the cell [20, 41, 42]. In contrast, anti-apoptotic members of the Bcl-2 gene family such as Bcl-2, Bcl-xl and Bfl-1(A1) form heterodimeric complexes with pro-apoptotic family members and thereby neutralize their activity [42–44]. Imbalances between the rates of synthesis and clearance of Aβ peptides and their pro-inflammatory and pro-oxidative effects, and also between pro-apoptotic and anti-apoptotic factions of the Bcl-2 gene family, are therefore important contributors to the onset, development and progression of degenerative mechanisms in neurological disease. Interestingly, in both in vitro and in vivo studies, antioxidants have beneficial effects in reducing markers for brain oxidation and apoptosis, suggesting that exogenously applied bioavailable factors can effectively moderate neural cell destruction and be part of a useful armamentarium in pharmacological strategy to treat neural degeneration [20, 45–50].

Alzheimer's Disease as an Inflammatory Brain Disease – DHA and Oxidative Stress

While the degree to which brain inflammation plays an initiator role in AD is controversial, there is abundant evidence that pathogenic inflammatory signaling contributes significantly to the maintenance and progression of the AD process. The enhancement in AD brain of ROS, activated microglia and astrocytes, complement proteins, pro-inflammatory cytokines such as IL-1β and TNF-α and their association with aggregated Aβ peptides and neuritic plaques suggests that early-to-late stage AD represents a progressive state of neural inflammation [19, 33, 34, 51–57]. A key genetic element that regulates the inducible generation of pro-inflammatory mediators, including prostaglandins, is COX-2, an oxido-reductase up-regulated in AD brain and a useful neocortical marker for the stage or degree of AD pathophysiological change [4, 19, 53, 58–61]. Free radicals and major pro-inflammatory cytokines in the brain such as IL-1β and TNF-α strongly activate both COX-2 and βAPP gene transcription in cultured brain cells and in models of brain injury that involve ischemia-reperfusion [54–62]. Recent findings that IL-1β can substitute for key aspects of hypoxia-mediated oxidative stress signaling further support a strong neurochemical connection between up-regulation of pro-inflammatory cytokine signaling, oxidative stress, apoptosis and neural cell death [5–8, 63–65]. AD brain can therefore be characterized biochemically by increases in the products and consequences of oxidative and inflammatory stress – accumulation of neurotoxic Aβ peptides, lipofuscin pigments, F4 neuroprostane (from non-enzymatically oxidized DHA), acute phase reactants and other components of the complement cascade, increases in hydroxynonenol (HNE), decreases in membrane fluidity, and depletion of DHA content [47, 58, 66].

DHA exerts anti-oxidative, anti-inflammatory and anti-apoptotic actions by reducing the cellular levels of ROS, in part by suppressing pro-inflammatory mediators and inducible COX-2 expression, and by maintaining higher levels of anti-oxidative enzyme activities such as those for glutathione [67–69]. Specific increases in HNE, a neurotoxic free radical aldehyde of fatty acid oxidation, may be one of the earliest biochemical markers for the development of AD [4–6, 65]. DHA treatment of cell cultures reduces HNE-induced oxidative stress and apoptosis [5, 6, 14, 65, 70]. Interestingly, COX-2 up-regulation in AD brain may have a direct bearing on γ-secretase activity and increased generation of amyloidogenic Aβ peptides, strengthening the pathological connection between brain inflammation and oxidative burden [19, 49, 50, 71]. Combined with extensive epidemiologic studies suggesting that non-steroidal anti-inflammatory drugs (NSAIDs), as inhibitors of inducible COX-2 activity, retard AD onset or severity, these data cumulatively suggest that inflammation-mediated oxidative stress and/or inflammatory cascades fuelled by oxidative stress are important factors that contribute to the progressive brain cell dysfunction and degeneration characteristic of AD brain [26, 33, 34, 72].

Therapeutic strategies aimed at effectively retarding Aβ peptide-, cytokine- and oxidation-induced brain cell stress are urgently needed to treat the insidious onset and progression of neurodegenerative disorders such as AD that have both oxidative stress and inflammatory components [4, 14, 17, 18, 49, 50]. The up-regulation of intrinsic, anti-apoptotic neurotrophic signals represents one such strategy. As further described below, DHA and NPD1 biosynthesis are key elements of a potent endogenous signaling system that effectively counteracts Aβ peptide and IL-1β-mediated oxidative stress, promoting neuroprotective signaling that supports brain and retinal cell function and survival [19, 38, 59–61, 73–75].

DHA in CNS Injury Oxidation and Oxygenation Pathways

As previously mentioned, DHA, the most abundant polyunsaturated fatty acid in the CNS, and obtained through the diet primarily from marine sources such as fish oil and algae, preferentially accumulates in the phospholipids of brain synaptic membranes and retinal photoreceptors. In rodent and non-human primate studies dietary deprivation of omega–3 fatty acids must be prolonged over one generation to reduce DHA content in the CNS. While this remarkably tenacious retention ability suggests that DHA is critical for neural and visual function, specific molecular mechanisms through which DHA elicits these positive, supportive bioactivities are just beginning to become understood. DHA incorporated into nuclear membranes and DHA exogenously applied to human neural cells in primary culture represses the expression of genes related to inflammation [4, 14, 38, 59–61, 76, 77]. Alterations in membrane architecture, function and fluidity coupled with specific repression of pro-inflammatory gene expression may contribute to the beneficial action of n–3 polyunsaturated fatty acids on cognition [57, 68, 69, 78]. The anti-inflammatory gene expression effects of DHA may arise in part through the inhibition of NF-κB-DNA binding response elements of the inducible nitric oxide synthase, COX-2 and other pro-inflammatory and/or pro-oxidative gene promoters [79–84].

Gene transcripts displaying changes in abundance in human fetal retinal explants supplemented with DHA encode for proteins involved in neurogenesis, neurotransmission, and the consolidation and refinement of synaptic connectivity [38, 85]. Because of the high concentration of DHA in the brain relative to other organs, DHA peroxidation is a major outcome of free radical-mediated oxidative brain injury induced by either acute trauma or more chronically through age-related neurodegenerative mechanisms. ROS directly attack membrane-esterified DHA in situ, generating an array of damaged pathogenic lipids and oxidized DHA intermediates [5, 6, 54, 65, 86, 87]. Lipid peroxidation is a self-propagating and self-sustaining neurodestructive process capable of extensive, progressive and prolonged neural tissue damage [5, 6, 16]. DHA esterified into phospholipids at the carbon two position of the glycerol backbone is liberated by phospholipase (PLA_2) to yield free DHA (fig. 1). The bioavailability of free unesterified DHA is a tightly regulated event and free DHA pools, normally at very low levels under basal conditions, become significantly increased during cerebral ischemia due to up-regulation of PLA_2 activity [54, 60, 61, 64]. Up-regulation of PLA_2 activity is also observed in Aβ peptide- and IL-1β-stressed human neural cells in primary culture and in AD neocortex and hippocampus [15, 18, 64, 88].

During oxidative stress, DHA may be oxidized non-enzymatically into F4-, D4-, E4-, A4- and J4-neuroprostanes, prostaglandin-like compounds formed independently of cyclooxygenase that further support oxidative stress [4, 14–16, 86, 87]. Synthesis of F4-neuroprostane-containing aminophospholipids may adversely affect neuronal function as a result of alterations they induce in the biophysical properties of neuronal plasma membranes [86, 87]. The abundance and speciation of F4

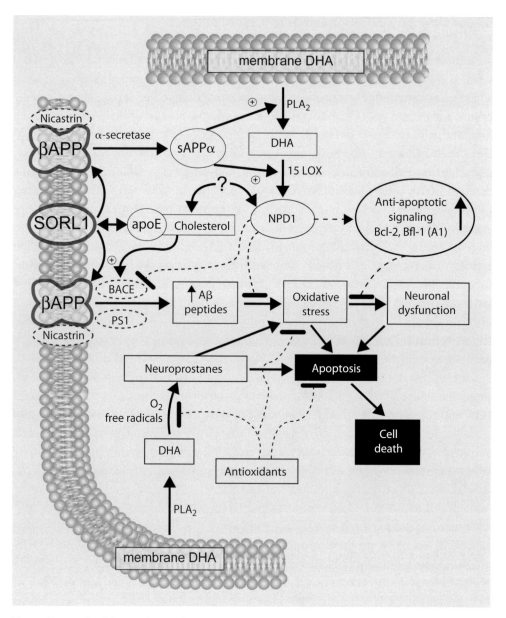

Fig. 1. Essentials of βAPP-Aβ peptide-DHA-NPD1 signaling, including enzymatic and non-enymatic processing pathways for DHA. DHA from the omega–3 essential fatty acid family preferentially accumulates within neuronal and retinal phospholipids of central nervous system membranes, concentrating specifically within neuronal synapses and retinal photoreceptors. Free DHA derived from membrane DHA stores (upper) is liberated via a stringently regulated phospholipase A_2 (PLA$_2$), and may subsequently be converted into the 10,17S-docosatriene neuroprotectin D1 (NPD1) through an enzyme-mediated lipoxygenation via a 15-lipoxygenase (15-LOX) or 15-LOX-like enzymes. The neurobiological activity of DHA-derived NPD1 in cultured human retinal pigment epithelial and human neural cells has been characterized as a potent cyto- and neuroprotective oxygenated lipid mediator [38, 59–61, 89, 73–75, 134, 135]. Membrane DHA (lower) is also rapidly oxidized non-enzymatically by molecular oxygen (O_2) and free radicals to form F4 neuroprostanes, a class of peroxidized lipids that further support oxidative stress and brain cell apoptosis leading to cellular dysfunction and cell death.

Lukiw

neuroprostanes and HNE, which reflect the general state of lipid peroxidation and oxidative stress, and may be useful biomarkers for the therapeutic efficacy of anti-oxidation drugs [5, 6, 11, 14, 16, 65, 86, 87].

Alternatively, membrane-esterified DHA can be liberated and oxygenated via enzymatic pathways, such as by tandem PLA_2-15-LOX action on free DHA, to generate the 10,17S-docosatriene or NPD1 (fig. 1). NPD1 elicits highly potent anti-oxidative and neuroprotective functions in brain and retinal cells [59–61, 73–75, 89]. The nature of the switch from membrane disruptive to neuroprotective roles for DHA, such as the generation of F4 neuroprostanes versus NPD1 and other DHA-derived neuroprotectins, is under intense research study. Changes in the redox balance of brain cells, modulated in part by bioavailable antioxidants and/or neurotoxic metal chelators, may affect the kinetics of these DHA-processing systems [17, 20].

β-Amyloid Precursor Protein Processing, DHA and Cholesterol

βAPP holoprotein, an ~110 kDa integral type-1 transmembrane glycoprotein and key player in AD neuropathology, is imbedded within lysosomal, Golgi, endoplasmic reticular, retinal and neuronal plasma membrane lipid bilayers, normally functioning in transport, intracellular contact and nuclear signaling [90–94]. βAPP can be sequentially processed via the β-amyloid cleavage enzyme (BACE; β-secretase), and subsequently by PS1/2 (γ-secretase), into ragged amyloidogenic Aβ peptides 37–43 amino acids in length, the most neurotoxic of which appear to be Aβ40 and Aβ42 peptides [23, 24, 95, 96]. Interestingly, the cleavage domains of βAPP targeted by β- and γ-secretase are membrane proximal, suggesting that βAPP-processing enzymes

Fig. 1 Continued These non-enzymatic reactions may be quenched by specific antioxidants and free radical scavengers [49, 50, 86, 87, 137]. The integral membrane protein β-amyloid precursor protein (βAPP) gives rise to sAPPα via a neurotrophic, non-amyloidogenic, α-secretase-mediated pathway that stimulates both PLA_2 and 15-LOX enzymes. Alternately, βAPP also generates neurotoxic Aβ peptides via a β-amyloid cleavage enzyme (BACE)-presenilin 1 (PS1) amyloidogenic pathway (β-γ secretase pathway) [23, 24, 103, 138]. The transmembrane protein nicastrin and the sorting receptor sortilin-1 (SORL1) direct trafficking of βAPP, and down-regulation of SORL1 may lead to activation of the amyloidogenic pathway and increased generation of Aβ peptides as is observed in AD brain [88]. SORL-1 interacts with the type E apolipoprotein carrier (apoE) which functions in part as the major cholesterol transporter in the brain [38, 97, 102]. Cholesterol also increases Aβ peptide production via stimulation of BACE and the β-γ secretase pathway [97, 103, 139–141]. 3-Hydroxy-3-methylglutaryl-coenzyme A reductase inhibitors (statins) both lower cholesterol and reduce intracellular and extracellular abundance of Aβ peptides in primary neuronal and neuronal-glial co-cultures and in clinical trials [109, 142–146]. Interactions between cholesterol, statins, DHA and NPD1 are not well understood although DHA supplementation in combination with statin therapy has shown significant health benefits in patients with hyperlipidemia, and demonstrate a further reduction of serum cholesterol than by statin treatment alone [147, 148].

operate directly at the membrane interface or within the membrane itself. The fatty acid composition of neuronal membranes, including DHA and cholesterol content, and cholesterol transporters, have direct bearing on whether βAPP is processed into neurotrophic or the more neurotoxic species (fig. 1) [97–102]. βAPP processing and Aβ peptides derived from βAPP in turn appear to be regulators of both lipid homeostasis and cholesterol biosynthesis [103–106]. DHA has been reported to suppress the age-related Aβ peptide shedding from human neural cells in primary culture [38], to repress Aβ peptide-related pathology in a Tg2576 transgenic cell model of AD [68], and to stimulate non-amyloidogenic βAPP processing and reduce both intracellular and extracellular levels of Aβ peptide in SH-SY5Y cells [107].

The effects of DHA and cholesterol on the activity of β-γ secretase enzymes are not well understood but are a tremendously active area of contemporary medical research. Initial interest in the cholesterol-βAPP-Aβ peptide connection came from the observation that cholesterol levels were found to positively correlate with Aβ peptide load in the brains of AD patients [57, 101, 108]. A class of inhibitors of the rate-limiting enzyme in cholesterol biosynthesis 3-hydroxy-3-methylglutaryl-coenzyme A reductase, collectively known as statins, have been repeatedly shown to lower serum cholesterol while reducing Aβ peptide abundance, both in vitro and in vivo [97, 103–109]. Cholesterol-rich regions of neuronal membranes known as lipid rafts appear to alter the distribution of βAPP-cleaving secretases within the membrane, resulting in production of the more amyloidogenic species of Aβ peptides and a decreased generation of the more neurotrophic forms of βAPP, such as the soluble sAPPα (see below, fig. 1) [38, 101, 108, 110, 111]. An unusual γ-secretase cleavage site within the hydrophobic trans-membrane domain of βAPP suggests that pathological events which alter or disorganize lipid bilayer structure or fluidity contribute to Aβ40 and Aβ42 peptide generation [98, 99, 111]. Cholesterol has significant biophysical effects on membrane lipid fluidity, curvature and the translocation, orientation or positioning of the βAPP holoprotein within lipid raft domains [101, 106, 112]. The neuronal membrane-enriched ATP-binding cassette transporters ABCA1 and ABCG1 play a significant role in the regulation of neuronal cholesterol trafficking and efflux, and in suppression of βAPP processing to generate Aβ peptides, hence their role in promoting cholesterol mobility remains an attractive Aβ peptide-reducing strategy [100, 113, 114]. Gross disorganization of the lipid bilayer and aberrant processing of βAPP may be further orchestrated by peroxidation of DHA, cholesterol, or by neurotoxic metal-ion catalyzed free radical damage to membrane lipid constituents [5, 6, 17, 20, 65]. While the interaction of cholesterol and statins with DHA are just beginning to become understood, DHA supplementation in combination with statin therapy demonstrates a significant enhancement in the reduction of serum cholesterol than is observed with statin treatment alone [cf. 147, 148].

Gene mutations in βAPP, BACE, PS1 or PS2 each drive the production of the more neurotoxic species of Aβ peptides but their individual contributions to neuronal plasma membrane dynamics and membrane biophysics remain elusive [29, 115–117]. The particularly neurotoxic peptide Aβ42, a 'sticky' 42-amino-acid self-aggregating peptide not only supports oxidative stress by contributing directly to neuronal dysfunction, apoptosis and eventual cell death, but are also 'secreted' into the extracellular space via the β-γ secretase pathway to trigger extraneuronal effects that support the extracellular generation of ROS [23, 24, 88, 97, 103, 118, 119]. While βAPP can generate toxic Aβ peptides, this integral membrane glycoprotein and can be alternatively processed via a membrane-bound α-secretase into a soluble form of APP (sAPPα), which is neuritogenic and neurotrophic. In fact, sAPPα supports normal neuronal function and also protects neurons from the toxicity of Aβ peptides [23, 24, 95, 96, 120]. A less abundant related protein, sAPPβ, cleaved by the proteolysis of βAPP by β-secretase, serves non-amyloidogenic functions [38, 51, 52]. A significant portion of the neuroprotective activity of DHA may be derived not only through its support of neural and retinal plasma membrane integrity and function, but also through its role as substrate for the generation of other oxygenated neuroprotective molecules. The roles of DHA and NPD1 in the membrane-bound enzymes involved in βAPP-processing pathways are just beginning to become understood. In APP/PS1 doubly transgenic mice, diets enriched in DHA were found to lower hippocampal Aβ peptide levels, and dietary supplementation with DHA in a triply transgenic AD mouse model reduced intraneuronal accumulation of Aβ peptide levels via a decrease in the steady-state levels of PS1 [98, 99, and unpubl. observations]. DHA has been found to attenuate both Aβ40 and Aβ42 peptide secretion in primary human neural cells, an effect accompanied by the formation of NPD1 [38, 59–61]. Neurotrophins such as pigment epithelium-derived factor (PEDF) induce concentration-dependent DHA-mediated NPD1 synthesis in retinal pigment endothelial cells. DHA and PEDF appear to synergistically modify the expression of Bcl-2 family members by activating anti-apoptotic proteins, by decreasing pro-apoptotic proteins, and by attenuating caspase-3 activation during oxidative stress [73–75, 121, 122]. DHA and NPD1 also induce a gene-expression program in human primary neural cells that up-regulates the production of anti-apoptotic Bcl-2 family members such as Bcl-2 and Bfl-1 (A1) that also promote neuronal cell survival. DHA and DHA-derived neuroprotectins are stimulated by sAPPα through up-regulation of PLA_2 and 15-LOX or 15-LOX-like activities. Specific direct actions of DHA or NPD1 on BACE (β-secretase) and/or PS1/PS2 (γ-secretase) activities, thereby down-regulating neurotoxic Aβ peptide production and subsequent ROS generation are currently not known.

Conclusion

The primary pathogenic events that initiate neurodegenerative disorders such as AD are multifaceted and multifactorial. Current clinical, epidemiological, molecular-genetic and neuropathological evidence suggests that this prototypic human neurodegenerative disease evolves from a complex interplay of genetic and environmental factors against a background of normal brain aging. Recent biochemical and epidemiological evidence suggests that dietary lipids such as cholesterol and DHA are causally involved in the aberrant neurochemical and physiological processes that initiate the neurodegenerative process [4, 10, 18, 19, 27, 39, 97, 123–127]. The hallmark pathological process in AD remains the progressive condensation and aggregation of fibrillar Aβ peptides into neuritic plaques that support oxidative stress, pro-inflammatory and pro-apoptotic signaling, resulting in neuronal dysfunction and irreversible loss of brain cell homeostasis. Mechanisms responsible for generating Aβ peptides, and their neurotoxic consequences such as driving brain cell oxidation, increase with age, and may potentially predispose aging humans to neurological dysfunction [23, 128–130]. The chronic nature of AD suggests that neuroprotective and survival factors are progressively lost, switching from an up-regulation in the expression of anti-apoptotic factors to increases in the expression of pro-apoptotic members of the Bcl-2 gene family [43, 44, 131, 132]. Unlike the actions of excessive cholesterol, the neuroprotective lipid DHA, and DHA-derived NPD1, decrease the rate of AB peptide generation, aggregation, and its consequences. DHA and NPD1 may also influence apoptosis-induced brain cell damage in part by shifting the balance from the expression of pro-apoptotic factors toward the expression of anti-apoptotic, survival-promoting members of the Bcl-2 gene family [38, 134–136].

Several important unanswered questions remain. The impact of DHA and NPD1 on the secretase-mediated cleavage mechanism of βAPP is still not well characterized. DHA and NPD1 as potential modulators of cholesterol biosynthesis, trafficking and apolipoprotein-mediated transport, βAPP processing, Aβ peptide speciation, generation and secretion during aging and in cytokine- and oxidation-stressed human brain cell models of AD are also not well understood [38, 98]. sAPPα, a modulator of DHA-derived NPD1 biosynthesis in cultured human neural cells and its bioactivity in young, adult and aging human brain, and in areas of the brain, such as the limbic system and association neocortex, targeted by AD neuropathology as compared with the relatively spared occipital cortex, is probably an important factor in modulating both DHA and NPD1 signaling. Further mechanistic studies on how DHA and NPD1 promotes neuroprotection through the up-regulation of anti-apoptotic Bcl-2 family proteins should further unravel how endogenously-derived lipid mediators promote brain cell survival that rally host defenses against oxidative stress and inflammation-triggered neuronal decline.

References

1   Beal MF: Mitochondria, free radicals, and neurodegeneration. Curr Opin Neurol 1996;6:661–666.
2   Pappolla MA, Omar RA, Kim KS, Robakis NK: Immunohistochemical evidence of oxidative stress in Alzheimer's disease. Am J Pathol 1992;140:621–628.
3   Pappolla MA, Chyan YJ, Omar RA, Hsiao K, Perry G, Smith MA, Bozner P: Evidence of oxidative stress and in vivo neurotoxicity of β-amyloid in a transgenic mouse model of Alzheimer's disease: a chronic oxidative paradigm for testing antioxidant therapies in vivo. Am J Pathol 1998;152:871–877.
4   Lukiw WJ, Bazan NG: Neuroinflammatory signaling up-regulation in Alzheimer's disease. Neurochem Res 2000;25:1173–1184.

5 Butterfield DA: Amyloid β-peptide (1–42)-induced oxidative stress and neurotoxicity: implications for neurodegeneration in Alzheimer's disease brain. Free Radic Res 2002;36:1307–1313.

6 Butterfield DA, Lauderback CM: Lipid peroxidation and protein oxidation in Alzheimer's disease brain: potential causes and consequences involving amyloid β-peptide-associated free radical oxidative stress. Free Radic Biol Med 2002;32:1050–1060.

7 Mattson MP: Oxidative stress, perturbed calcium homeostasis, and immune dysfunction in Alzheimer's disease. J Neurovirol 2002;8:539–550.

8 Mattson MP, Culmsee C, Yu ZF, Camandola S: Roles of nuclear factor-κB in neuronal survival and plasticity. J Neurochem 2000;74:443–456.

9 Aliev G, Smith MA, Obrenovich ME, de la Torre JC, Perry G: Role of vascular hypoperfusion-induced oxidative stress and mitochondria failure in the pathogenesis of Alzheimer disease. Neurotox Res 2003;5:491–504.

10 Chaney MO, Baudry J, Esh C, Childress J, Luehrs DC, Kokjohn TA, Roher AE: A beta, aging, and Alzheimer's disease: a tale, models, and hypotheses. Neurol Res 2003;25:581–589.

11 Fam SS, Morrow JD: The isoprostanes: unique products of arachidonic acid oxidation – a review. Curr Med Chem 2003;10:1723–1740.

12 Lynch AM, Moore M, Craig S, Lonergan PE, Martin DS, Lynch MA: Analysis of interleukin-1β-induced cell signaling activation in rat hippocampus following exposure to gamma irradiation. Protective effect of eicosapentaenoic acid. J Biol Chem 2003;278: 51075–51084.

13 Brigelius-Flohe R, Banning A, Kny M, Bol GF: Redox events in interleukin-1 signaling. Arch Biochem Biophys 2004;423:66–73.

14 Leuner K, Hauptmann S, Abdel-Kader R, Scherping I, Keil U, Strosznajder JB, Eckert A, Muller WE: Mitochondrial dysfunction: the first domino in brain aging and Alzheimer's disease? Antioxid Redox Signal 2007;9:1659–1675.

15 Lukiw WJ: Gene expression profiling in fetal, aged and Alzheimer hippocampus – a continuum of stress-related signaling. Neurochem Res 2004;29: 1287–1297.

16 Montine KS, Quinn JF, Zhang J, Fessel JP, Roberts LJ 2nd, Morrow JD, Montine TJ: Isoprostanes and related products of lipid peroxidation in neurodegenerative diseases. Chem Phys Lipids 2004;128:117–124.

17 Alexandrov PN, Zhao Y, Pogue AI, Tarr MA, Kruck TP, Percy ME, Cui JG, Lukiw WJ: Synergistic effects of iron and aluminum on stress-related gene expression in primary human neural cells. J Alzheimers Dis 2005;8:117–127.

18 Zhao Y, Cui JG, Lukiw WJ: Natural secretory products of human neural and microvessel endothelial cells: implications in pathogenic 'spreading' and Alzheimer's disease. Mol Neurobiol 2006;34:181–192.

19 Lukiw WJ, Bazan NG: Survival signalling in Alzheimer's disease. Biochem Soc Trans 2006;34: 1277–1282.

20 Castellani RJ, Moreira PI, Liu G, Dobson J, Perry G, Smith MA, Zhu X: Iron: the redox-active center of oxidative stress in Alzheimer disease. Neurochem Res 2007;32:1640–1645.

21 Nunomura A, Perry G, Aliev G, Hirai K, Takeda A, Balraj EK, Jones PK, Ghanbari H, Wataya T, Shimohama S, Chiba S, Atwood CS, Petersen RB, Smith MA: Oxidative damage is the earliest event in Alzheimer disease. J Neuropathol Exp Neurol 2001; 60:759–767.

22 Cui JG, Hill JM, Zhao Y, Lukiw WJ: Expression of inflammatory genes in the primary visual cortex of late-stage Alzheimer's disease. Neuroreport 2007;18: 115–119.

23 Selkoe D, Kopan R: Notch and presenilin: regulated intramembrane proteolysis links development and degeneration. Annu Rev Neurosci 2003;26:565–597.

24 Selkoe DJ: American College of Physicians; American Physiological Society. Alzheimer disease: mechanistic understanding predicts novel therapies. Ann Intern Med 2004;140:627–638.

25 Cacabelos R, Fernandez-Novoa L, Lombardi V, Corzo L, Pichel V, Kubota Y: Cerebrovascular risk factors in Alzheimer's disease: brain hemodynamics and pharmacogenomic implications. Neurol Res 2003;25:567–580.

26 Fitzpatrick AL, Kuller LH, Ives DG, Lopez OL, Jagust W, Breitner JC, Jones B, Lyketsos C, Dulberg C: Incidence and prevalence of dementia in the Cardiovascular Health Study. J Am Geriatr Soc 2004;52:195–204.

27 Iadecola C: Neurovascular regulation in the normal brain and in Alzheimer's disease. Nat Rev Neurosci 2004;5:347–360.

28 Hoozemans JJ, Chafekar SM, Baas F, Eikelenboom P, Scheper W: Always around, never the same: pathways of amyloid β-induced neurodegeneration throughout the pathogenic cascade of Alzheimer's disease. Curr Med Chem 2006;13:2599–2605.

29 Sidera C, Parsons R, Austen B: Proteolytic cascade in the amyloidogenesis of Alzheimer's disease. Biochem Soc Trans 2004;32:33–36.

30 Hashimoto M, Hossain S, Shimada T, Shido O: Docosahexaenoic acid-induced protective effect against impaired learning in amyloid β-infused rats is associated with increased synaptosomal membrane fluidity. Clin Exp Pharmacol Physiol 2006;33: 934–939.

31 Koo EH: The β-amyloid precursor protein and Alzheimer's disease: does the tail wag the dog? Traffic 2002;3:763–770.

32 Greenberg SM: Cerebral amyloid angiopathy and vessel dysfunction. Cerebrovasc Dis 2002;13(suppl 2):42–47.

33 McGeer EG, McGeer PL: Inflammatory processes in Alzheimer's disease. Prog Neuropsychopharmacol Biol Psychiatry 2003;27:741–749.

34 McGeer PL, Rogers J, McGeer EG: Inflammation, anti-inflammatory agents and Alzheimer disease: the last 12 years. J Alzheimers Dis 2006;9:271–276.

35 Raina AK, Zhu X, Shimohama S, Perry G, Smith MA: Tipping the apoptotic balance in Alzheimer's disease: the abortosis concept. Cell Biochem Biophys 2003;39:249–255.

36 Monji A, Utsumi H, Ueda T, Imoto T, Yoshida I, Hashioka S, Tashiro K, Tashiro N: Amyloid-β-protein (25–35)-associated free radical generation is strongly influenced by the aggregational state of the peptides. Life Sci 2002;70:833–841.

37 Hajimohamadreza I, Treherne JM: The role of apoptosis in neurodegenerative diseases. Prog Drug Res 1997;48:55–98.

38 Lukiw WJ, Cui JG, Marcheselli VL, Bodker M, Botkjaer A, Gotlinger K, Serhan CN, Bazan NG: A role for docosahexaenoic acid-derived neuroprotectin D1 in neural cell survival and Alzheimer disease. J Clin Invest 2005;115:2774–2783.

39 Lukiw WJ, Pappolla M, Pelaez RP, Bazan NG: Alzheimer's disease – a dysfunction in cholesterol and lipid metabolism. Cell Mol Neurobiol 2005;25:475–483.

40 Frebel K, Wiese S: Signalling molecules essential for neuronal survival and differentiation. Biochem Soc Trans 2006;34:1287–1290.

41 Lang-Rollin IC, Rideout HJ, Noticewala M, Stefanis L: Mechanisms of caspase-independent neuronal death: energy depletion and free radical generation. J Neurosci 2003;23:11015–11025.

42 Culmsee C, Landshamer S: Molecular insights into mechanisms of the cell death program: role in the progression of neurodegenerative disorders. Curr Alzheimer Res 2006;3:269–283.

43 Kirkin V, Joos S, Zornig M: The role of Bcl-2 family members. Biochim Biophys Acta 2004;1644:229–249.

44 Zhu X, Wang Y, Ogawa O, Lee HG, Raina AK, Siedlak SL, Harris PL, Fujioka H, Shimohama S, Tabaton M, Atwood CS, Petersen RB, Perry G, Smith MA: Neuroprotective properties of Bcl-w in Alzheimer disease. J Neurochem 2004;89:1233–1240.

45 Djaldetti R, Lev N, Melamed E: Neuroprotection in progressive brain disorders. Israeli Med Assoc J 2003;5:576–880.

46 Waldmeier PC: Prospects for antiapoptotic drug therapy of neurodegenerative diseases. Prog Neuropsychopharmacol Biol Psychiatry 2003;27:303–321.

47 Huang X, Moir RD, Tanzi RE, Bush AI, Rogers JT: Redox-active metals, oxidative stress, and Alzheimer's disease pathology. Ann NY Acad Sci 2004;1012:153–163.

48 Facheris M, Beretta S, Ferrarese C: Peripheral markers of oxidative stress and excitotoxicity in neurodegenerative disorders: tools for diagnosis and therapy? J Alzheimers Dis 2004;6:177–184.

49 Boedker M, Boetkjaer A, Bazan NG, Cui JG, Zhao Y, Pelaez RP, Lukiw WJ: Budesonide epimer R, LAU-8080 and phenyl butyl nitrone synergistically repress cyclooxygenase-2 induction in [IL-1β + Aβ42]-stressed human neural cells. Neurosci Lett 2005;380:176–180.

50 Boetkjaer A, Boedker M, Cui JG, Zhao Y, Lukiw WJ: Synergism in the repression of COX-2- and TNF-α induction in platelet activating factor-stressed human neural cells. Neurosci Lett 2007;426:59–63.

51 Hong S, Gronert K, Devchand PR, Moussignac RL, Serhan CN: Novel docosatrienes and 17S-resolvins generated from docosahexaenoic acid in murine brain, human blood, and glial cells. Autacoids in anti-inflammation. J Biol Chem 2003;278:14677–14687.

52 Hong HS, Hwang EM, Sim HJ, Cho HJ, Boo JH, Oh SS, Kim SU, Mook-Jung I: Interferon-γ stimulates β-secretase expression and sAPPβ production in astrocytes. Biochem Biophys Res Commun 2003;307:922–927.

53 Hoozemans J, Veerhuis R, Rozemuller A, Eikelenboom P: The pathological cascade of Alzheimer's disease: the role of inflammation and its therapeutic implications. Drugs Today 2002;38: 429–443.

54 Zhang R, Brennan ML, Shen Z, MacPherson JC, Schmitt D, Molenda CE, Hazen SL: Myeloperoxidase functions as a major enzymatic catalyst for initiation of lipid peroxidation at sites of inflammation. J Biol Chem 2002;277:46116–46122.

55 Bazan NG, Birkle DL, Reddy TS: Docosahexaenoic acid (22:6,n–3) is metabolized to lipoxygenase reaction products in the retina. Biochem Biophys Res Commun 1984;125:741–747.

56 Bazan NG, Colangelo V, Lukiw WJ: Prostaglandins and other lipid mediators in Alzheimer's disease. Prostaglandins Other Lipid Mediat 2002;68–69: 197–210.

57 Reid PC, Urano Y, Kodama T, Hamakubo T: Alzheimer's disease: cholesterol, membrane rafts, isoprenoids and statins. J Cell Mol Med 2007;11:383–392.

58 Bazan NG, Lukiw WJ: Cyclooxygenase-2 and presenilin-1 gene expression induced by interleukin-1β and amyloid β42 peptide is potentiated by hypoxia in primary human neural cells. J Biol Chem 2002;277:30359–30367.

59 Bazan NG: Synaptic lipid signaling: significance of polyunsaturated fatty acids and platelet-activating factor. J Lipid Res 2003;44:2221–2233.

60 Bazan NG: Cell survival matters: docosahexaenoic acid signaling, neuroprotection and photoreceptors. Trends Neurosci 2006;29:263–271.

61 Bazan NG: Omega–3 fatty acids, pro-inflammatory signaling and neuroprotection. Curr Opin Clin Nutr Metab Care 2007;10:136–141.

62 Lahiri DK, Chen D, Vivien D, Ge YW, Greig NH: Role of cytokines in the gene expression of amyloid β-protein precursor: identification of a 5'-UTR-binding nuclear factor and its implications in Alzheimer's disease. J Alzheimers Dis 2003;5:81–90.

63 Stiehl DP, Jelkmann W, Wenger RH, Hellwig-Burgel T: Normoxic induction of the hypoxia-inducible factor 1α by insulin and interleukin-1β involves the phosphatidylinositol 3-kinase pathway. FEBS Lett 2002;512:157–162.

64 Sun GY, Xu J, Jensen MD, Simonyi A: Phospholipase A$_2$ in the central nervous system: implications for neurodegenerative diseases. J Lipid Res 2004;45:205–213.

65 Poon HF, Calabrese V, Scapagnini G, Butterfield DA: Free radicals: key to brain aging and heme oxygenase as a cellular response to oxidative stress. J Gerontol Biol Sci Med Sci 2004;59:478–493.

66 Barnham KJ, Masters CL, Bush AI: Neurodegenerative diseases and oxidative stress. Nat Rev Drug Discov 2004;3:205–214.

67 Kim H-Y, Akbar M, Lau A, Edsall L: Inhibition of neuronal apoptosis by docosahexaenoic acid (22:6, n–3). Role of phosphatidylserine in antiapoptotic effect. J Biol Chem 2000;275:35215–35223.

68 Cole GM, Frautschy SA: Docosahexaenoic acid protects from amyloid and dendritic pathology in an Alzheimer's disease mouse model. Nutr Health 2006; 18:249–259.

69 Kim YJ, Chung HY: Antioxidative and anti-inflammatory actions of docosahexaenoic acid and eicosapentaenoic acid in renal epithelial cells and macrophages. J Med Food 2007;10:225–231.

70 Pfrommer CA, Erl W, Weber PC: Docosahexaenoic acid induces ciap1 mRNA and protects human endothelial cells from stress-induced apoptosis. Am J Physiol Heart Circ Physiol 2006;290: H2178–H2186.

71 Qin W, Ho L, Pompl PN, Peng Y, Zhao Z, Xiang Z, Robakis NK, Shioi J, Suh J, Pasinetti GM: Cyclooxygenase (COX)-2 and COX-1 potentiate β-amyloid peptide generation through mechanisms that involve γ-secretase activity. J Biol Chem 2003;278:50970–50977.

72 Fujiwara Y, Yokoyama M, Sawada R, Seyama Y, Ishii M, Tsutsumi S, Aburatani H, Hanaka S, Itakura H, Matsumoto A: Analysis of the comprehensive effects of polyunsaturated fatty acid on mRNA expression using a gene chip. J Nutr Sci Vitaminol (Tokyo) 2003;49:125–132.

73 Mukherjee PK, Marcheselli VL, Serhan CN, Bazan NG: Neuroprotectin D1: a docosahexaenoic acid-derived docosatriene protects human retinal pigment epithelial cells from oxidative stress. Proc Natl Acad Sci USA 2004;101:8491–8496.

74 Mukherjee PK, Marcheselli VL, Barreiro S, Hu J, Bok D, Bazan NG: Neurotrophins enhance retinal pigment epithelial cell survival through neuroprotectin D1 signaling. Proc Natl Acad Sci USA 2007;104:13152–13157.

75 Mukherjee PK, Marcheselli VL, de Rivero Vaccari JC, Gordon WC, Jackson FE, Bazan NG: Photoreceptor outer segment phagocytosis attenuates oxidative stress-induced apoptosis with concomitant neuroprotectin D1 synthesis. Proc Natl Acad Sci USA 2007; 104:13158–13163.

76 Chapkin RS, Davidson LD, Davidson LA: Phospholipid molecular species composition of mouse liver nuclei. Influence of dietary n–3 fatty acid ethyl esters. Biochem J 1992;287:237–240.

77 Lau FC, Shukitt-Hale B, Joseph JA: Nutritional intervention in brain aging: reducing the effects of inflammation and oxidative stress. Subcell Biochem 2007;42:299–318.

78 Puskas LG, Kitajka K, Nyakas C, Barcelo-Coblijn G, Farkas T: Short-term administration of omega–3 fatty acids from fish oil results in increased transthyretin transcription in old rat hippocampus. Proc Natl Acad Sci USA 2003;100:1580–1585.

79 Kielar ML, Jeyarajah DR, Penfield JG, Lu CY: Docosahexaenoic acid decreases IRF-1 mRNA and thus inhibits activation of both the IRF-E and NF-κD response elements of the iNOS promoter. Transplantation 2000;69:2131–2137.

80 Lukiw WJ, Pelaez RP, Martinez J, Bazan NG: Budesonide epimer R or dexamethasone selectively inhibit platelet-activating factor-induced or interleukin- 1β-induced DNA binding activity of cis-acting transcription factors and cyclooxygenase-2 gene expression in human epidermal keratinocytes. Proc Natl Acad Sci USA 1998;95: 3914–3919.

81 Lukiw WJ, LeBlanc HJ, Carver LA, McLachlan DRC, Bazan NG: Run on transcription in human neocortical nuclei. J Mol Neurosci 1998;11:67–78.

82 Lukiw WJ, Rogaev EI, Bazan NG: Potential of transcriptional coordination of nine genes associated with Alzheimer's disease. Alzheimer Rep 2000;3: 231–242.

83 Lukiw WJ, Gordon WC, Rogaev EI, Thompson H, Bazan NG: Presenilin-2 expression up-regulation in a model of retinopathy of prematurity and pathoangiogenesis. Neuroreport 2001;12:53–57.

84 Lukiw WJ, Ottlecz A, Lambrou G, Grueninger M, Finley J, Thompson HW, Bazan NG: Coordinate activation of HIF-1 and NF-κB DNA binding and COX-2 and VEGF expression in retinal cells by hypoxia. Invest Ophthalmol Vis Sci 2003;44:4163–4170.

85 Rojas CV, Martinez JI, Flores I, Hoffman DR, Uauy R: Gene expression analysis in human fetal retinal explants treated with docosahexaenoic acid. Invest Ophthalmol Vis Sci 2003;44:3170–3177.

86 Roberts LJ 2nd, Montine TJ, Markesbery WR, Tapper AR, Hardy P, Chemtob S, Dettbarn WD, Morrow JD: Formation of isoprostane-like compounds (neuroprostanes) in vivo from docosahexaenoic acid. J Biol Chem 1998;273: 13605–13612.

87 Roberts LJ 2nd, Fessel JP, Davies SS: The biochemistry of the isoprostane, neuroprostane, and isofuran pathways of lipid peroxidation. Brain Pathol 2005; 15:143–148.

88 Zhao Y, Cui JG, Lukiw WJ: Reduction of sortilin-1 in Alzheimer hippocampus and in cytokine-stressed human brain cells. Neuroreport 2007;18:1187–1191.

89 Marcheselli VL, Hong S, Lukiw WJ, Tian XH, Gronert K, Musto A, Hardy M, Gimenez JM, Chiang N, Serhan CN, Bazan NG: Novel docosanoids inhibit brain ischemia-reperfusion-mediated leukocyte infiltration and pro-inflammatory gene expression. J Biol Chem 2003;278:43807–43817.

90 Scott BL, Bazan NG: Membrane docosahexaenoate is supplied to the developing brain and retina by the liver. Proc Natl Acad Sci USA 1989;86:2903–2907.

91 Van Broeck B, Van Broeckhoven C, Kumar-Singh S: Current insights into molecular mechanisms of Alzheimer disease and their implications for therapeutic approaches. Neurodegener Dis 2007;4:349–365.

92 Mirra SS, Heyman A, McKeel D, Sumi SM, Crain BJ, Brownlee LM, Vogel FS, Hughes, JP, van Belle G, Berg L: The Consortium to Establish a Registry for Alzheimer's Disease (CERAD). Part II. Standardization of the neuropathologic assessment of AD. Neurology 1991;41:479–486.

93 Casserly I, Topol E: Convergence of atherosclerosis and Alzheimer's disease: inflammation, cholesterol, and misfolded proteins. Lancet 2004;363:1139–1146.

94 Shie FS, LeBoeur RC, Jin LW: Early intraneuronal Aβ deposition in the hippocampus of APP transgenic mice. Neuroreport 2003;14:123–129.

95 Guo Q, Sopher BL, Furukawa K, Pham DG, Robinson N, Martin GM, Mattson MP: Alzheimer's presenilin mutation sensitizes neural cells to apoptosis induced by trophic factor withdrawal and amyloid β-peptide: involvement of calcium and oxyradicals. J Neurosci 1997;17:4212–422.

96 Guo Q, Robinson N, Mattson MP: Secreted β-amyloid precursor protein counteracts the proapoptotic action of mutant presenilin-1 by activation of NF-κB and stabilization of calcium homeostasis. J Biol Chem 1998;273:12341–12351.

97 Lukiw WJ: Cholesterol and 24S-hydroxycholesterol trafficking in Alzheimer's disease. Expert Rev Neurother 2006;6:683–693.

98 Oksman M, Iivonen H, Hogyes E, Amtul Z, Penke B, Leenders I, Broersen L, Lutjohann D, Hartmann T, Tanila H: Impact of different saturated fatty acid, polyunsaturated fatty acid and cholesterol containing diets on β-amyloid accumulation in APP/PS1 transgenic mice. Neurobiol Dis 2006;23:563–572.

99 Green KN, Martinez-Coria H, Khashwji H, Hall EB, Yurko-Mauro KA, Ellis L, LaFerla FM: Dietary docosahexaenoic acid and docosapentaenoic acid ameliorate amyloid-β and τ pathology via a mechanism involving presenilin 1 levels. J Neurosci 2007; 27:4385–4395.

100 Tansley GH, Burgess BL, Bryan MT, Su Y, Hirsch-Reinshagen V, Pearce J, Chan JY, Wilkinson A, Evans J, Naus KE, McIsaac S, Bromley K, Song W, Yang HC, Wang N, DeMattos RB, Wellington CL: The cholesterol transporter ABCG1 modulates the subcellular distribution and proteolytic processing of β-amyloid precursor protein. J Lipid Res 2007; 48:1022–1034.

101 Cheng H, Vetrivel KS, Gong P, Meckler X, Parent A, Thinakaran G: Mechanisms of disease: new therapeutic strategies for Alzheimer's disease-targeting APP processing in lipid rafts. Nat Clin Pract Neurol 2007;3:374–382.

102 Hirsch-Reinshagen V, Wellington CL: Cholesterol metabolism, apolipoprotein E, adenosine triphosphate-binding cassette transporters, and Alzheimer's disease. Curr Opin Lipidol 2007;18:325–332.

103 Grimm MO, Grimm HS, Hartmann T: Amyloid β as a regulator of lipid homeostasis. Trends Mol Med 2007;13:337–344.

104 Zinser EG, Hartmann T, Grimm MO: Amyloid β-protein and lipid metabolism. Biochim Biophys Acta 2007;1768:1991–2001.

105 Wirths O, Thelen KM, Lutjohann D, Falkai P, Bayer TA: Altered cholesterol metabolism in APP695-transfected neuroblastoma cells. Brain Res 2007; 1152:209–214.

106 Grimm MO, Tschape JA, Grimm HS, Zinser EG, Hartmann T: Altered membrane fluidity and lipid raft composition in presenilin-deficient cells. Acta Neurol Scand Suppl 2006;185:27–32.

107 Sahlin C, Pettersson FE, Nilsson LN, Lannfelt L, Johansson AS: Docosahexaenoic acid stimulates non-amyloidogenic APP processing resulting in reduced Aβ levels in cellular models of Alzheimer's disease. Eur J Neurosci 2007;26:882–889.

108 Wolozin B: Cholesterol and the biology of Alzheimer's disease. Neuron 2004;41:7–10.

109 Fassbender K, Simons M, Bergmann C, Stroick M, Lutjohann D, Keller P, Runz H, Kuhl S, Bertsch T, von Bergmann K, Hennerici M, Beyreuther K, Hartmann T: Simvastatin strongly reduces levels of Alzheimer's disease β-amyloid peptides Aβ42 and Aβ40 in vitro and in vivo. Proc Natl Acad Sci USA 2001;98:5856–5861.

110 Cordy JM, Hooper NM, Turner AJ: The involvement of lipid rafts in Alzheimer's disease. Mol Membr Biol 2006;23:111–122.

111 Gamerdinger M, Clement AB, Behl C: Cholesterol-like effects of selective cyclooxygenase inhibitors and fibrates on cellular membranes and amyloid-β production. Mol Pharmacol 2007;72:141–151.

112 Carter CJ: Convergence of genes implicated in Alzheimer's disease on the cerebral cholesterol shuttle: APP, cholesterol, lipoproteins, and atherosclerosis. Neurochem Int 2007;50:12–38.

113 Famer D, Meaney S, Mousavi M, Nordberg A, Bjorkhem I, Crisby M: Regulation of α- and β-secretase activity by oxysterols: cerebrosterol stimulates processing of APP via the α-secretase pathway. Biochem Biophys Res Commun 2007; 359:46–50.

114 Kim WS, Rahmanto AS, Kamili A, Rye KA, Guillemin GJ, Gelissen IC, Jessup W, Hill AF, Garner B: Role of ABCG1 and ABCA1 in regulation of neuronal cholesterol efflux to apolipoprotein E discs and suppression of amyloid-β peptide generation. J Biol Chem 2007;282:2851–2861.

115 Thinakaran G: Metabolism of presenilins. J Mol Neurosci 2001;17:183–192.

116 Murphy MP, Das P, Nyborg AC, Rochette MJ, Dodson MW, Loosbrock NM, Souder TM, McLendon C, Merit SL, Piper SC, Jansen KR, Golde TE: Overexpression of nicastrin increases Aβ production. FASEB J 2003;17:1138–1140.

117 Jankowsky JL, Fadale DJ, Anderson J, Xu GM, Gonzales V, Jenkins NA, Copeland NG, Lee MK, Younkin LH, Wagner SL, Younkin SG, Borchelt DR: Mutant presenilins specifically elevate the levels of the 42 residue β-amyloid peptide in vivo: evidence for augmentation of a 42-specific γ-secretase. Hum Mol Genet 2004;13:159–170.

118 Tong L, Thornton PL, Balazs R, Cotman CW: Beat-amyloid-(1–42) impairs activity-dependent cAMP-response element-binding protein signaling in neurons at concentrations in which cell survival Is not compromised. J Biol Chem 2001;276:17301–17306.

119 Turner RS, Suzuki N, Chyung AS, Younkin SG, Lee VM: Amyloids β40 and β42 are generated intracellularly in cultured human neurons and their secretion increases with maturation. J Biol Chem 1996; 271:8966–8970.

120 Barger SW, Mattson MP: Participation of gene expression in the protection against amyloid β-peptide toxicity by the β-amyloid precursor protein. Ann NY Acad Sci 1996;777:303–309.

121 Gordon WC, Bazan NG: Docosahexaenoic acid utilization during rod photoreceptor cell renewal. J Neurosci 1990;10:2190–2202.

122 Gamoh S, Hashimoto M, Sugioka K, Shahdat Hossain M, Hata N, Misawa Y, Masumura S: Chronic administration of docosahexaenoic acid improves reference memory-related learning ability in young rats. Neuroscience 1999;93:237–241.

123 Girouard H, Iadecola C: Neurovascular coupling in the normal brain and in hypertension, stroke, and Alzheimer disease. J Appl Physiol 2006;100:328–335.

124 Colangelo V, Schurr J, Ball MJ, Pelaez RP, Bazan NG, Lukiw WJ: Gene expression profiling of 12,633 genes in Alzheimer hippocampal CA1: transcription and neurotrophic factor down-regulation and up-regulation of apoptotic and pro-inflammatory signaling. J Neurosci Res 2002;70:462–473.

125 Cutler RG, Kelly J, Storie K, Pedersen WA, Tammara A, Hatanpaa K, Troncoso JC, Mattson MP: Involvement of oxidative stress-induced abnormalities in ceramide and cholesterol metabolism in brain aging and Alzheimer's disease. Proc Natl Acad Sci USA 2004;101:2070–2075.

126 Grant WB: Dietary links to Alzheimer's Disease: 1999 update. J Alzheimers Dis 1999;1:197–201.

127 Vaya J, Schipper HM: Oxysterols, cholesterol homeostasis, and Alzheimer disease. J Neurochem 2007;102:1727–1737.

128 Fukumoto H, Rosene DL, Moss MB, Raju S, Hyman BT, Irizarry MC: Beta-secretase activity increases with aging in human, monkey, and mouse brain. Am J Pathol 2004;164:719–725.

129 Flood DG, Reaume AG, Dorfman KS, Lin YG, Lang DM, Trusko SP, Savage MJ, Annaert WG, De Strooper B, Siman R, Scott RW: FAD mutant PS-1 gene-targeted mice: increased Aβ, 42 and Aβ deposition without APP overproduction. Neurobiol Aging 2002;23:335–348.

130 Cui JG, Kuroda H, Chandrasekharan NV, Pelaez RP, Dimmons DL, Bazan NG, Lukiw WJ: Cyclo-oxygenase-3 gene expression in Alzheimer hippocampus and in stressed human neural cells. Neurochem Res 2004;29:1731–1737.

131 Tarte K, Jourdan M, Veyrune JL, Berberich I, Fiol G, Redal N, Shaughnessy J, Klein B: The Bcl-2 family member Bfl-1/A1 is strongly repressed in normal and malignant plasma cells but is a potent anti-apoptotic factor for myeloma cells. Br J Haematol 2004;125:373–382.

132 Akhtar RS, Ness JM, Roth KA: Bcl-2 family regulation of neuronal development and neurodegeneration. Biochim Biophys Acta 2004;1644:189–203.

133 Metcalfe AD, Hunter HR, Bloor DJ, Lieberman BA, Picton HM, Leese HJ, Kimber SJ, Brison DR: Expression of 11 members of the Bcl-2 family of apoptosis regulatory molecules during human pre-implantation embryo development and fragmentation. Mol Reprod Dev 2004;68:35–50.

134 Serhan CN, Clish CB, Brannon J, Colgan S, Chiang N, Gronert K: Anti-microinflammatory lipid signals generated from dietary n–3 fatty acids via cyclooxygenase-2 and transcellular processing: a novel mechanism for NSAID and n–3 PUFA therapeutic actions. J Exp Med 2000;192:1197–1204.

135 Serhan CN, Hong S, Gronert K, Colgan SP, Devchand PR, Mirick G, Moussignac RL: Resolvins: a family of bioactive products of omega–3 fatty acid transformation circuits initiated by aspirin treatment that counter proinflammation signals. J Exp Med 2002;196:1025–1037.

136 Graham SH, Chen J, Clark RS. Bcl-2 family gene products in cerebral ischemia and traumatic brain injury. J Neurotrauma 2000;17:831–841.

137 Markesbery WR, Kryscio RJ, Lovell MA, Morrow JD: Lipid peroxidation is an early event in the brain in amnestic mild cognitive impairment. Ann Neurol 2005;58:730–735.

138 Frears ER, Stephens DJ, Walters CE, Davies H, Austen BM: The role of cholesterol in the biosynthesis of β-amyloid. Neuroreport 1999;10:1699–1705.

139 Schenk D: Alzheimer's disease: a partner for presenilin. Nature 2002;407:48–54.

140 Takeda K, Araki W, Tabira T: Enhanced generation of intracellular Aβ42 amyloid peptide by mutation of presenilins PS1 and PS2. Eur J Neurosci 2004;19: 258–264.

141 Mattson MP, Mattson EP: Amyloid peptide enhances nail rusting: novel insight into mechanisms of aging and Alzheimer's disease. Ageing Res Rev 2002;1: 327–330.

142 Stein TD, Johnson JA: Genetic programming by the proteolytic fragments of the amyloid precursor protein: somewhere between confusion and clarity. Rev Neurosci 2003;14:317–341.

143 Simons M, Keller P, De Strooper B, Beyreuther K, Dotti CG, Simons K. Cholesterol depletion inhibits the generation of β-amyloid in hippocampal neurons. Proc Natl Acad Sci USA 1998;95:6460–6464.

144 Notkola IL, Sulkava R, Pekkanen J, Erkinjuntti T, Ehnholm C, Kivinen P, Tuomilehto J, Nissinen A: Serum total cholesterol, apolipoprotein E ε4 allele, and Alzheimer's disease. Neuroepidemiology 1998;17:14–20.

145 Webster NJ, Green KN, Peers C, Vaughan PF: Altered processing of amyloid precursor protein in the human neuroblastoma SH-SY5Y by chronic hypoxia. J Neurochem 2002;83:1262–1271.

146 Bodovitz S, Klein WL: Cholesterol modulates α-secretase cleavage of amyloid precursor protein. J Biol Chem 1996;271:4436–4440.

147 Martin RE: Docosahexaenoic acid decreases phospholipase A_2 activity in the neurites/nerve growth cones of PC12 cells. J Neurosci Res 1998;54:805–813.

148 Meyer BJ, Hammervold T, Rustan AC, Howe PR: Dose-dependent effects of docosahexaenoic acid supplementation on blood lipids in statin-treated hyperlipidaemic subjects. Lipids 2007;42:109–115.

Walter J. Lukiw, BS, MS, PhD
LSU Neuroscience Center of Excellence and Department of Ophthalmology
Louisiana State University Health Sciences Center
2020 Gravier Street, Suite 904, New Orleans, LA 70112-2272 (USA)
Tel. +1 504 599 0842, Fax +1 504 568-5801, E-Mail wlukiw@lsuhsc.edu

Simopoulos AP, Bazan NG (eds): Omega-3 Fatty Acids, the Brain and Retina.
World Rev Nutr Diet. Basel, Karger, 2009, vol 99, pp 71–96

Administration of Docosahexaenoic Acid, Uridine and Choline Increases Levels of Synaptic Membranes and Dendritic Spines in Rodent Brain

Richard J. Wurtman[a] · Mehmet Cansev[a,b] · Toshimasa Sakamoto[a] · Ismail H. Ulus[a,b]

[a]Department of Brain and Cognitive Sciences, Massachusetts Institute of Technology, Cambridge, Mass., USA, and [b]Department of Pharmacology and Clinical Pharmacology, Uludag University Medical School, Gorukle, Bursa, Turkey

That docosahexaenoic acid (DHA), an omega–3 polyunsaturated fatty acid (PUFA), can affect brain function and behavior no longer is controversial: deficiencies in this compound are associated with impairments in cognitive development, correctable by its repletion [1] and the consumption of DHA or fish oil by humans reportedly slows cognitive decline in the aged [2] and in subjects with early Alzheimer's disease [3] and promotes mental development in infants [4]. Some of DHA's effects on brain have been shown to occur with 'physiologic' doses which raise its plasma concentrations significantly but keep them within their normal range [5]; others probably are pharmacologic. Some are shared with eicosapentaenoic acid (EPA), another omega–3 PUFA, or with the omega–6 fatty acid arachidonic acid (AA), and others with both or neither of these compounds.

In general, nutrients and drugs that modify brain function or behavior tend to do so by affecting synaptic transmission [6]: they modulate the quantities of particular neurotransmitter molecules within synaptic clefts, or act directly on the transmitter's receptors or on downstream signal-transduction molecules. Is this also the case for DHA? Hypotheses attempting to explain how DHA affects brain function have, in general, been based on its incorporation into membrane phospholipids and consequent effects on membrane fluidity [7]; on proteins affecting transcription (RXR [8]) or neurite outgrowth (syntaxin-3 [9]); on increasing phosphatidylserine (PS) production [10]; on suppression of neuronal apoptosis [11]; or on the neuroprotective actions of its product 10,17S-docosatriene [12]. Little has been known concerning possible changes DHA might produce in synaptic transmission.

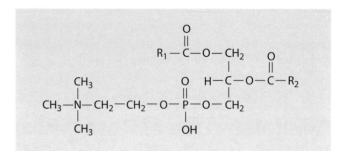

Fig. 1. Structure of phosphatidylcholine.

Now it can be stated that DHA does indeed affect important components of brain neurotransmission: it increases the synthesis and levels of phosphatides, the main constituents of synaptic membranes, and of specific pre- and postsynaptic proteins [13, 14], and it promotes the formation of dendritic spines [15], where most excitatory synaptic transmission takes place. In doing these things, DHA acts in concert with two other circulating compounds, uridine and choline [13]. Like DHA, these compounds also cross the blood-brain barrier (BBB) via specific transport mechanisms and also affect the substrate saturation of the enzymes that utilize them for synthesizing phosphatides. The effects of administering all three phosphatide precursors together tend to be greater than the summed effects of giving each alone. Both uridine (via its product uridine-5′-triphosphate [UTP]) and DHA may also promote membrane phosphatide synthesis by interacting with specific neuronal proteins, such as the P2Y receptor for UTP [16] and syntaxin-3 for DHA [9].

This article summarizes available information concerning mechanisms by which DHA affects synaptic membrane levels, synapse formation, and brain neurotransmission. Because DHA's effects on synaptic membrane depend to such a great extent on its interactions with brain uridine and choline, the article also describes the metabolism of these compounds in some detail.

Biosynthesis of Membrane Phosphatides

All cells utilize DHA and other fatty acids, uridine, and choline to form the phosphatide subunits (e.g. phosphatidylcholine [PC]) (fig. 1) which, when aggregated, constitute the major components of their membranes. PC, the principal subunit in brain, is synthesized from these precursors by the cytidinediphosphocholine (CDP-choline) cycle or 'Kennedy cycle' [17] (fig. 2). PC, in turn, provides the phosphocholine moiety for synthesizing sphingomyelin (SM), another major choline-containing brain phospholipid. The phosphatide phosphatidylethanolamine (PE) also is synthesized via the Kennedy cycle, utilizing ethanolamine instead of choline, while the third major structural phosphatide, PS, is produced by exchanging a serine molecule for the choline in PC or the ethanolamine in PE [18].

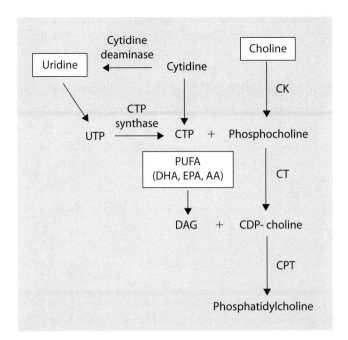

Fig. 2. Phosphatidylcholine (PC) biosynthesis via the Kennedy cycle [17]. In rats, cytidine is the major circulating pyrimidine [95]; in humans [19] and gerbils [20] the primary circulating pyrimidine is uridine. Only small amounts of circulating cytidine are converted to brain CTP, since the blood-brain barrier (BBB) high-affinity transporter for pyrimidines (CNT2) has a very low affinity for cytidine [96–98]; uridine, in contrast, readily enters the brain via CNT2, yielding UTP which can be converted to CTP by CTP synthase [89]. CTP then reacts with phosphocholine to form CDP-choline, which combines with diacylglycerol (DAG), preferentially species containing PUFAs like DHA, EPA or AA to form PC. Boxes indicate the compounds that are obtained from the circulation. Synthesis of PE via the Kennedy cycle utilizes ethanolamine instead of choline [data from 14].

The CDP-choline cycle involves three sequential enzymatic reactions (fig. 2). In the first, catalyzed by choline kinase (CK), a monophosphate is transferred from ATP to the hydroxyl oxygen of the choline, yielding phosphocholine. The second, catalyzed by CTP:phosphocholine cytidylyltransferase (CT), transfers cytidylylmonophosphate (CMP) from cytidine-5′-triphosphate (CTP) to the phosphorus of phosphocholine, yielding cytidylyldiphosphocholine (also known as CDP-choline or as citicoline). As discussed below, much of the CTP that the human brain uses for this reaction derives from circulating uridine [19]. The third and last reaction, catalyzed by CDP-choline:1,2-diacylglycerol cholinephosphotransferase (CPT), bonds the phosphocholine of CDP-choline to the hydroxyl group on the 3-carbon of diacylglycerol (DAG), yielding the PC. All three precursors of PC must be obtained entirely or in large part from the circulation, and because the PC-synthesizing enzymes that act on all three have low affinities for them, blood levels of all three can affect the overall rate of PC synthesis [13, 20].

Thus, choline administration increases brain phosphocholine levels in rats [21] and humans [22], because CK's K_m for choline (2.6 mM [23]) is much higher than usual

Table 1. Effects of UMP-containing diet and/or DHA on brain phospholipid levels [data from 13]

Treatments	Total PL	PC	PE	SM	PS	PI
Control diet + Vehicle	351	152	65	45	33	21
UMP diet + Vehicle	367	171*	84*	52	35	31**
Control diet + DHA	392	185*	78*	56*	39	32**
UMP diet + DHA	442***	220***	113***	73***	46***	36***

Groups of 8 gerbils were given either a control or a UMP-containing (0.5%) diet, and received orally (by gavage) DHA (300 mg/kg; in a vehicle of 5% gum Arabic solution) or just its vehicle for 28 days. On the 29th day their brains were harvested and assayed for phospholipids. *$p < 0.05$; **$p < 0.01$, and ***$p < 0.001$ compared with values from Control diet + Vehicle group. Data are presented as nmol/mg protein.

brain choline levels (30–60 µM) [24–26]. Most commonly the second, CT-catalyzed reaction is most rate-limiting in PC synthesis, either because not all of the CT enzyme is fully activated by being attached to a cellular membrane [27] or because local CTP concentrations are insufficient to saturate the CT [26]. Thus, when brain CTP levels are increased by giving animals uridine [20], CTP's circulating precursor in human blood [19], PC synthesis is accelerated [20]. The activity of CPT and the extent to which this enzyme is saturated with DAG can also control the overall rate of PC synthesis, as has been shown, for example, in permeabilized HeLa cells exposed to glycerol-3-phosphate and acyl-CoA [28], or in PC12 cells extending neurites after exposure to the nerve growth factor (NGF) [29]: in PC-12 cells, NGF increased DAG levels 5-fold, CPT activity by 70%, and the incorporation of choline into PC by 2-fold. As discussed below, DAG species containing DHA or other PUFAs on the middle carbon apparently are preferentially utilized for phosphatide synthesis compared with the amounts utilized for producing triglycerides [30]. (This does not explain, of course, why giving DHA and presumably increasing levels of DHA-containing DAG would also increase the levels of PC in a cell, e.g. in table 1).

If rodents are given a standard diet that also contains both choline and uridine (as its monophosphate, UMP) and, by gavage, DHA, brain PC synthesis rapidly increases [13, 20], and absolute levels of PC per cell (DNA) or per mg protein increase substantially (e.g., by 40–50% after several weeks of daily treatment [13] (table 1). This treatment also increases the levels of each of the other principal membrane phosphatides (table 1), as well as those of particular proteins known to be localized within synaptic membranes (for example, synapsin-1 [31], PSD-95 [32] and syntaxin-3 [9]), but not the ubiquitously-distributed brain protein β-tubulin (fig. 3) [13, 14]. As discussed below, treatment with DHA, UMP and choline also promotes the formation of dendritic spines in adult gerbil hippocampus [15] (see section 6), and improves hippocampus-dependent cognitive behaviors in rats reared in a socially-deprived

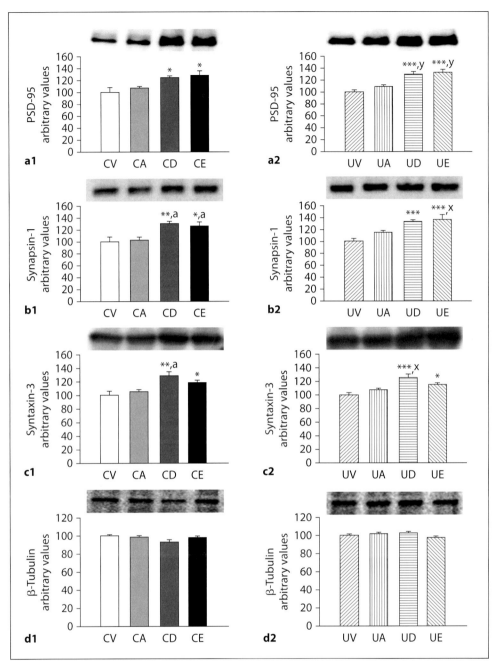

Fig. 3. Effects of AA, DHA or EPA, alone or in combination with a UMP-supplemented diet, on levels of the pre- or postsynaptic proteins PSD-95 (**a1**, **a2**); synapsin-1 (**b1**, **b2**) and syntaxin-3 (**c1**, **c2**). CV = Control diet + vehicle; CA = control diet + AA; CD = control diet + DHA; CE = control diet + EPA; UV = UMP-supplemented diet + vehicle; UA = UMP-supplemented diet + AA; UD = UMP-supplemented diet + DHA; UE = UMP-supplemented diet + EPA. *p < 0.05; **p < 0.01, and ***p < 0.001 compared with CV, and ᵃp < 0.05 compared with CA on the left-sided columns (**a1**, **b1**, **c1**) using one-way ANOVA. *p < 0.05; **p < 0.01, and ***p < 0.001 compared with UV, and ˣp < 0.05 and ʸp < 0.01 compared with UA on the right-sided columns (**a2**, **b2**, **c2**) using one-way ANOVA [data from 14].

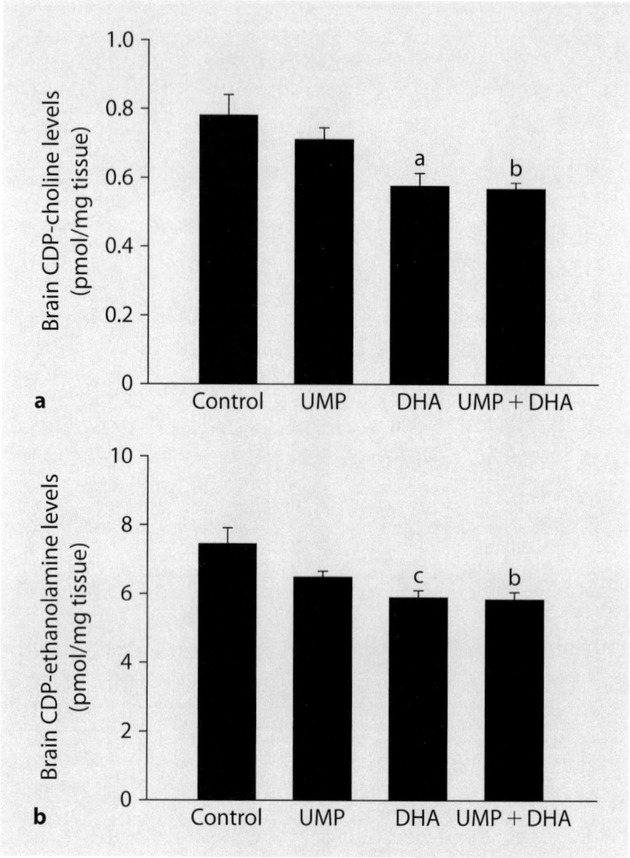

Fig. 4. Effects of DHA on brain CDP-choline or CDP-ethanolamine levels. Groups of 8 gerbils received either a control or a UMP-containing (0.5%) diet and, by gavage, DHA (300 mg/kg; in a vehicle of 5% gum Arabic solution) or just its vehicle, for 28 days. On the 29th day their brains were harvested and assayed for (**a**) CDP-choline or (**b**) CDP-ethanolamine. [a]$p < 0.05$ and [c]$p < 0.01$ when compared with the values for control diet + vehicle group; [b]$p < 0.05$ when compared with values for UMP diet + vehicle group [data from 13].

environment [33] (see section 7). Thus, the production, levels, and functional properties of PC, other phosphatides, and proteins in brain membranes, are found to depend to a surprising extent on blood levels of PC's three circulating precursors. Providing supplemental UMP or DHA without the other also increases brain phosphatide levels, but by less than when all three precursors are presented. (Choline is included in all of the diets.)

In studies designed to affirm that the increases in brain phosphatide levels caused by giving DHA, with or without UMP, reflect actual increases in phosphatide synthesis (and not, for example, inhibition of phosphatide degradation), brain levels of CDP-choline and CDP-ethanolamine, the immediate precursors of PC and PE, have also been measured. It was postulated that if DHA acted by generating more DHA-containing DAG, and if this compound then combined with endogenous CDP-choline or CDP-ethanolamine to form additional PC or PE, then DHA administration might concurrently reduce brain CDP-choline and CDP-ethanolamine levels while increasing those of PC and PE. This expectation was confirmed [13] among animals receiving DHA, or DHA + UMP; CDP-choline and CDP-ethanolamine levels fell significantly while those of PC and PE rose (fig. 4).

Properties of the Enzymes That Mediate Brain Phosphatide Synthesis

As discussed above, the ability of each of the circulating phosphatide precursors to affect the overall rate of phosphatide synthesis results from the relatively low affinities of these enzymes for their substrates. This unusual property is discussed below.

Choline Kinase
The synthesis of PC (fig. 2) is initiated by the phosphorylation of choline, in which, as described above, CK (EC 2.7.1.32) catalyzes the transfer of a monophosphate group from ATP to the hydroxyl oxygen of the choline. In some neurons choline is also used for synthesizing the neurotransmitter acetylcholine (ACh), a process catalyzed by choline acetyltransferase (ChAT), which mediates the transfer of an acetyl group from acetyl-CoA to the hydroxyl oxygen of the choline. The ACh is then stored, largely within synaptic vesicles, for future release. Like CK, ChAT has a very low affinity for its choline substrate [34, 35]. The K_m's of these enzymes in brain (which describe the choline concentrations at which the enzymes operate at only half-maximal velocity) are reportedly 2.6 mM [23] and 540 μM [36], respectively, whereas brain choline levels are only about 30–60 μM [24–26]. Hence, the rates of both phosphocholine and ACh synthesis are highly responsive to treatments which raise or lower brain choline levels.

The ability of choline administration to increase the synthesis and brain levels of phosphocholine was first noted in 1982 [21] and its similar effect on ACh in 1975 [37, 38]. It had previously been shown that the production of another brain neurotransmitter, serotonin, was increased among animals receiving physiologic doses of its circulating precursor, tryptophan [39, 40]. This was shown to be because tryptophan hydroxylase, the enzyme that determines the overall rate at which tryptophan is converted to serotonin, has a very low affinity for this substrate. Inasmuch as the affinities for choline of CK and ChAT had also been found, in in vitro studies, to be low, it seemed reasonable to enquire as to whether choline availability could also control the syntheses of phosphocholine or ACh.

Even though brain choline concentrations shared with those of tryptophan the ability to control the rates at which the precursor is used for neurotransmitter synthesis, choline and tryptophan differed in an important respect: although both are used by certain neurons for two purposes – tryptophan for conversion to serotonin and incorporation into proteins, and choline for conversion to ACh and incorporation into phospholipids – in the case of tryptophan these two processes are segregated into different parts of the neuron, the nerve terminal and perikaryon, whereas for choline both can take place within the nerve terminal inasmuch as that structure contains both ChAT and CK. Hence, the acetylation and phosphorylation of choline sometimes compete for available substrate [41, 42]: When cholinergic neurons are forced to fire frequently and maintain the rapid release of ACh, choline's incorporation into PC decreases [41] and the breakdown of membrane PC increases ('autocannibalism'), liberating additional choline for ACh synthesis [43–45]. However, when the utilization of choline to form PC is increased (by providing supplemental uridine and an omega–3 fatty acid, as described above), ACh synthesis is not diminished, probably because so little choline is used in cholinergic neurons for phosphatide formation, relative to the amount needed for ACh synthesis [42].

CTP: Phosphocholine Cytidylyltransferase
CTP: phosphocholine cytidylyltransferase (CT; EC 2.7.7.15) catalyzes the condensation of CTP and phosphocholine to form CDP-choline (fig. 2). CT is present in both the soluble and particulate fractions of the cell [46]; the cytosolic form is reportedly inactive and the membrane-bound form active [27, 47]. Increases in the association of CT with membranes reportedly correlate with increases in CT activity and in the net synthesis of PC in vitro [48–50]. Some other lipids (e.g. PS) [51] and DAG [48, 52] also stimulate the translocation of CT from the cytosol to membranes in vitro, thereby activating the enzyme. However, translocation is clearly not the sole mechanism for CT activation, inasmuch as increases in the activity of membrane-bound CT often do not correlate with decreases in that of the cytosolic enzyme [53] (as would be expected if translocation were the only means whereby CT become activated). The phosphorylation state of CT may also be important [54] as well as the enzyme's substrate saturation with CTP and perhaps with phosphocholine, as described below.

CT has been purified to homogeneity [55], and has been cloned from rat liver [56] and from a human erythroleukemic cell line [57]. The purified form exists as an elongated dimer [58]. Mammalian CT proteins contain four functional domains: an N-terminal nuclear targeting sequence, a catalytic domain, a membrane-lipid binding domain, and a C-terminal phosphorylation domain. The K_m's of CT for CTP and phosphocholine in brains of laboratory rodents and humans are reportedly 1–1.3 mm and 0.30–0.31 mm [26, 59], respectively, while brain levels of these compounds are only 70–110 μm [20, 60, 61] and 0.32–0.69 mm [21, 25, 62] respectively. Hence, brain CT normally is highly unsaturated with CTP, and only about half-saturated with phosphocholine in vivo, suggesting that its degrees of substrate saturation, particularly with CTP, exert important limiting roles in PC synthesis. In fact, treatments that increase cellular CTP (e.g. administration of a uridine or cytidine source) have been shown to enhance CDP-choline and PC synthesis in poliovirus-infected HeLa cells [63]; undifferentiated PC12 cells [64, 65]; slices of rat corpus striatum [66], and gerbil brain in vivo [20].

CDP-Choline: 1,2-Diacylglycerol Cholinephosphotransferase
CDP-choline:1,2-diacylglycerol cholinephosphotransferase (CPT; EC 2.7.8.2) catalyzes the final reaction in the Kennedy cycle; it transfers the phosphocholine moiety from CDP-choline to DAG, thus yielding PC (fig. 2). CPT, an integral membrane protein, is present primarily in the endoplasmic reticulum [67]. The enzyme protein has been solubilized and partially purified from microsomes of rat liver [68, 69], rat

brain [70] and hamster liver [71]. A human cDNA has been isolated which codes for an enzyme with both cholinephotransferase and ethanolamine-phosphotrans-ferase (EPT) activities (hCEPT1 [72]), and a different human cDNA has also been isolated, the product of which exhibits only cholinephotransferase-specific activity (hCPT1 [73]). CPT may be a reversible enzyme, synthesizing CDP-choline from PC and CMP in microsomal preparations from liver [74, 75] or brain [76–78].

The choline phosphotransferase reaction also is unsaturated with the enzyme's substrates: its K_m values for CDP-choline and DAG in rat liver are 200 and 150 μM [79] respectively, while the concentrations of these compounds in liver are approximately 40 μM [80] and 300 μM [81]. (A DAG concentration of at least 1,000 μM thus would probably be needed to saturate the enzyme.) Brain CDP-choline and DAG levels are even lower, i.e., about 10–30 μM [20, 82] and 75 μM [61], respectively. Levels of cellular DAG have been shown to limit PC synthesis in permeabilized HeLa cells [28], cultured rat hepatocytes [83], and PC12 cells (described above) [29]. None of these studies distinguished between the enzyme which acts on both choline and etha-nolamine (PECT1) and the enzyme that acts only on choline (PCT1). A more recent report, using cloning and expression methods, described the K_m of human PECT1 for CDP-choline, as being 36 μM [84], which would probably still be too high for the enzyme to be saturated with this substrate in brain. The K_m of PCT for its sub-strates might also be affected by the fatty acid composition of the DAG molecule; for example, incubating mouse liver microsomes with DAG molecules that contained two oleic acids (1,2-dioleoyl-sn-glycerol [Di-C18:1 (cis-9)]) rather than two palmitic acids (1,2-dipalmitoyl-sn-glycerol [Di-C16:0]), increased its K_m's for DAG from 86 ± 6 to 1,860 ± 39 μM and its K_m for CDP-choline from 41 ± 2 to 1,000 ± 141 μM [85]. Hence the enzyme's affinity for its substrates declined by 20- to 25-fold. Apparently no data are available demonstrating that fatty acids (e.g., DHA) most able to promote PC synthesis [86] do so because they enhance cellular levels of DAG species which CPT binds most effectively or on which it has greatest catalytic activity.

Uptake of Uridine into Brain and Its Conversion to UTP and CTP
Since brain uridine can, by elevating CTP levels, modulate the effect of DHA on syn-aptic membrane formation, the enzymes and uptake proteins that mediate blood uri-dine's effect on brain CTP are discussed here.

Uridine and cytidine are transported across cell membranes, including the BBB, via two families of transport proteins, i.e. the Na^+-independent, low-affinity, equili-brative transporters (ENT1 and ENT2) [87] and the Na^+-dependent, high-affinity, concentrative (CNT1, CNT2, and CNT3) [88] nucleoside transporters [89]. The two ENT proteins, which transport uridine and cytidine with similar affinities, have been cloned from rat [90] and mouse [91]. Inasmuch as their K_m values for the pyrimi-dines are in the high micromolar range (100–800 μM [92]) they probably mediate BBB pyrimidine uptake only when plasma levels of uridine and cytidine have been elevated experimentally. In contrast, CNT2, which transports both the pyrimidine uridine and such purines as adenosine, probably do mediate uridine transport across the BBB under physiologic conditions. K_m values for the binding of uridine and adenosine to this protein (which has been cloned from rat BBB [93]) are in the low micromolar range (9–40 μM in kidney, intestine, spleen, liver, macrophage and monocytes [94]), while plasma uridine levels are subsaturating, i.e. 0.9–3.9 μM in rats [95], 3.1–4.9 μM in humans [95], and around 6.5 μM in gerbils [20]. Cytidine has not been thought to be a substrate for CNT2 [88], however recent studies suggest that CNT2 can also transport this compound, but with a much lower affinity than that for uridine [96–98].

It should be noted that, while both of the pyrimidines, uridine and cytidine, are present in the blood of laboratory rats, human blood contains unmeasurably low quantities of cytidine [95] even among individuals consuming a cytidine source like oral CDP-choline [19]; the cytidine is quantitatively deaminated to uridine in the human liver. Hence circulating uridine, and not cytidine, is the precursor of the brain CTP utilized for phosphatide synthesis. Gerbil blood contains both pyrimidines, but proportionately less cytidine than blood of rats; hence, gerbils are often used as a model for studying the effects of exogenous uridine sources on the human brain [99].

Like other circulating compounds, pyrimidines may also be taken up into brain via the epithelium of the choroid plexus (CP) and the ENT1, ENT2 and CNT3 transporters [87, 88]; all of these proteins have been found in CP epithelial cells of rats [90, 100, 101] and rabbits [102, 103]. However, the surface area of BBB is probably 1,000 times that of the CP epithelium (i.e., 21.6 vs. 0.021 m^2 in humans [104]), hence the BBB is the major locus at which circulating uridine enters the brain.

Uridine and cytidine are converted to their respective nucleotides by successive phosphorylations catalyzed by various kinases. Uridine-cytidine kinase (UCK) (ATP:uridine 5′-phosphotransferase, EC 2.7.1.48) phosphorylates uridine and cytidine to form UMP and CMP, respectively [105–107]. Several different forms of UCK exist, possibly as isoenzymes [108, 109]. Humans have two such isoenzymes, UCK1 and UCK2, both of which have been cloned [110, 111]. UMP-CMP kinase (UMP-CMPK) (ATP:CMP phosphotransferase, EC 2.7.4.14) [112–114] then converts UMP or CMP to UDP or CDP. These nucleotides in turn are further phosphorylated to UTP and CTP, by nucleoside diphosphate kinases (NDPK) (nucleoside triphosphate:nucleoside diphosphate phosphotransferase, EC 2.7.4.6) [115, 116]. mRNAs for UCK1 [111] and UMP-CMPK [117] have been described in brain [118, 119], as has NDPK activity.

Various interconversions between uridine and cytidine, and between their respective nucleotides, are known to occur in mammalian cells. Cytidine and CMP can be deaminated to uridine and UMP [120], while UTP is aminated to CTP by CTP synthase (UTP:ammonia ligase [ADP-forming], EC 6.3.4.2) [121, 122]. This enzyme acts by transferring an amide nitrogen from glutamine to the C-4 position of UTP, thus forming CTP [123]. CTP synthase activity has been demonstrated in rat brain [124].

All of the enzymes described above apparently are unsaturated with their respective nucleosides or nucleotides in brain and other tissues. For example, the K_m's for uridine and cytidine of UCK prepared from various tissues varied between 33 and 270 μM [106, 107, 125, 126], and the K_m for uridine of recombinant enzyme cloned from mouse brain was 40 μM [127, 128]. Brain uridine and cytidine levels are about 22–46 pmol/mg wet weight [20, 129] and 6–43 pmol/mg wet weight [20, 130], respectively. Hence, the syntheses of UTP and CTP, and the subsequent syntheses of brain PC and PE via the Kennedy pathway, depend on available levels of their pyrimidine substrates. Indeed, increasing the supply of uridine or cytidine to neuronal cells, in vitro [16, 65, 66] or in vivo [20, 99], enhanced the phosphorylation of uridine and cytidine, and elevated levels of UTP, CTP, and CDP-choline.

Availability of DHA and Other PUFAs to Brain Cells

As discussed extensively elsewhere in this volume, the omega–3 PUFAs DHA and EPA, and the omega–6 fatty acid AA are essential for humans and other animals, and thus must be obtained from the diet either as such or as their also-essential precursors, α-linolenic acid (ALA) and linoleic acid (LA).

Although the processes by which circulating PUFAs are taken up into the brain and, subsequently, into brain cells await full characterization, they are thought to include both simple diffusion (also termed 'flip-flop' [131]) and protein-mediated transport [132]. One such transport protein (B-FATP) [133] has been cloned [134]. DHA, EPA and AA are then transported from the brain's ECF into cells, and can be activated to their corresponding CoA species (e.g., docosahexaenoyl-CoA; eicosapentaenoyl-CoA; arachidonoyl-CoA) and acylated to the sn-2 position of DAG [135] to form PUFA-rich DAG species [136, 137]. DHA is acylated by a specific acyl-CoA synthetase, Acsl6 [138] which exhibits a low affinity for this substrate (K_m = 26 μM [139] relative to usual brain DHA levels (1.3–1.5 μM) [140]). Hence, treatments that raise blood DHA levels rapidly increase its uptake into and retention by brain cells.

EPA can be acylated to DAG by the Acyl-CoA synthetase [141] or it can be converted to DHA by brain astrocytes [142], allowing its effects on brain phosphatides and synaptic proteins, described below, to be mediated by DHA itself. Exogenously administered AA, like DHA, is preferentially incorporated into brain phosphatides [143, 144], as well as into other lipids, e.g. the plasmalogens [145, 146]. AA shares with DHA the ability to activate syntaxin-3 [9], however, as described below, its oral administration to laboratory rodents apparently does not promote synaptic membrane synthesis nor dendritic spine formation.

DHA and AA are major components of brain membrane phospholipids [147]. While AA is widespread through the brain and is abundant in phosphatidylinositol (PI) and PC, DHA is concentrated in synaptic regions of gray matter [148] and is especially abundant in PE and PS [149]. In contrast, EPA is found only in trace amounts in brain phosphatides, mostly in PI [150]. No significant differences have been described between the relative proportions of ingested omega–3 and omega–6 PUFAs that actually enter the systemic circulation [151, 152]. Moreover, the rates at which radioactively-labeled DHA and AA are taken up into brain and incorporated into phospholipids following systemic injections also are similar [143, 153]. (To our knowledge, no study has compared the brain uptake of EPA with that of another PUFA in rodents or humans, however exogenously administered EPA does increase brain EPA levels in vivo [154].) On the other hand, the half-lives of the omega–3 PUFAs in the blood (20 ± 5.2 h for DHA and 67 ± 14 h for EPA [155]) are substantially higher than that for AA (3.8 s [156]). Similarly, the half-life of DHA in brain PC (22.4 ± 2.9 h), but not in PI or PE, is much longer than that of AA (3.79 ± 0.12 h) [157]. Thus, a considerable proportion of AA may be cleared from plasma or oxidized before it is utilized for PC synthesis, or, once incorporated into phosphatides, may be liberated by hydrolysis (mediated by phospholipase A_2 [158]), and then oxidized.

It should be noted that the ability of orally-administered DAG, given daily for several weeks, to increase brain phosphatide levels does not necessarily imply that, concurrent with such increases, the quantities of DHA in the phosphatides, relative to those of other fatty acids, also are increased. Indeed this has not been demonstrated.

Effects of DHA and Other PUFAs on Synaptic Protein and Phosphatide Levels in Gerbils

In experiments designed to compare the effects of administering each of the three PUFAs, DHA, EPA, or AA, on brain phosphatide levels, animals received 300 mg/kg daily by gavage of one of the fatty acids for 4 weeks, with or without dietary UMP and with choline as noted previously. Giving DHA without uridine increased PC, PI, PE and PS levels significantly, by 18, 20, 22, and 28% respectively (table 2), throughout the brain (e.g. in cortex, striatum, hippocampus, brain stem and cerebellum) (table 3). Giving EPA also increased brain PE, PS, and PI levels significantly, by 21, 24 and 27%, respectively (table 2). In contrast, AA administration failed to affect brain levels of any of the phosphatides (table 2) [14].

Consuming the UMP-supplemented diet alone increased brain PS and PC levels significantly (by 15 and 16%, respectively) (table 2) compared with those in control gerbils. Among gerbils receiving both UMP and DHA, brain PC, PE, PS, and PI levels rose significantly by 12, 26, 34, and 38%, respectively (table 2). Similarly, among gerbils receiving both UMP and EPA, brain PC, PE, PS, and PI levels rose significantly by 13, 30, 41 and 56%, respectively (table 2). In contrast, giving UMP with AA failed to increase levels of any brain phosphatide above those found in gerbils receiving UMP alone (table 2). Total brain phospholipid levels were also elevated significantly, by 16 and 23% following treatment with UMP + DHA, or with UMP + EPA, respectively (table 2), but not by treatment with UMP + AA [14]. Essentially similar results

Table 2. Effects of various PUFAs, given with a control diet (**a**) or a UMP-supplemented diet (**b**), on gerbil brain phosphatide levels [data from 14]

a

	Total PL	PC	PE	PS	PI
Control diet + Vehicle	322	113	63	251	15
Control diet + AA	326	114	65	281	16
Control diet + DHA	344	133*	77*	32***	18*
Control diet + EPA	347	125	76*	31**	19**, a
UMP diet[1] + Vehicle	332	131*	701	29*	16

Groups of gerbils were given a control diet, and received by gavage AA, DHA, or EPA (each 300 mg/kg; in a vehicle of 5% gum Arabic solution) or just its vehicle for 28 days. On the 29th day their brains were harvested and assayed for phosphatides as described in the text. Data are given as means ± SEM. *p < 0.05; **p < 0.01, and ***p < 0.001 compared to Control diet + Vehicle group, and [a]p < 0.05 compared to Control diet + AA group by one-way ANOVA.
[1]Data from gerbils receiving the UMP diet but no PUFAs are included in table 2a to illustrate that uridine alone also affects phosphatide levels. Data are presented as nmol/mg protein.

b

	Total PL	PC	PE	PS	PI
UMP diet + Vehicle	332	131	70	29	16
UMP diet + AA	379	132	81	31	20
UMP diet + DHA	384*	147**, y	88**	39**	22**
UMP diet + EPA	407***	148**, y	91***	41**, x	25***

Groups of gerbils were given a UMP-containing (0.5%) diet, and received by gavage AA, DHA, or EPA (each 300 mg/kg; in a vehicle of 5% gum Arabic solution) or just its vehicle for 28 days. On the 29th day their brains were harvested and assayed for phosphatides as described in the text. Data are given as means ± SEM. *p < 0.05; **p < 0.01, and ***p < 0.001 compared to Control diet + Vehicle group, and [x]p < 0.05 and [y]p < 0.01 compared to UMP diet + AA group by one-way ANOVA.

were obtained whether data were expressed per μg DNA or per mg protein (data not shown).

Giving gerbils, as above, DHA or EPA alone significantly increased brain levels of the postsynaptic density protein PSD-95, by 24 or 28% (fig. 3a1). When this treatment was combined with dietary UMP the observed increases in PSD-95 were 29 or 33% greater than those found after UMP supplementation alone (fig. 3a2). AA failed to affect brain PSD-95 levels either when given alone or in combination with the UMP-supplemented diet (fig. 3a). Similar to PSD-95, levels of synapsin-1, a presynaptic vesicular protein, were also significantly increased, by 31 or 27% respectively, by DHA or EPA treatment alone (fig. 3b1) or by 33 or 36% when the PUFA was combined with

Table 3. Effects of giving UMP-supplemented diet (0.5%) and DHA (300 mg/kg) on phosphatide levels in different gerbil brain regions [data from 14]

	Cortex	Striatum	Hippocampus	Brain Stem	Cerebellum
Total PL					
Control diet + Vehicle	267	265	264	450	270
UMP diet + DHA	316**	339***	314**	521**	317**
PC					
Control diet + Vehicle	94	100	102	114	98
UMP diet + DHA	122***	126*	117***	139***	111***
PE					
Control diet + Vehicle	58	60	61	117	64
UMP diet + DHA	80**	85***	81***	156***	85***
PS					
Control diet + Vehicle	24	24	24	30	24
UMP diet + DHA	30***	29*	28***	35***	29**
PI					
Control diet + Vehicle	10.6	7.6	8.8	9.3	10.4
UMP diet + DHA	13.2**	11.9***	11***	11.8*	11.5*

Groups of gerbils were given a UMP-containing (0.5%) diet and, received by gavage, DHA (300 mg/kg; in a vehicle of 5% gum Arabic solution) or just the vehicle, for 28 days. On the 29th day various brain regions were harvested and assayed for phosphatides as described in the text. Data are presented as nmol/mg protein. $*p < 0.05$; $**p < 0.01$, and $***p < 0.001$ compared to Control diet + Vehicle group using Student's t test.

UMP (fig. 3b2). Again, AA failed to affect brain synapsin-1 levels when given alone or in combination or concurrently with a UMP-supplemented diet (fig. 3b).

Also similarly to PSD-95 and synapsin-1, brain levels of syntaxin-3, a plasma membrane SNARE (soluble *N*-thylmaleimidesensitive-factor attachment protein receptor) protein which reportedly mediates the stimulation by PUFAs of neurite outgrowth [9], and exocytosis [159], in cultured cells, were significantly increased in animals receiving DHA or EPA by 29 or 19%, respectively (fig. 3c1); whether or not they also received UMP, but AA was without effect alone or in combination with UMP (fig. 3c).

None of the PUFA, given alone or with UMP, changed brain levels of the structural protein β-tubulin, perhaps reflecting its ubiquity in brain; hence, β-tubulin was used as the loading control for Western blot assays of synaptic proteins (fig. 3d).

The mechanism that allows the omega–3 fatty acids DHA and EPA, but not the omega–6 fatty acid AA to increase synaptic membrane is unclear. As discussed above, exogenously administered AA, like DHA, is preferentially incorporated into brain phosphatides [143, 144], as well as into other brain lipids (e.g. the plasmalogens [145, 146]), and AA shares with DHA the ability to activate syntaxin-3 in vitro [9].

Mechanisms that could underlie the differential effects of omega–3 and omega–6 PUFAs on membrane synthesis might include, among others, different efficacies for their uptakes into brain or their acylation; different half-lives in the circulation; different affinities for enzymes that control their incorporation into DAG and phosphatides (apparently not the case [14]; differences in the rates at which the PUFAs are removed from phosphatides by deacylation; the differential activation of genes encoding proteins needed for membrane synthesis [5], or the tendency of AA to be incorporated into phospholipids by the acylation of 1-acyl-2-lyso-snglycerophospholipids, not via the Kennedy cycle [160].

Effects of DHA and Other PUFAs on Dendritic Spine Formation and Synaptogenesis

Dendritic spines are small membranous protrusions extending from postsynaptic dendrites in neurons most of which eventually form synapses with presynaptic axon terminals. The dendritic spines compartmentalize postsynaptic responses, and their numbers are thought to reflect the density of excitatory synapses within regions of the central nervous system [161–163]. Oral supplementation with DHA to adult gerbils increases the number of dendritic spines in the hippocampus, particularly if the animals are also supplemented with UMP (fig. 5). This effect is associated with parallel increases in levels of membrane phosphatides and of various pre- and postsynaptic hippocampus proteins, as described above. Oral DHA may thus increase the number of brain synapses, particularly when co-administered with UMP [15].

Gerbils that received daily doses of DHA for 4 weeks (100 or 300 mg/kg, by gavage) exhibited increased dendritic spine density (i.e. the number of spines per length of dendrite) in CA1 pyramidal neurons (fig. 6); the increases were 12% ($p = 0.04$) with the 100 mg/kg/day dose, and 18% ($p < 0.01$) with the 300 mg/kg/day dose. These effects were amplified when gerbils received both DHA (300 mg/kg/day, by gavage, as above) and UMP (0.5%, via the standard choline-containing diet) for 4 weeks, DHA supplementation alone increasing spine density by 19% ($p < 0.04$; fig. 5) and administration of both precursors did so by 36%, or approximately double the increase produced by DHA alone ($p = 0.008$) (fig. 5). (Giving UMP alone did not affect dendritic spine density significantly (fig. 5), however it did increase spine density when all dendritic protrusions were included for statistical analysis, including the filopodia, which are precursor forms of dendritic spines.) The effect on dendritic spine density of giving both DHA and UMP was already apparent after 1 week of treatment ($p = 0.02$), and continued for as long as animals were treated (4 weeks) (fig. 5). DHA + UMP did not affect the length nor width of individual dendritic spines, only their number.

In the above experiments the increases in hippocampal phospholipids after DHA alone were: PC 8%, PE 26%, PS 75%, and PI 29% (all $p < 0.5$ except for PC), and after

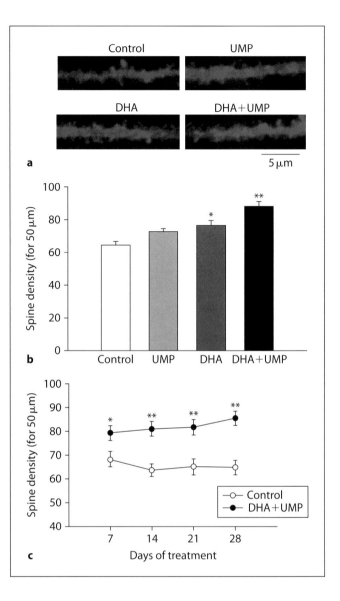

Fig. 5. Effects of DHA, alone or in combination with a UMP-supplemented diet, on dendritic spine formation in adult gerbil hippocampus. Animals received UMP (0.5%), DHA (300 mg/kg) or both daily for 4 weeks; control gerbils received neither. **a** Apical dendrites of CA1 pyramidal neurons. **b** Animals supplemented with DHA exhibited a significant increase in spine density (by 19%, *p = 0.004 vs. Control); those receiving both DHA and UMP exhibited a greater increase (by 36%, **p < 0.01 vs. Control or by 17%, p = 0.008 vs. DHA). n = 20–25 neurons from 4 animals per group. One-way ANOVA followed by Tukey's test. **c** The effect of DHA + UMP on spine density was apparent by 1 week after the start of the treatment. The treated groups received both UMP (0.5%) and DHA (300 mg/kg) daily for 1, 2, 3 or 4 weeks; the control groups were given only a regular diet. n = 12–20 neurons from 2 animals per group. Two-way ANOVA followed by Tukey's test. *p = 0.02; **p < 0.01 [data from 15].

DHA + UMP were: PC 28%, PE 59%, PS 160%, and PI 100% (all p < 0.01 vs. their controls). Comparable increases were noted in the pre- and postsynaptic proteins examined in the contralateral hippocampus of the same animals. Expression levels of PSD-95 [164] and GluR-1 [165, 166] are known to be highly associated with the growth of dendritic spines, and also with the intensity of the physiological responses of the postsynaptic neurons. Synapsin-1, on the other hand, is expressed in presynaptic terminals, and apparently anchors synaptic vesicles to the actin cytoskeleton for exocytosis or synaptogenesis [167, 168]. The increases in PSD-95, synapsin-1, and GluR-1 (the metabotropic glutamate receptor subunit) after treatment with DHA alone were 42, 37, and 29% (all p ≤ 0.05), while the increases after treatment with

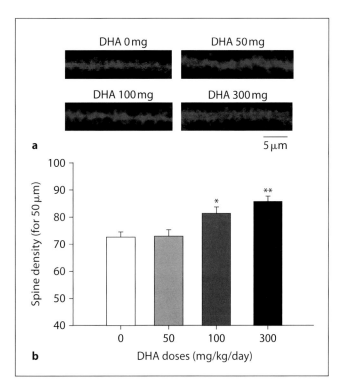

Fig. 6. Effects of oral supplementation with various doses of DHA on dendritic spine density in adult gerbil hippocampus. Animals were supplemented with 0, 50, 100 or 300 mg/kg of DHA daily for 4 weeks. **a** Apical dendrites of CA1 pyramidal neurons. **b** Animals supplemented with 100 or 300 mg/kg/day showed increased spine density: a 12% increase after the 100 mg/kg/day dose (*p = 0.04) and an 18% increase after the 300 mg/kg/day dose (**p < 0.01 vs. 0 mg/kg/day). n = 16–20 neurons from 2 animals per group [data from 15].

DHA + UMP were by 44, 57, and 37%, respectively (all p < 0.01). Treatment with DHA or with DHA + UMP also elevated brain levels of actin, a cytoskeletal protein which can directly regulate the morphology of dendritic spines and which is implicated in such manifestations of synaptic plasticity as long-term potentiation (LTP) and depression (LTD) [161–163, 166, 169]. Actin levels rose by 60% after DHA, and by 88% in animals receiving DHA + UMP.

In contrast, levels of β-tubulin, a cytoskeletal protein that is not specifically localized within synaptic structures, were unaffected by the treatments [15].

Oral supplementation with AA failed to affect dendritic spine density in the CA1 region of the adult gerbil hippocampus even though, like DHA, AA does affect synaptic plasticity in cultured neurons [170–172]. As described above, AA also failed to affect hippocampal levels of phosphatides or of synaptic proteins [15].

The mechanisms through which DHA, with or without uridine, increases dendritic spine formation may also involve presynaptic processes. Results from various model systems indicate that both DHA [9, 173, 174] and uridine [16, 175, 176] can promote axonal growth and exocytosis in cultured cells. As mentioned previously, DHA can activate the SNARE protein syntaxin-3 [9] while uridine, through UTP, can activate P2Y receptors [16], which are expressed in hippocampal neurons [177] and are implicated in presynaptic induction of LTP [178]. Formation of dendritic spines and synaptogenesis in mammalian brains can be induced or initiated by presynaptic neurons, and this process may involve calcium [161–163, 179]. The increases in spine density with DHA and UMP treatment (fig. 5) may thus result from potentiation of pre- or postsynaptic mechanisms.

Effects of Uridine on Neurotransmitter Release

Consumption by rats of a diet containing uridine (as UMP) and choline can increase dopamine (DA) and ACh levels in, and – as assessed using in vivo microdialysis – their release from, corpus striatum neurons. Apparently no data are available on the effects on neurotransmitter production or release of giving DHA alone or with the other two phosphatide precursors. Dietary supplementation of aged male Fischer 344 rats with 2.5% UMP for 6 weeks, ad libitum, increased the release of striatal DA that was evoked by potassium-induced depolarization from $283 \pm 9\%$ in control rats to $341 \pm 21\%$ in those receiving the UMP ($p < 0.05$) [175]. In general, each animal's DA release correlated with its striatal DA content, measured postmortem. The levels of neurofilament-70 and neurofilament-M proteins, two markers of neurite outgrowth, were also increased after UMP treatment, to $182 \pm 25\%$ of control levels for the neurofilament-70 ($p < 0.05$) and to $221 \pm 34\%$ ($p < 0.01$) for the neurofilament-M [175].

In a similar microdialysis study, ACh release, basally as well as after administration of atropine (a muscarinic antagonist which blocks inhibitory presynaptic cholinergic receptors), was found to be enhanced following UMP consumption. Among aged animals consuming a UMP-containing diet (2.5%, w/w) for 1 or 6 weeks, baseline ACh levels in striatal microdialysates rose from 73 to 148 fmol/min after 1 week of treatment ($p < 0.05$), and to 197 fmol/min after 6 weeks ($p < 0.05$) [176]. Dietary UMP (0.5%, 1 week) also amplified the increase in ACh release caused by giving atropine (10 μM, via the artificial CSF); atropine alone increased ACh concentrations from 81 to 386 fmol/min in control rats and from 127 to 680 fmol/min in those consuming UMP ($p < 0.05$). Young rats eating the UMP-containing diet exhibited similar responses. These data suggest that giving a uridine source may enhance some cholinergic functions, perhaps by increasing synaptic membrane or the ACh stored in synaptic vesicles.

Additional evidence that treatment with UMP alone or with UMP + DHA can affect brain neurotransmission comes from a few behavioral studies [33, 180]. Among socially-impoverished rats DHA (300 mg/kg by gavage) or DHA + dietary UMP (0.5%) treatment for 4 weeks reversed the deficits in hippocampal-dependent learning and memory performance [33] (fig. 7). Similarly, chronic dietary administration of UMP (0.1%) alone for 3 months also ameliorated this impairment among the impoverished rats [180]. Since in these small studies both UMP alone and UMP + DHA completely restored learning and memory in the socially-impoverished animals, these data do not allow comparisons to be made on the relative efficacies of the two treatments.

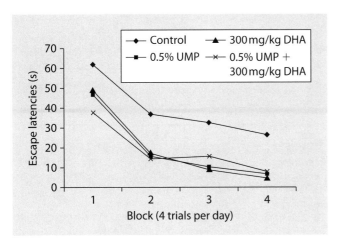

Fig. 7. Rats were allowed to eat 16% protein chow, or the same diet supplemented with 0.5% UMP and/or by gavage 300 mg/kg DHA. Rats began to eat the UMP-supplemented chow, and to receive the daily gavage of DHA, at approximately 4 weeks of age, 4 weeks prior to testing in a water maze, which continued throughout testing. Also beginning at 4 weeks of age and continuing for a duration of 4 weeks, rats were placed in impoverished conditions (IC). Impoverished conditions required that rats be housed individually without toys, and exercised 3 times a week for 15 min in an empty room to avoid weight gain. Following exposure to 4 weeks of impoverished environmental conditions, rats' learning and memory was tested using the hidden version of the Morris water maze (8 animals in each group) [data from 33].

Conclusions

Brain phosphatide synthesis requires three circulating compounds: DHA, uridine, and choline. Administration of these compounds orally increases the levels of phosphatides in brain cells, and also those of synaptic proteins and the numbers of dendritic spines; EPA but not AA reproduces these effects of DHA. This treatment may thus enhance neurotransmission.

Administering these phosphatide precursors may be useful in clinical situations in which the number of particular brain synapses and/or neurons is inadequate because of a disease process (e.g. neurodegenerative disorders like Alzheimer's or Parkinson's diseases) or a developmental disturbance (e.g. prematurity). In some of these situations patients already may be treated with supplemental DHA [3, 181]. Available data suggest that the beneficial effects of giving this PUFA will be enhanced if patients also receive adequate amounts of uridine. (They may also benefit from supplemental choline, although at least in infants, plasma choline levels are already manifold higher than they are in adults [182, 183], and breast milk is particularly rich in choline sources [183].) Clinical testing will be needed to determine whether this approach is effective.

Acknowledgements

Studies in the authors' laboratories described in this review were supported in part by the National Institute of Mental Health (MH-28783) and the Center for Brain Sciences and Metabolism Charitable Trust.

References

1 Moriguchi T, Salem N Jr: Recovery of brain docosahexaonate leads to recovery of spatial task performance. J Neurochem 2003;87:297–309.

2 Schaefer EJ, Bongard V, Beiser AS, Lamon-Fava S, Robinson SJ, Au R, Tucker KL, Kyle DJ, Wilson PW, Wolf PA: Plasma phosphatidylcholine docosahexaenoic acid content and risk of dementia and Alzheimer disease: the Framingham Heart Study. Arch Neurol 2006;63:1545–1550.

3 Freund-Levi Y, Eriksdotter-Jonhagen M, Cederholm T, Basun H, Faxen-Irving G, Garlind A, Vedin I, Vessby B, Wahlund LO, Palmblad J: Omega–3 fatty acid treatment in 174 patients with mild to moderate Alzheimer disease: OmegAD study: a randomized double-blind trial. Arch Neurol 2006;63:1402–1408.

4 Birch EE, Garfield S, Hoffman DR, Uauy R, Birch DG: A randomized clinical trial of early dietary supply of long-chain polyunsaturated fatty acids and mental development in term infants. Dev Med Child Neurol 2000;42:174–181.

5 Kothapalli KSD, Anthony JC, Pan BS, Hsieh AT, Nathanielsz PW, Brenna JT: Differential cerebral cortex transcriptomes of baboon neonates consuming moderate and high docosahexaenoic acid formulas. PLoS ONE 2007;2:e370.

6 Cooper JR, Bloom FE, Roth RH: The Biochemical Basis of Neuropharmacology, ed 8. New York, Oxford University Press, 2003.

7 Hashimoto M, Hossain S, Shimada T, Shido O: Docosahexaenoic acid-induced protective effect against impaired learning in amyloid β-infused rats is associated with increased synaptosomal membrane fluidity. Clin Exp Pharmacol Physiol 2006;33:934–939.

8 Mata de Urquiza A, Liu S, Sjoberg M, Zetterstrom RH, Griffiths W, Sjovall J, Perlmann T: Docosahexaenoic acid, a ligand for the retinoid X receptor in mouse brain. Science 2000;290:2140–2144.

9 Darios F, Davletov B: Omega–3 and omega–6 fatty acids stimulate cell membrane expansion by acting on syntaxin-3. Nature 2006;440:813–817.

10 Kim H-Y: Novel metabolism of docosahexaenoic acid in neural cells. J Biol Chem 2007;282:18661–18665.

11 Akbar M, Calderon F, Wen Z, Kim HY: Docosahexaenoic acid: a positive modulator of Akt signaling in neuronal survival. Proc Natl Acad Sci USA 2005;102:10858–10863.

12 Hong S, Gronert K, Devchand PR, Moussignac RL, Serhan CN: Novel docosatrienes and 17S-resolvins generated from docosahexaenoic acid in murine brain, human blood, and glial cells. Autacoids in anti-inflammation. J Biol Chem 2003;278:14677–14687.

13 Wurtman RJ, Ulus IH, Cansev M, Watkins CJ, Wang L, Marzloff G: Synaptic proteins and phospholipids are increased in gerbil brain by administering uridine plus docosahexaenoic acid orally. Brain Res 2006;1088:83–92.

14 Cansev M, Wurtman RJ: Chronic administration of docosahexaenoic acid or eicosapentaenoic acid, but not arachidonic acid, alone or in combination with uridine, increases brain phosphatide and synaptic protein levels in gerbils. Neuroscience 200724;148:421–431.

15 Sakamoto T, Cansev M, Wurtman RJ: Oral supplementation with docosahexaenoic acid and uridine 5′-monophosphate increases dendritic spine density in adult gerbil hippocampus. Brain Res 2007;1182:50–59.

16 Pooler AM, Guez DH, Benedictus R, Wurtman RJ: Uridine enhances neurite outgrowth in nerve growth factor-differentiated pheochromocytoma cells. Neuroscience 2005;134:207–214.

17 Kennedy EM, Weiss SB: The function of cytidine coenzymes in the biosynthesis of phospholipids. J Biol Chem 1956;222:193–214.

18 Sastry PS: Lipids of nervous tissue: composition and metabolism. Prog Lipid Res 1985;24:69–176.

19 Wurtman RJ, Regan M, Ulus I, Yu L: Effect of oral CDP-choline on plasma choline and uridine levels in humans. Biochem Pharmacol 2000;60:989–992.

20 Cansev M, Watkins CJ, van der Beek EM, Wurtman RJ: Oral Uridine 5′ monophosphate (UMP) increases brain CDP-choline levels in gerbils. Brain Res 2005;1058:101–108.

21 Millington WR, Wurtman RJ: Choline administration elevates brain phosphorylcholine levels. J Neurochem 1982;38:1748–1752.

22 Babb SM, Ke Y, Lange N, Kaufman MJ, Renshaw PF, Cohen BM: Oral choline increases choline metabolites in human brain. Psychiatry Res 2004;130:1–9.

23 Spanner S, Ansell GB: Choline kinase and ethanolamine kinase activity in the cytosol of nerve endings from rat forebrain. Biochem J 1979;178:753–760.

24 Stavinoha WB, Weintraub ST: Choline content of rat brain. Science 1974;183:964–965.

25 Klein J, Gonzales R, Koppen A, Loffelholz K: Free choline and choline metabolites in rat brain and body fluids: sensitive determination and implications for choline supply to the brain. Neurochem Int 1993;22:293–300.

26 Ross BM, Moszczynska A, Blusztajn JK, Sherwin A, Lozano A, Kish SJ: Phospholipid biosynthetic enzymes in human brain. Lipids 1997;32:351–358.

27 Vance DE, Pelech SL: Enzyme translocation in the regulation of phosphatidylcholine biosynthesis. Trends Biochem Sci 1984;9:17–20.

28 Lim P, Cornell R, Vance DE: The supply of both CDP-choline and diacylglycerol can regulate the rate of phosphatidylcholine synthesis in HeLa cells. Biochem Cell Biol 1986;64:692–698.

29 Araki W, Wurtman RJ: Control of membrane phosphatidylcholine synthesis by diacylglycerol levels in neuronal cells undergoing neurite outgrowth. Proc Natl Acad Sci USA 1997;94:11946–11950.

30 Marszalek JR, Lodish HF: Docosahexaenoic acid, fatty acid-interacting proteins, and neuronal function: breast milk and fish are good for you. Annu Rev Cell Dev Biol 2005;21:633–657.

31 Ferreira A, Rapoport M: The synapsins: beyond the regulation of neurotransmitter release. Cell Mol Life Sci 2002;59:589–595.

32 Fujita A, Kurachi Y: SAP family proteins. Biochem Biophys Res Commun 2000;269:1–6.

33 Holguin S, Huang Y, Liu J, Wurtman RJ: Chronic Administration of DHA and UMP Improves The Impaired Memory of Environmentally Impoverished Rats. Behav Brain Res 2008;191:11–16.

34 Hersh LB: Kinetic studies of the choline acetyltransferase reaction using isotope exchange at equilibrium. J Biol Chem 1982;257:12820–12834.

35 Tucek S: The synthesis of acetylcholine: twenty years of progress. Prog Brain Res 1990;84:467–477.

36 Rossier J: Acetyl-coenzyme A and coenzyme A analogues. Their effects on rat brain choline acetyltransferase. Biochem J 1977;165:321–326.

37 Cohen EL, Wurtman RJ: Brain acetylcholine: Increase after systemic choline administration. Life Sci 1975;16:1095–1102.

38 Haubrich DR, Wang PFL, Wedeking PW: Distribution and metabolism of intravenously administered choline[methyl-^{3}H] and synthesis in vivo of acetylcholine in various tissues of guinea pigs. J Pharmacol Exp Ther 1975;193:246–255.

39 Fernstrom JD, Wurtman RJ: Brain serotonin content: physiological dependence on plasma tryptophan levels. Science 1971;173:149–152.

40 Cansev M, Wurtman RJ: Aromatic amino acids in the brain; in Lajtha A (ed): Amino Acids and Peptides in the Nervous System. Handbook of Neurochemistry and Molecular Neurobiology. Berlin, Springer, 2007, vol 6, pp 59–99.

41 Farber SA, Savci V, Wei A, Slack BE, Wurtman RJ: Choline's phosphorylation in rat striatal slices is regulated by the activity of cholinergic neurons. Brain Res 1996;723:90–99.

42 Ulus IH, Watkins CJ, Cansev M, Wurtman RJ: Cytidine and uridine increase striatal CDP-choline levels without decreasing acetylcholine synthesis or release. Cell Mol Neurobiol 2006;26:563–577.

43 Maire J-C, Wurtman RJ: Effects of electrical stimulation and choline availability on the release and contents of acetylcholine and choline in superfused slices from rat striatum. J Physiol 1985;80:189–195.

44 Blusztajn JK, Holbrook PG, Lakher M, Liscovitch M, Maire JC, Mauron C, Richardson UI, Tacconi M, Wurtman RJ: 'Autocannibalism' of membrane choline-phospholipids: physiology and pathology. Psychopharmacol Bull 1986;22:781–786.

45 Ulus IH, Wurtman RJ, Mauron C, Blusztajn JK: Choline increases acetylcholine release and protects against the stimulation-induced decrease in phosphatide levels within membranes of rat corpus striatum. Brain Res 1989;484:217–227.

46 Wilgram GF, Kennedy EP: Intracellular distribution of some enzymes catalyzing reactions in the biosynthesis of complex lipids. J Biol Chem 1963;238:2615–2619.

47 Tronchere H, Record M, Terce F, Chap H: Phosphatidylcholine cycle and regulation of phosphatidylcholine biosynthesis by enzyme translocation. Biochim Biophys Acta 1994;1212:137–151.

48 Sleight R, Kent C: Regulation of phosphatidylcholine biosynthesis in cultured chick embryonic muscle treated with phospholipase C. J Biol Chem 1980;255:10644–10650.

49 Sleight R, Kent C: Regulation of phosphatidylcholine biosynthesis in mammalian cells. I. Effects of phospholipase C treatment on phosphatidylcholine metabolism in Chinese hamster ovary cells and LM mouse fibroblasts. J Biol Chem 1983;258:824–830.

50 Pelech SL, Cook HW, Paddon HB, Vance DE: Membrane-bound CTP:phosphocholine cytidylyltransferase regulates the rate of phosphatidylcholine synthesis in HeLa cells treated with unsaturated fatty acids. Biochim Biophys Acta 1984;795:433–440.

51 Cornell RB, Northwood IC: Regulation of CTP:phosphocholine cytidylyltransferase by amphitropism and relocalization. Trends Biochem Sci 2000;25:441–447.

52 Utal AK, Jamil H, Vance DE: Diacylglycerol signals the translocation of CTP:choline-phosphate cytidylyltransferase in HeLa cells treated with 12-O- tetradecanoylphorbol-13-acetate. J Biol Chem 1991;266:24084–24091.

53 Weinhold PA, Charles L, Rounsifer ME, Feldman DA: Control of phosphatidylcholine synthesis in Hep G2 cells. Effect of fatty acids on the activity and immunoreactive content of choline phosphate cytidylyltransferase. J Biol Chem 1991;266:6093–6100.

54 Watkins JD, Kent C: Regulation of CTP: phosphocholine cytidylyltransferase activity and subcellular location by phosphorylation in Chinese hamster ovary cells. The effect of phospholipase C treatment. J Biol Chem 1991;266:21113–21117.

55 Weinhold PA, Rounsifer ME, Feldman DA: The purification and characterization of CTP: phosphorylcholine cytidylyltransferase from rat liver. J Biol Chem 1986;261:5104–5110.

56 Kalmar GB, Kay RJ, Lachance A, Aebersold R, Cornell RB: Cloning and expression of rat liver CTP: phosphocholine cytidylyltransferase: an amphipathic protein that controls phosphatidylcholine synthesis. Proc Natl Acad Sci USA 1990;87:6029–6033.

57 Kalmar GB, Kay RJ, Lachance A, Cornell RB: Primary structure and expression of a human CTP:phosphocholine cytidylyltransferase. Biochim Biophys Acta 1994;1219:328–334.

58 Cornell R: Chemical cross-linking reveals a dimeric structure for CTP:phosphocholine cytidylyltransferase. J Biol Chem 1989;264:9077–9082.

59 Mages F, Rey C, Fonlupt P, Pacheco H: Kinetic and biochemical properties of CTP:choline-phosphate cytidylyltransferase from the rat brain. Eur J Biochem 1988;178:367–372.

60 Mandel P, Edel-Harth S: Free nucleotides in the rat brain during post-natal development. J Neurochem 1966;13:591–595.

61 Abe K, Koqure K, Yamomoto H, Imazawa M, Miyamoto K: Mechanism of arachidonic acid liberation during ischemia in gerbil cerebral cortex. J Neurochem 1987;48:503–509.

62 Nitsch RM, Blusztajn JK, Pittas AG, Slack BE, Growdon JH, Wurtman RJ: Evidence for a membrane defect in Alzheimer disease brain. Proc Natl Acad Sci USA 1992;89:1671–1675.

63 Choy PC, Paddon HB, Vance DE: An increase in cytoplasmic CTP accelerates the reaction catalyzed by CTP:phosphocholine cytidylyltransferase in poliovirus-infected HeLa cells. J Biol Chem 1980;255:1070–1073.

64 Lopez G, Coviella I, Wurtman RJ: Enhancement by cytidine of membrane phospholipid synthesis. J Neurochem 1992;59:338–343.

65 Richardson UI, Watkins CJ, Pierre C, Ulus IH, Wurtman RJ: Stimulation of CDP-choline synthesis by uridine or cytidine in PC12 rat pheochromocytoma cells. Brain Res 2003;971:161–167.

66 Savci V, Wurtman RJ: Effect of cytidine on membrane phospholipid synthesis in rat striatal slices. J Neurochem 1995;64:378–384.

67 Coleman R, Bell RML: Phospholipid synthesis in isolated fat cells. Studies of microsomal diacylglycerol cholinephosphotransferase and diacylglycerol ethanolaminephosphotransferase activities. J Biol Chem 1977;252:3050–3056.

68 Kanoh H, Ohno K: Solubilization and purification of rat liver microsomal 1,2-diacylglycerol: CDP-choline cholinephosphotransferase and 1,2-diacylglycerol: CDP-ethanolamine ethanolaminephosphotransferase. Eur J Biochem 1976;66:201–210.

69 Ishidate K, Matsuo R, Nakazawa Y: CDP-choline:1,2-diacylglycerol cholinephosphotransferase from rat liver microsomes. I. Solubilization and characterization of the partially purified enzyme and the possible existence of an endogenous inhibitor. Lipids 1993;28:89–96.

70 Roberti R, Vecchini A, Freysz L, Masoom M, Binaglia L: An improved procedure for the purification of ethanolaminephosphotransferase. Reconstitution of the purified enzyme with lipids. Biochim Biophys Acta 1989;1004:80–88.

71 O K-M, Choy PC: Solubilization and partial purification of cholinephosphotransferase in hamster tissues. Lipids 1990;25:122–124.

72 Henneberry AL, McMaster CR: Cloning and expression of a human choline/ethanolaminephosphotransferase: synthesis of phosphatidylcholine and phosphatidylethanolamine. Biochem J 1999;339:291–298.

73 Henneberry AL, Wistow G, McMaster CR: Cloning, genomic organization, and characterization of a human cholinephosphotransferase. J Biol Chem 2000;275:29808–29815.

74 Kanoh H, Ohno K: Utilization of endogenous phospholipids by the back-reaction of CDP-choline (-ethanolamine): 1,2-diglyceride choline (ethanolamine)-phosphotransferase in rat liver microsomes. Biochim Biophys Acta 1973;306:207–217.

75 Kanoh H, Ohno K: Studies on 1,2-diglycerides formed from endogenous lecithins by the back-reaction of rat liver microsomal cdpcholine: 1,2-diacylglycerol cholinephosphotransferase. Biochim Biophys Acta 1973;326:17–25.

76 Goracci G, Francescangeli E, Horrocks LA, Porcelatti G: The reverse reaction of cholinephosphotransferase in rat brain microsomes. A new pathway for degradation of phosphatidylcholine. Biochim Biophys Acta 1981;664:373–379.

77 Goracci G, Francescangeli E, Horrocks LA, Porcelatti G: A comparison of the reversibility of phosphoethanolamine transferase and phosphocholine transferase in rat brain microsomes. Biochim Biophys Acta 1986;876:387–391.

78 Roberti R, Mancini A, Freysz L, Binaglia L: Reversibility of the reactions catalyzed by cholinephosphotransferase and ethanolaminephosphotransferase solubilized from rat-brain microsomes. Biochim Biophys Acta 1992;1165:183–188.

79 Cornell RB: Cholinephosphotransferase from mammalian sources. Methods Enzymol 1992;209:267–272.

80 Korniat EK, Beeler DA: Water-soluble phospholipid precursor pool-sizes in quick-frozen and unfrozen rat livers. Anal Biochem 1975;69:300–305.

81 Turinsky J, Bayly BP, O'Sullivan DM: 1,2-Diacylglycerol and ceramide levels in rat liver and skeletal muscle in vivo. Am J Physiol 1991;261:E620–E627.

82 Alberghina M, Viola M, Giuffrida AM: Pool size of CDP-choline in the brain, heart, and lung of normal hypoxic guinea pigs. J Neurosci Res 1981;6:719–722.

83 Jamil H, Utal AK, Vance DE: Evidence that cyclic AMP-induced inhibition of phosphatidylcholine biosynthesis is caused by a decrease in cellular diacylglycerol levels in cultured rat hepatocytes. J Biol Chem 1992;267:1752–1760.

84 Wright MM, McMaster CR: PC and PE synthesis: mixed micellar analysis of the cholinephosphotransferase and ethanolaminephosphotransferase activities of human choline/ethanolamine phosphotransferase 1 (CEPT1). Lipids 2002;37:663–672.

85 Mantel CR, Schultz AR, Miyazawa K, Broxmeyer HE: Kinetic selectivity of cholinephosphotransferase in mouse liver: the K_m for CDP-choline depends on diacylglycerol structure. Biochem J 1993;289:815–820.

86 Richardson UI, Wurtman RJ: Polyunsaturated fatty acids regulate phosphatidylcholine synthesis in PC12 cells. Biochim Biophys Acta 2007;1771:558–563.

87 Baldwin SA, Beal PR, Yao SYM, King AE, Cass CE, Young JD: The equilibrative nucleoside transporter family, SLC29. Pflügers Arch 2004;447:735–743.

88 Gray JH, Owen RP, Giacomini KM: The concentrative nucleoside transporter family, SLC28. Pflügers Arch 2004;447:728–734.

89 Cansev M: Uridine and cytidine in the brain: their transport and utilization. Brain Res Brain Res Rev 2006;52:389–397.

90 Redzic ZB, Biringer J, Barnes K, Baldwin SA, Al-Sarraf H, Nicola PA, Young JD, Cass CE, Barrand MA, Hlandky SB: Polarized distribution of nucleoside transporters in rat brain endothelial and choroid plexus epithelial cells. J Neurochem 2005;94:1420–1426.

91 Murakami H, Ohkura A, Takanaga H, Matsuo H, Koyabu N, Naito M, Tsuruo T, Ohtani H, Sawada Y: Functional characterization of adenosine transport across the BBB in mice. Int J Pharm 2005;290:37–44.

92 Pastor-Anglada M, Felipe A, Casado FJ: Transport and mode of action of nucleoside derivatives used in chemical and antiviral therapies. Trends Pharmacol Sci 1998;19:424–430.

93 Li JY, Boado RJ, Pardridge WM: Cloned blood-brain barrier adenosine transporter is identical to the rat concentrative Na$^+$ nucleoside cotransporter CNT2. J Cereb Blood Flow Metab 2001;21:929–936.

94 Griffith DA, Jarvis SM: Nucleoside and nucleobase transport systems of mammalian cells. Biochim Biophys Acta 1996;1286:153–181.

95 Traut TW: Physiological concentrations of purines and pyrimidines. Mol Cell Biochem 1994;140:1–22.

96 Larrayoz IM, Fernandez-Nistal A, Garces A, Gorraitz E, Lostao MP: Characterization of the rat Na$^+$/nucleoside cotransporter 2 (rCNT2) and transport of nucleoside-derived drugs using electrophysiological methods. Am J Physiol 2006;291:C1395–C1404.

97 Nagai K, Nagasawa K, Koma M, Hotta A, Fujimoto S: Cytidine is a novel substrate for wild-type concentrative nucleoside transporter 2. Biochem Biophys Res Commun 2006;347:439–443.

98 Nagai K, Nagasawa K, Koma M, Kihara Y, Fujimoto S: Contribution of an unidentified sodium-dependent nucleoside transport system to the uptake and cytotoxicity of anthracycline in mouse M5076 ovarian sarcoma cells. Biochem Pharmacol 2006;71:565–573.

99 Cansev, M, Wurtman RJ: Exogenous cytidine-5′-diphosphocholine increases brain cytidine-5′-diphosphocholine levels in gerbils. J Neurochem 2005;94(suppl 2):105–106.

100 Anderson CM, Xiong W, Geiger JD, Young JD, Cass CE, Baldwin SA, Parkinson FE: Distribution of equilibrative, nitrobenzylthioinosine-insensitive nucleoside transporters (ENT1) in rat brain. J Neurochem 1999;73:867–873.

101 Anderson CM, Baldwin SA, Young JD, Cass CE, Parkinson FE: Distribution of mRNA encoding a nitrobenzylthioinosine-insensitive nucleoside transporter (ENT2) in rat brain. Brain Res Mol Brain Res 1999;70:293–297.

102 Wu X, Yuan G, Brett CM, Hui AC, Giacomini KM: Sodium-dependent nucleoside transport in choroid plexus from rabbit. Evidence for a single transporter for purine and pyrimidine nucleosides. J Biol Chem 1992;267:8813–8818.

103 Wu X, Gutierrez MM, Giacomini KM: Further characterization of the sodium-dependent nucleoside transporter (N3) in choroid plexus from rabbit. Biochim Biophys Acta 1994;1191:190–196.

104 Pardridge WM: Invasive brain drug delivery; in Pardridge WM (ed): Brain Drug Targeting: The Future of Brain Drug Development. Cambridge/UK, Cambridge University Press, 2001, pp 13–35.

105 Canellakis ES: Pyrimidine metabolism. II. Enzymatic pathways of uracil anabolism. J Biol Chem 1957; 227:329–338.

106 Skold O: Uridine kinase from Erlich ascites tumor: purification and properties. J Biol Chem 1960; 235: 3273–3279.

107 Orengo A: Regulation of enzymic activity by metabolites. I. Uridine-cytidine kinase of Novikoff ascites rat tumor. J Biol Chem 1969;244:2204–2209.

108 Krystal G, Webb TE: Multiple forms of uridine kinase in normal and neoplastic rat liver. Biochem J 1971;124:943–947.

109 Absil J, Tuilie M, Roux J-M: Electrophoretically distinct forms of uridine kinase in the rat. Tissue distribution and age-dependence. Biochem J 1980; 185:273–276.

110 Koizumi K, Shimamoto Y, Azuma A, Wataya Y, Matsuda A, Sasaki T, Fukushima M: Cloning and expression of uridine/cytidine kinase cDNA from human fibrosarcoma cells. Int J Mol Med 2001;8: 273–278.

111 Van Rompay AR, Norda A, Linden K, Johansson M, Karlsson A: Phosphorylation of uridine and cytidine analogs by two human uridine-cytidine kinases. Mol Pharmacol 2001;59:1181–1186.

112 Hurwitz J: The enzymatic incorporation of ribonucleotides into polydeoxynucleotide material. J Biol Chem 1959;234:2351–2358.

113 Sugino Y, Teraoka H, Shimono H: Metabolism of deoxyribonucleotides. I. Purification and properties of deoxycytidine monophosphokinase of calf thymus. J Biol Chem 1966;241:961–969.

114 Ruffner BW, Anderson EP: Adenosine triphosphate: uridine monophosphate-cytidine monophosphate phosphotransferase from *Tetrahymena pyriformis*. J Biol Chem 1969;244:5994–6002.

115 Berg P, Joklik WK: Enzymatic phosphorylation of nucleoside diphosphates. J Biol Chem 1954;210:617–672.

116 Parks RE Jr, Agarwal RP: Nucleoside diphosphokinases; in Boyer PD (ed): The Enzymes. New York, Academic Press, 1973, pp 307–333.

117 Van Rompay AR, Johansson M, Karlsson A: Phosphorylation of deoxycytidine analog monophosphates by UMP-CMP kinase: molecular characterization of the human enzyme. Mol Pharmacol 1999;56:562–569.

118 Langen H, Berndt P, Roder D, Cairns N, Lubec G, Fountoulakis M: Two-dimensional map of human brain proteins. Electrophoresis 1999;20:907–916.

119 Kim SH, Fountoulakis M, Cairns NJ, Lubec G: Human brain nucleoside diphosphate kinase activity is decreased in Alzheimer's disease and Down syndrome. Biochem Biophys Res Commun 2002; 296:970–975.

120 Wang TP, Sable HZ, Lampen JO: Enzymatic deamination of cytosine nucleosides. J Biol Chem 1950; 184:17–28.

121 Lieberman I: Enzymatic amination of uridine triphosphate to cytidine triphosphate. J Biol Chem 1956;222:765–775.

122 Hurlbert RB, Kammen HO: Formation of cytidine nucleotides from uridine nucleotides by soluble mammalian enzymes: requirements for glutamine and guanosine nucleotides. J Biol Chem 1960;235: 443–449.

123 Zalkin H: CTP synthase. Methods Enzymol 1985; 113:282–287.

124 Genchev DD, Mandel P: CTP synthetase activity in neonatal and adult rat brain. J Neurochem 1974;22: 1027–1030.

125 Anderson EP: Nucleoside and nucleotide kinases; in Boyer PD (ed.): The Enzymes. New York, Academic Press, 1973, pp 49–96.

126 Greenberg N, Schumm DE, Webb TE: Uridine kinase activities and pyrimidine nucleoside phosphorylation in fluoropyrimidine-sensitive and -resistant cell lines of the Novikoff hepatoma. Biochem J 1977;164:379–387.

127 Ropp PA, Traut TW: Cloning and expression of a cDNA encoding uridine kinase from mouse brain. Arch Biochem Biophys 1996;336:105–112.

128 Ropp PA, Traut TW: Uridine kinase: altered enzyme with decreased affinities for uridine and CTP. Arch Biochem Biophys 1998;359:63–68.

129 Mascia L, Cotrufo T, Cappiello M, Ipata PL: Ribose 1-phosphate and inosine activate uracil salvage in rat brain. Biochim Biophys Acta 1999;1472:93–98.

130 Peters GJ, van Groeningen CJ, Laurensse EJ, Lankelma J, Leyva A, Pinedo HM: Uridine-induced hypothermia in mice and rats in relation to plasma and tissue levels of uridine and its metabolites. Cancer Chemother Pharmacol 1987;20:101–108.

131 Kamp F, Westerhoff HV, Hamilton JA: Movement of fatty acids, fatty acid analogues, and bile acids across phospholipid bilayers. Biochemistry 1993;32:11074–11086.

132 Abumrad NA, Park JH, Park CR: Permeation of long-chain fatty acid into adipocytes. Kinetics, specificity, and evidence for involvement of a membrane protein. J Biol Chem 1984;259:8945–8953.

133 Chmurzynska A: The multigene family of fatty acid-binding proteins: function, structure and polymorphism. J Appl Genet 2006;47:39–48.

134 Shimizu F, Watanabe TK, Shinomiya H, Nakamura Y, Fujiwara T: Isolation and expression of a cDNA for human brain fatty acid-binding protein (B-FABP). Biochim Biophys Acta 1997;1354:24–28.

135 Robinson PJ, Noronha J, DeGeorge JJ, Freed LM, Nariai T, Rapoport SI: A quantitative method for measuring regional in vivo fatty-acid incorporation into and turnover within brain phospholipids: review and critical analysis. Brain Res Brain Res Rev 1992;17:187–214.

136 Bazan NG: Supply of n–3 polyunsaturated fatty acids and their significance in the central nervous system; in Wurtman RJ, Wurtman JJ (eds): Nutrition and the Brain. New York, Raven Press, 1990, vol 8, pp 1–24.

137 Thies F, Pillon C, Moliere P, Lagarde M, Lecerf J: Preferential incorporation of sn-2 lysoPC DHA over unesterified DHA in the young rat brain. Am J Physiol 1994;267:R1273–R1279.

138 Marszalek JR, Kitidis C, DiRusso CC, Lodish HF: Long-chain acyl-CoA synthetase 6 preferentially promotes DHA metabolism. J Biol Chem 2005;280:10817–10826.

139 Reddy TS, Sprecher P, Bazan NG: Long-chain acyl-coenzyme A synthetase from rat brain microsomes. Kinetic studies using [$1-^{14}$C]docosahexaenoic acid substrate. Eur J Biochem 1984;145:21–29.

140 Contreras MA, Greiner RS, Chang MC, Myers CS, Salem N Jr, Rapoport SI: Nutritional deprivation of α-linolenic acid decreases but does not abolish turnover and availability of unacylated docosahexaenoic acid and docosahexaenoyl-CoA in rat brain. J Neurochem 2000;75:2392–2400.

141 Neufeld EJ, Wilson DB, Sprecher H, Majerus PW: High affinity esterification of eicosanoid precursor fatty acids by platelets. J Clin Invest 1983;72:214–220.

142 Moore SA, Yoder A, Murphy S, Dutton GR, Spector AA: Astrocytes, not neurons, produce docosahexaenoic acid (22:6ω–3) and arachidonic acid (20:4ω–6). J Neurochem 1991;56:518–524.

143 DeGeorge JJ, Nariai T, Yamazaki S, Williams WM, Rapoport SI: Arecoline-stimulated brain incorporation of intravenously administered fatty acids in unanesthetized rats. J Neurochem 1991;56:352–355.

144 Sarda N, Gharib A, Moliere P, Grange E, Bobillier P, Lagarde M: Docosahexaenoic acid (cervonic acid) incorporation into different brain regions in the awake rat. Neurosci Lett 1991;123:57–60.

145 Farooqui AA, Horrocks LA: Plasmalogens, phospholipase A₂, and docosahexaenoic acid turnover in brain tissue. J Mol Neurosci 2001;16:263–272.

146 Nagan N, Zoeller RA: Plasmalogens: biosynthesis and functions. Prog Lipid Res 2001;40:199–229.

147 O'Brien JS, Sampson EL: Fatty acid and fatty aldehyde composition of the major brain lipids in normal human gray matter, white matter, and myelin. J Lipid Res 1965;6:545–551.

148 Breckenridge WC, Gombos G, Morgan IG: The lipid composition of adult rat brain synaptosomal plasma membranes. Biochim Biophys Acta 1972; 266:695–707.

149 Svennerholm L: Distribution and fatty acid composition of phosphoglycerides in normal human brain. J Lipid Res 1968;9:570–579.

150 Hicks AM, DeLong CJ, Thomas MJ, Samuel M, Cui Z: Unique molecular signatures of glycerophospholipid species in different rat tissues analyzed by tandem mass spectrometry. Biochim Biophys Acta 2006; 1761:1022–1029.

151 Carlier H, Bernard A, Caselli C: Digestion and absorption of polyunsaturated fatty acids. Reprod Nutr Dev 1991;31:475–500.

152 Bezard J, Blond JP, Bernard A, Clouet P: The metabolism and availability of essential fatty acids in animal and human tissues. Reprod Nutr Dev 1994;34: 539–568.

153 Rapoport SI, Chang MCJ, Spector AA: Delivery and turnover of plasma-derived essential PUFAs in mammalian brain. J Lipid Res 2001;42:678–685.

154 Philbrick DJ, Mahadevappa VG, Ackman RG, Holub BJ: Ingestion of fish oil or a derived n–3 fatty acid concentrate containing eicosapentaenoic acid affects fatty acid compositions of individual phospholipids of rat brain, sciatic nerve and retina. J Nutr 1987; 117:1663–1670.

155 Pawlosky RJ, Hibbeln JR, Novotny JA, Salem N Jr: Physiological compartmental analysis of α-linolenic acid metabolism in adult humans. J Lipid Res 2001; 42:1257–1265.

156 Zhou L, Vessby B, Nilsson A: Quantitative role of plasma free fatty acids in the supply of arachidonic acid to extrahepatic tissues in rats. J Nutr 2002;132: 2626–2631.

157 Rapoport SI: In vivo approaches and rationale for quantifying kinetics and imaging brain lipid metabolic pathways. Prostaglandins Other Lipid Mediat 2005;77:185–196.

158 Strokin M, Sergeeva M, Reiser G: Docosahexaenoic acid and arachidonic acid release in rat brain astrocytes is mediated by two separate isoforms of phospholipase A₂ and is differently regulated by cyclic AMP and Ca²⁺. Br J Pharmacol 2003;139:1014–1022.

159 Teng FYH, Wang Y, Tang BL: The syntaxins. Genome Biol 2001;2:3012–3017.

160 Lands WEM, Inoue M, Sugiura Y, Okuyama H: Selective incorporation of polyunsaturated fatty acids into phosphatidylcholine by rat liver microsomes. J Biol Chem 1982;257:14968–14972.

161 Matus A: Actin-based plasticity in dendritic spines. Science 2000;290:754–758.

162 Hering H, Sheng M: Dendritic spines: structure, dynamics and regulation. Nat Rev Neurosci 2001;2:880–888.

163 Nimchinsky EA, Sabatini BL, Svoboda K: Structure and function of dendritic spines. Annu Rev Physiol 2002;64:313–353.

164 El-Husseini AE, Schnell E, Chetkovich DM, Nicoll RA, Bredt DS: PSD-95 involvement in maturation of excitatory synapses. Science 2000;290:1364–1368.

165 Kasai H, Matsuzaki M, Noguchi J, Yasumatsu N, Nakahara H: Structure-stability-function relationships of dendritic spines. Trends Neurosci 2003;26:360–368.

166 Matsuzaki M, Honkura N, Ellis-Davies GC, Kasai H: Structural basis of long-term potentiation in single dendritic spines. Nature 2004;429:761–766.

167 Greengard P, Valtorta F, Czernik AJ, Benfenati F: Synaptic vesicle phosphoproteins and regulation of synaptic function. Science 1993;259:780–785.

168 Ziv NE, Garner CC: Cellular and molecular mechanisms of presynaptic assembly. Nat Rev Neurosci 2004;5:385–399.

169 Matus A: Growth of dendritic spines: a continuing story. Curr Opin Neurobiol 2005;15:67–72.

170 Williams JH, Errington ML, Lynch MA, Bliss TVP: Arachidonic acid induces a long-term activity-dependent enhancement of synaptic transmission in the hippocampus. Nature 1989;341:739–742.

171 Ramakers GM, Storm JFA: Postsynaptic transient K^+ current modulated by arachidonic acid regulates synaptic integration and threshold for LTP induction in hippocampal pyramidal cells. Proc Natl Acad Sci USA 2002;99:10144–10149.

172 Feinmark SJ, Begum R, Tsvetkov E, Goussakov I, Funk CD, Siegelbaum SA, Bolshakov VY: 12-Lipoxygenase metabolites of arachidonic acid mediate metabotropic glutamate receptor-dependent long-term depression at hippocampal CA3-CA1 synapses. J Neurosci 2003;23:11427–11435.

173 Ikemoto A, Kobayashi T, Watanabe S, Okuyama H: Membrane fatty acid modifications of PC12 cells by arachidonate or docosahexaenoate affect neurite outgrowth but not norepinephrine release. Neurochem Res 1997;22:671–678.

174 Calderon F, Kim H-Y: Docosahexaenoic acid promotes neurite growth in hippocampal neurons. J Neurochem 2004;90:979–988.

175 Wang L, Pooler AM, Albrecht MA, Wurtman RJ: Dietary uridine 5′-monophosphate supplementation increases potassium-evoked dopamine release and promotes neurite outgrowth in aged rats. J Mol Neurosci 2005;27:137–145.

176 Wang L, Albrecht MA, Wurtman RJ: Dietary supplementation with uridine 5′-monophosphate (UMP), a membrane phosphatide precursor, increases acetylcholine level and release in striatum of aged rat. Brain Res 2007;1133:42–48.

177 Abbracchio MP, Burnstock G, Boeynaems J-M, Barnard EA, Boyer JL, Kennedy C, Knight GE, Fumagalli M, Gachet C, Jacobson KA, Weisman GA: International Union of Pharmacology LVIII: update on the P2Y G protein-coupled nucleotide receptors: from molecular mechanisms and pathophysiology to therapy. Pharmacol Rev 2006;58:281–341.

178 Price GD, Robertson SJ, Edwards FA: Long-term potentiation of glutamatergic synaptic transmission induced by activation of presynaptic P2Y receptors in the rat medial habenula nucleus. Eur J Neurosci 2003;17:844–850.

179 Yuste R, Bonhoeffer T: Genesis of dendritic spines: insights from ultrastructural and imaging studies. Nat Rev Neurosci 2004;5:24–34.

180 Teather LA, Wurtman RJ: Chronic administration of UMP ameliorates the impairment of hippocampal-dependent memory in impoverished rats. J Nutr 2006;136:2834–2837.

181 Fleith M, Clandinin MT: Dietary PUFA for preterm and term infants: Review of clinical studies. Crit Rev Food Sci Nutr 2005;45:205–229.

182 Zeisel SH, Epstein MF, Wurtman RJ: Elevated choline concentration in neonatal plasma. Life Sci 1980;26:1827–1831.

183 Ilcol YO, Ozbek R, Hamurtekin E, Ulus IH: Choline status in newborns, infants, children, breast-feeding women, breast-fed infants and human breast milk. J Nutr Biochem 2005;16:489–499.

Richard J. Wurtman
MIT, 43 Vassar St., Building 46, Room 5023b
Cambridge, MA 02139 (USA)
Tel. +1 617 253 6731, Fax +1 617 253 6882, E-Mail dick@mit.edu

Simopoulos AP, Bazan NG (eds): Omega-3 Fatty Acids, the Brain and Retina.
World Rev Nutr Diet. Basel, Karger, 2009, vol 99, pp 97–104

An Assessment of Dietary Docosahexaenoic Acid Requirements for Brain Accretion and Turnover during Early Childhood

Kevin B. Hadley · Alan S. Ryan · Edward B. Nelson · Norman Salem

Martek Biosciences Corp., Columbia, Md., USA

Brain development begins shortly after conception. In humans, the brain approaches adult mass within the first 2 years of life. Within this time, the foundation for the neural circuitry of the brain is established. As the body's central command center, the brain is responsible for orchestrating physiological actions in response to environmental stimuli. Normal brain operation is therefore critical for optimizing survivability in the animal kingdom and socioeconomic potential for humans. Early access to an adequate supply of substrates for neural development is a key requirement for preventing irreversible cognitive deficits [1–3].

The omega–3 and omega–6 long-chain polyunsaturated fatty acids (LC-PUFAs) docosahexaenoic acid (DHA, 22:6n–3) and arachidonic acid (AA, 20:4n–6) are the major n–3 and n–6 PUFAs in the membrane structural lipids of the white and gray matter of the brain, and retina [4, 5]. In humans, AA is present throughout the gray and white matter of the brain at the sn-2 position of phosphatidylinositol and phosphatidylethanolamine [6]. DHA is highly enriched in the synaptic regions of gray matter [7] at the sn-2 position of phosphatidylethanolamine and phosphatidylserine [6]. In nervous tissue, both DHA and AA serve as precursors of signal mediators [8, 9]. They are also needed for vesicle fusion [10] and synaptic neurotransmission [11]. In addition, DHA affects several aspects of brain development and function. In particular, neuron proliferation [12], gene expression [13], size [14, 15], connectivity [16, 17], synapse turnover [18], neurotransmitter levels [19, 20], and survivability [21]. The effects of DHA on neural activities ultimately influence cognition [22] and behavior [23, 24].

LC-PUFAs are synthesized from the respective essential fatty acid precursors, α-linolenic (ALA) and linoleic acid. In humans, ALA to DHA conversion efficiency is estimated to be less than 1% [25]. Therefore, in periods of rapid brain growth [26],

Table 1. Brain weight and content of DHA by age [data from 26]

Age years	Days post-conception	Brain weight g	Brain concentration of DHA, nmol/g	Total brain DHA (calculated, mg)
–0.028	Beginning of 3rd trimester	99	2,826	92
0 (birth)	104	413	5,292	718
0.44	160.60	756	7,255	1,802
1.15	420	1,100	8,714	3,149
2.28	832	1,180	9,669	3,748

adequate dietary LC-PUFA supplementation is needed in order to obtain the minimal levels required to support optimal neurological development [27, 28]. For this reason numerous investigators have sought to determine the dietary requirement for DHA during infancy and throughout life [27, 29–31]. A number of studies have considered dietary DHA requirements based upon brain accretion rates of DHA [32], tissue concentration [33], and turnover or metabolism of DHA in the brain [31]. Initial estimates by Cunnane et al. [27] indicated that during the first 6 months of life, DHA accumulates in the brain at a rate of about 10 mg/day in breast-fed infants. They proposed that in order to support this rate of accretion or accumulation, a minimum dietary intake of 20 mg/day of DHA is needed. The accretion rate of dietary DHA in the brains of infants was therefore estimated to be about 50% of intake [27]. Based on isotope tracer information from neonatal primates, Su et al. [29, 30] reported a much lower estimate for the rate of DHA accretion. According to their estimate, only 1.7% of dietary DHA is accumulated in the primate brain, whereas only 0.23% of brain DHA accretion was attributable to conversion of its precursor, ALA. In another study, Rapoport et al. [31, 34] described aspects of human brain metabolism for both DHA and AA (20:4n–6). These authors considered rates and mechanisms of incorporation of these LC-PUFAs from plasma to replace the amounts lost by turnover. However, dietary requirements and accretion rates for specific age groups were not reported.

In the present assessment, we consider the data for DHA accretion, concentration, and turnover from previously published studies and propose a general model for human brain DHA homeostasis. An estimate for the dietary requirement of DHA during early childhood (1–2 years of age) is provided.

Methods

DHA Content in the Brain
Based on autopsy information, Martinez [26] reported the amount of DHA (nmol/g) present in the brain at different ages (e.g., third trimester to 2.28 years of age, table 1). From the third trimester of life to 2.3 years of age there is about a 12-fold increase in brain size [35], and the concentration of

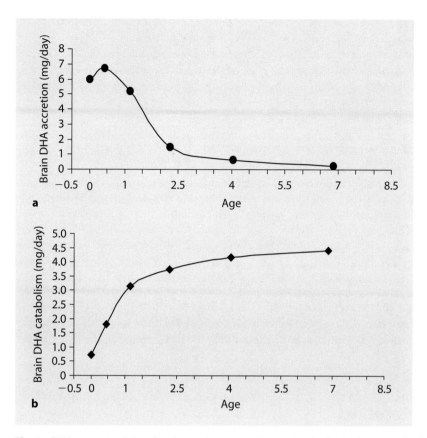

Fig. 1. DHA accretion (**a**) and estimated turnover (**b**) rate by the brain during early development.

DHA increases from 2,826 to 9,669 nmol/g [26]. To provide an estimate of the daily accretion of DHA between 1 and 2 years of age as described below, we used the information for children 1.15 and 2.28 years of age as provided by Martinez [26] (fig. 1a).

Total brain DHA for a typical 1-year-old was determined to be 3.15 g by using the molecular weight of 329 g/mol for DHA, and a brain weight of 1,100 g (table 1) (8,714 nmol × 329 ng/nmol × 10^{-6} = 2.86 mg DHA/g brain tissue; 2.86 mg DHA × 1,100 g brain = 3.2 g DHA). Total brain DHA for a 2-year-old was estimated similarly by using a brain weight of 1,180 g to calculate 3.75 g at 2.28 years of age. The amount of DHA accumulated daily in the brain between 1.15 and 2.28 years is 1.46 mg/day (3.75–3.15 g = 0.6 g or 600 mg; 832–420 days = 412 days; 600 mg/412 day = 1.46 mg DHA/day).

DHA Turnover in the Brain
In addition to the content of DHA in the brain, information about daily turnover is needed to assess DHA uptake by the brain. Turnover is defined as the quantity of unesterified DHA lost to efflux or catabolism by the brain, and is equivalent to the amount incorporated from circulation for adults [31]. Incorporation data from recently reported radioisotope-labeling studies [36] and the total content of brain DHA calculated above were used. To measure incorporation, an adult human male was administered radiolabeled DHA [36]. An accretion rate of 4.6 mg/day (14 μmol/day) was reported [36]. Incorporation at this rate for a 1,500 g brain containing 4,773 mg (9.7 μmol/g) of

DHA, according to Rapoport's described method [31] was then used. From this, an estimated turn-over of 0.1%/day was derived [(14 μmol/1,500 g/day)/9.7 μmol/g] ×100).

Assuming a constant turnover throughout this time period, the estimated rate of DHA turnover for a 1- to 2-year-old child with a total amount of 3.75 g of DHA in the brain is 3.75 mg/day (0.001/day × 3.75 g) (fig. 1b).

Daily Dietary Requirement of DHA during Early Childhood
The dietary requirement of DHA is the sum of two components: daily accretion (1.45 mg/day) and turnover, i.e. catabolism (3.75 mg/day). Thus, during the period of about 1–2 years of age, 5.2 mg/day of DHA (1.45 mg + 3.75 mg/day) is needed by the brain.

Dietary DHA is available to the brain from either circulating preformed DHA or from the conversion of ALA to DHA. Following absorption, hepatic metabolism and redistribution determine LC-PUFA availability for other tissues via the circulation [37]. In the liver, 50–80% of the ALA from the diet undergoes β-oxidation [38]. In contrast, preformed dietary DHA bypasses the β-oxidation pathway and is much more bioavailable for accretion by various tissues relative to ALA derived DHA [39].

In the USA, the average intake of ALA is ~700 mg/day between 1 and 3 years of age [40]. Assuming that only 0.23% [29, 41] (0.0023 × 700 mg/day = 1.6 mg/day) of this amount is available for use by the brain, the remaining 3.6 mg/day (5.2–1.6 mg/day) must be provided by preformed dietary DHA. Because only 1.7% of dietary preformed DHA reaches the brain [29, 41], 212 mg/day (3.6 mg/day/0.017) is necessary to maintain DHA homeostasis in the brain between 1 and 2 years of age.

Discussion and Conclusions

Our calculations show that 212 mg/day of DHA is required to support the net require-ment composed of brain accretion and catabolism components of 5.2 mg/day of DHA between 1 and 2 years of age. Notably, the value for brain DHA accretion and turn-over that this estimate is based on is nearly identical to the estimate of about 5 mg/day previously reported by Cunnane et al. [27]. During perinatal development, brain growth is rapid and DHA plays an important role in cognitive function and visual acuity [42]. Additional amounts of DHA may be needed to prevent potential losses due to disease, infection, surgery, undernutrition or other conditions that adversely affect metabolism [27, 34].

A recommended dietary intake has not been established for DHA. Instead, rec-ommendations at present have been based on adequate intake values established for ALA, the precursor of DHA. The Institute of Medicine (IOM) recommends that dietary intake of the omega–3 LC-PUFAs DHA and/or eicosapentaenoic acid make up 10% of the adequate intake of ALA [43]. Accordingly, the current IOM recom-mendation for DHA for the 1- to 3-year-old child is only 70 mg/day. Notably, the fact that eicosapentaenoic acid does not accumulate in the brain of humans [26] and primates [30, 44] is not mentioned in the IOM report [43]. Recommendations by an expert panel indicated that an intake level of 0.35% DHA, or about 80–200 mg/day, was adequate between birth and 6 months of age [45]. The World Health Organization recommends 20 mg/kg/day of DHA for term infants based on neurological benefits [46]. In terms of dietary intake, this amounts to 172–248 mg/day for infants between the 5th and 95th percentile of body weight at 1 year of age, a level that is in agreement with the daily recommendation provided here.

Presently, the amounts of DHA added to commercially available infant formulas are based upon median LC-PUFA concentrations in Western human milk [47]. As a result, dietary concentrations of DHA in infant formulas range from 0.15 to 0.32%, or 8.1–17 mg DHA/100 kcal. Throughout the world, DHA intake by nursing infants varies widely because of differences in maternal dietary habits and access to DHA-enriched foods [47]. The mean DHA content of human milk in Japan is close to 1% compared to only 0.06% availability for nursing infants in Pakistan [48]. From this it is clear that nutrient availability in breast milk depends largely upon environmental resources. Based upon the rate of DHA accretion by the brain during the early phases of development [26] a dietary DHA requirement near 1% has been estimated by this assessment.

Other sources of LC-PUFAs for infant brain development include tissue stores and synthesis. Careful estimates indicate that in term infants peripheral body compartments are used as reserves to support brain substrate requirements when the availability of preformed DHA is inadequate [27]. Indeed, a recent study of deuterated EFA metabolism showed evidence of DHA efflux from certain tissue reserves and concomitant maintenance by the brain, retina, and other high priority systems [49]. Human infants are capable of synthesizing DHA from ALA [50]. Recent studies indicate that neonatal DHA synthesis levels of ~12 mg/kg/day are reduced to about 2 mg/kg/day as toddler age nears [51]. However, the preponderance of evidence supports a wide gap between DHA accrual by the brain due primarily to endogenous synthesis, versus preformed dietary sources [52–55]. Ultimately, the combination of limited synthesis and storage capacities by peripheral tissues necessitates preformed DHA in the diet in order to maintain circulating levels [28, 56]. In the USA, the transition from breast milk to complementary foods typically occurs between 4 and 6 months of age. Infants are typically weaned long before the brain growth spurt has been completed. DHA intake by children between 7 months and 3 years old is about 30 mg/day [57]. This amount is less than one-third of the dietary intake level from human milk, at 6 months of age.

In order to provide adequate DHA for the growing infant brain, requirements based upon brain metabolism and function are needed. Evidence of this has recently been demonstrated in non-human primates by a nearly 3-fold higher dietary DHA requirement to saturate DHA levels in the cerebral cortex, relative to mother-reared controls (63 vs. 21.3 mg DHA/100 kcal) [24]. However, the potential health benefits gained from nutritional DHA seems to persist well beyond early infancy [25–29]. In fact, a recently reported clinical study, preterm infants supplemented with 1% DHA showed improved neurodevelopment after 18 months relative to those supplied with 0.2–0.3% [58].

To better define dietary DHA requirements for optimal brain and neurophysiological health, more information about DHA concentration in the brain and overall metabolism during growth and development is necessary. Additional autopsy analyses of tissue DHA, and brain DHA uptake and turnover studies using radiotracers and other techniques are needed for accurately estimating dietary requirements for humans.

In this assessment, data for brain metabolism of DHA was derived from human and animal models. This was obviously due to technical limitations related to characterizing LC-PUFA metabolism and distribution in different tissues in humans. Other considerations include the use of data from adults for estimating DHA turnover. Reports of the DHA content in the adult brain indicate values of 4.6–5.3 g [31, 34, 59]. There are many possible reasons to explain this variation of DHA content. Since ideal DHA accumulation levels in the adult human brain have not been identified, the significance of these amounts is unknown. Moreover, studies of DHA metabolism by the human brain should be accompanied by information about biomarkers of DHA status. Such information is indeed relevant due to potential influences on the rate of DHA, and possibly total 22-carbon LC-PUFA, turnover [60]. A clearer understanding of each of these factors is important to facilitate determination of metabolic requirements for DHA by humans.

The model presented here for the dietary requirement of DHA during 1–2 years of age is based on the physiological demands of the brain rather than on an estimate derived from the caloric contribution of ALA or LC-PUFA status. The limited conversion of ALA to DHA necessitates the use of pre-formed dietary DHA. A recommendation for DHA intended for normal brain development should reflect physiological requirements throughout life. According to our estimates, 212 mg/day of dietary preformed DHA are required to support DHA accretion and turnover in the brain during (between 1 and 2 years of age) early childhood. More work is needed in this area, in order to better understand the nutritional LC-PUFA needs of the growing brain.

References

1 Beard JL, Connor JR: Iron status and neural functioning. Annu Rev Nutr 2003;23:41–58.

2 Grantham-McGregor S, Ani C: A review of studies on the effect of iron deficiency on cognitive development in children. J Nutr 2001;131:649S–68S.

3 Lozoff B: Perinatal iron deficiency and the developing brain. Pediatr Res 2000;48:137–139.

4 O'Brien JS, Sampson EL: Fatty acid and fatty acid aldehyde composition of the major brain lipids in normal human gray matter, white matter, and myelin. J Lipid Res 1965;6:545–551.

5 Salem N Jr: Omega–3 fatty acids: molecular and biochemical aspects; in Spiller J, Scala GA (eds): Current Topics in Nutrition and Disease. New York, Liss, 1989, pp 109–228.

6 Svennerholm L: Distribution and fatty acid composition of phosphoglycerides in normal human brain. J Lipid Res 1968;9:570–579.

7 Breckenridge WC, Gombos G, Morgan IG: The lipid composition of adult rat brain synaptosomal plasma membranes. Biochim Biophys Acta 1972;266:695–707.

8 Stillwell W, Shaikh SR, Zerouga M, Siddiqui R, Wassall SR: Docosahexaenoic acid affects cell signaling by altering lipid rafts. Reprod Nutr Dev 2005;45:559–579.

9   Sang N, Chen C: Lipid signaling and synaptic plasticity. Neuroscientist 2006;12:425–434.

10 Darios F, Davletov B: Omega-3 and omega-6 fatty acids stimulate cell membrane expansion by acting on syntaxin-3. Nature 2006;440:813–817.

11 Lesa GM, Palfreyman M, Hall DH, et al: Long chain polyunsaturated fatty acids are required for efficient neurotransmission in C. elegans. J Cell Sci 2003;116: 4965–4975.

12 Coti Bertrand P, O'Kusky JR, Innis SM: Maternal dietary (n–3) fatty acid deficiency alters neurogenesis in the embryonic rat brain. J Nutr 2006;136: 1570–1575.

13 Rao JS, Ertley RN, Lee HJ, et al: n–3 polyunsaturated fatty acid deprivation in rats decreases frontal cortex BDNF via a p38 MAPK-dependent mechanism. Mol Psychiatry 2007;12:36–46.

14 Ahmad A, Moriguchi T, Salem N: Decrease in neuron size in docosahexaenoic acid-deficient brain. Pediatr Neurol 2002;26:210–218.

15 Ahmad A, Murthy M, Greiner RS, Moriguchi T, Salem N Jr: A decrease in cell size accompanies a loss of docosahexaenoate in the rat hippocampus. Nutr Neurosci 2002;5:103–113.

16 Sakamoto T, Cansev M, Wurtman RJ: Oral supplementation with docosahexaenoic acid and uridine 5′-monophosphate increases dendritic spine density in adult gerbil hippocampus. Brain Res 2007; 1182:50–59.

17 Marszalek JR, Kitidis C, Dararutana A, Lodish HF: Acyl-CoA synthetase-2 overexpression enhances fatty acid internalization and neurite outgrowth. J Biol Chem 2004;279:23882–23891.

18 Wurtman RJ, Ulus IH, Cansev M, Watkins CJ, Wang L, Marzloff G: Synaptic proteins and phospholipids are increased in gerbil brain by administering uridine plus docosahexaenoic acid orally. Brain Res 2006;1088:83–92.

19 Vancassel S, Leman S, Hanonick L, et al: n–3 polyunsaturated fatty acid supplementation reverses stress-induced modifications on brain monoamine levels in mice. J Lipid Res 2008;49:340–348.

20 Chalon S: Omega-3 fatty acids and monoamine neurotransmission. Prostaglandins Leukot Essent Fatty Acids 2006;75:259–269.

21 Bazan NG: Cell survival matters: docosahexaenoic acid signaling, neuroprotection and photoreceptors. Trends Neurosci 2006;29:263–271.

22 Birch EE, Garfield S, Castaneda Y, Hughbanks-Wheaton D, Uauy R, Hoffman D: Visual acuity and cognitive outcomes at 4 years of age in a double-blind, randomized trial of long-chain polyunsaturated fatty acid-supplemented infant formula. Early Hum Dev 2007;83:279–284.

23 Ng KF, Innis SM: Behavioral responses are altered in piglets with decreased frontal cortex docosahexaenoic acid. J Nutr 2003;133:3222–3227.

24 Vancassel S, Blondeau C, Lallemand S, et al: Hyperactivity in the rat is associated with spontaneous low level of n–3 polyunsaturated fatty acids in the frontal cortex. Behav Brain Res 2007;180:119–126.

25 Williams CM, Burdge G: Long-chain n–3 PUFA: plant vs. marine sources. Proc Nutr Soc 2006;65:42–50.

26 Martinez M: Polyunsaturated fatty acids in the developing human brain, red cells and plasma: influence of nutrition and peroxisomal disease. World Rev Nutr Diet. Basel, Karger, 1994, vol 75, pp 70–78.

27 Cunnane SC, Francescutti V, Brenna JT, Crawford MA: Breast-fed infants achieve a higher rate of brain and whole-body docosahexaenoate accumulation than formula-fed infants not consuming dietary docosahexaenoate. Lipids 2000;35:105–111.

28 Jackson KA, Gibson RA: Weaning foods cannot replace breast milk as sources of long-chain polyunsaturated fatty acids. Am J Clin Nutr 1989;50:980–982.

29 Su HM, Bernardo L, Mirmiran M, et al: Bioequivalence of dietary α-linolenic and docosahexaenoic acids as sources of docosahexaenoate accretion in brain and associated organs of neonatal baboons. Pediatr Res 1999;45:87–93.

30 Su HM, Bernardo L, Mirmiran M, Ma XH, Nathanielsz PW, Brenna JT: Dietary 18:3n–3 and 22:6n–3 as sources of 22:6n–3 accretion in neonatal baboon brain and associated organs. Lipids 1999;34: S347–S350.

31 Rapoport SI, Chang MC, Spector AA: Delivery and turnover of plasma-derived essential PUFAs in mammalian brain. J Lipid Res 2001;42:678–685.

32 Cunnane SC: Application of new methods and analytical approaches to research on polyunsaturated fatty acid homeostasis. Lipids 2001;36:975–979.

33 Martinez M: Tissue levels of polyunsaturated fatty acids during early human development. J Pediatr 1992;120:S129–S138.

34 Rapoport SI: What are the normal rates of human brain metabolism of arachidonic and docosahexaenoic acids, and what may happen when their metabolic balance is altered by dietary n–3 PUFA deprivation? ISSFAL Australia, 2006, p 143.

35 Matsuzawa J, Matsui M, Konishi T, et al: Age-related volumetric changes of brain gray and white matter in healthy infants and children. Cereb Cortex 2001;11:335–342.

36 Rapoport SI, Rao JS, Igarashi M: Brain metabolism of nutritionally essential polyunsaturated fatty acids depends on both the diet and the liver. Prostaglandins Leukot Essent Fatty Acids 2007;77:251–261.

37 Scott BL, Bazan NG: Membrane docosahexaenoate is supplied to the developing brain and retina by the liver. Proc Natl Acad Sci USA 1989;86:2903–2907.

38 Lin YH, Salem N Jr: Whole-body distribution of deuterated linoleic and α-linolenic acids and their metabolites in the rat. J Lipid Res 2007;48:2709–2724.

39 Su HM, Huang MC, Saad NM, Nathanielsz PW, Brenna JT: Fetal baboons convert 18:3n–3 to 22:6n–3 in vivo: a stable isotope tracer study. J Lipid Res 2001;42:581–586.

40 Food and Nutrition Board, Institute of Medicine Panel on Macronutrients ScotSEoDRI: Dietary Reference Intakes for Energy, Carbohydrate, Fiber, Fat, Fatty Acids, Cholesterol, Protein, and Amino Acids. Washington, National Academies Press, 2005.

41 Su HM, Bernardo L, Mirmiran M, Ma XH, Nathanielsz PW, Brenna JT: Dietary 18:3n–3 and 22:6n–3 as sources of 22:6n–3 accretion in neonatal baboon brain and associated organs. Lipids 1999; 34(suppl):S347–S350.

42 Innis SM: Dietary (n–3) fatty acids and brain development. J Nutr 2007;137:855–859.

43 Dietary Reference Intakes for Energy – Summary 2005.

44 Su HM, Huang MC, Saad NM, Nathanielsz PW, Brenna JT: Fetal baboons convert 18:3n–3 to 22:6n–3 in vivo. A stable isotope tracer study. J Lipid Res 2001;42:581–586.

45 Simopoulos A, Leaf, A, Salem, N: Workshop on the Essentiality of and Recommended Dietary Intakes for Omega-6 and Omega-3 Fatty Acids. International Society for the Study of Fatty Acids and Lipids, August 2007.

46 Report of a Joint Expert Consultation: Fats and Oils in Human Nutrition. Rome, WHO/FAO, 1994, pp 49–55.

47 Makrides M, Neumann MA, Gibson RA: Effect of maternal docosahexaenoic acid supplementation on breast milk composition. Eur J Clin Nutr 1996;50: 352–357.

48 Brenna JT, Varamini B, Jensen RG, Diersen-Schade DA, Boettcher JA, Arterburn LM: Docosahexaenoic and arachidonic acid concentrations in human breast milk worldwide. Am J Clin Nutr 2007;85: 1457–1464.

49 Demar JC Jr, Dimartino C, Baca AW, Lefkowitz W, Salem N Jr: Effect of dietary docosahexaenoic acid on biosynthesis of docosahexaenoic acid from α-linolenic acid in young rats. J Lipid Res 2008;49: 1963–1980.

50 Salem N Jr, Wegher B, Mena P, Uauy R: Arachidonic and docosahexaenoic acids are biosynthesized from their 18-carbon precursors in human infants. Proc Natl Acad Sci USA 1996;93:49–54.

51 Carnielli VP, Simonato M, Verlato G, et al: Synthesis of long-chain polyunsaturated fatty acids in preterm newborns fed formula with long-chain polyunsaturated fatty acids. Am J Clin Nutr 2007;86:1323–1330.

52 Jamieson EC, Farquharson J, Logan RW, et al: Infant cerebellar gray and white matter fatty acids in relation to age and diet. Lipids 1999;34:1065–1071.

53 Farquharson J, Cockburn F, Patrick WA, Jamieson EC, Logan RW: Infant cerebral cortex phospholipid fatty-acid composition and diet. Lancet 1992;340: 810–813.

54 Diau GY, Hsieh AT, Nagy SA, Wijendran V, Nathanielsz PW, JTB: The influence of long chain polyunsaturate supplementation on docosahexaenoic acid and arachidonic acid in baboon neonate central nervous system. BMC Med 2005;3: 1–12.

55 Sarkadi-Nagy E, Wijendran V, Diau GY, et al: Formula feeding potentiates docosahexaenoic and arachidonic acid biosynthesis in term and preterm baboon neonates. J Lipid Res 2004;45:71–80.

56 Hoffman DR, Theuer RC, Castaneda YS, et al: Maturation of visual acuity is accelerated in breast-fed term infants fed baby food containing DHA-enriched egg yolk. J Nutr 2004;134:2307–2313.

57 Institute of Medicine of the National Academies: Dietary Reference Intakes: Energy, Carbohydrate, Fiber, Fatty Acids, Cholesterol, Protein, and Amino Acids. Washington, National Academies Press, 2002.

58 Makrides M, Gibson RA, Collins CT, McPhee AJ: The DINO trial outcomes: does high-dose dietary docosahexaenoic acid improve the neurodevelopmental outcome of preterm infants? Kansas City, International Society for the Study of Fatty Acids and Lipids, 2008.

59 Martinez M: Severe deficiency of docosahexaenoic acid in peroxisomal disorders: a defect of Δ4 desaturation? Neurology 1990;40:1292–1298.

60 DeMar JC Jr, Ma K, Bell JM, Rapoport SI: Half-lives of docosahexaenoic acid in rat brain phospholipids are prolonged by 15 weeks of nutritional deprivation of n–3 polyunsaturated fatty acids. J Neurochem 2004;91:1125–1137.

Kevin B. Hadley, PhD
Martek Biosciences Corp.
6840 Dobbin Road, Columbia, MD 21045 (USA)
Tel. +1 443 542 2582, Fax +1 410 997 7789, E-Mail khadley@martek.com

Simopoulos AP, Bazan NG (eds): Omega-3 Fatty Acids, the Brain and Retina.
World Rev Nutr Diet. Basel, Karger, 2009, vol 99, pp 105–158

Variation in Lipid-Associated Genes as They Relate to Risk of Advanced Age-Related Macular Degeneration

John Paul SanGiovanni · Sonia Mehta · Sonul Mehta

aNational Eye Institute, Clinical Trials Branch, National Institutes of Health, Bethesda, Md.;
bScheie Eye Institute, Department of Ophthalmology, University of Pennsylvania, Philadelphia, Pa., and
cDepartment of Ophthalmology, Georgetown University and Washington Hospital Center,
Washington, D.C., USA

Conceptual Basis of Inquiry: Points at Which Gene Variants May Impact Lipid Age-Related Macular Degeneration Relationships

Age-related macular degeneration (AMD) is a major cause of visual impairment and blindness in people of Western European ancestry [1]. Approximately 3.4 million, 1.8 million, and 130 thousand people are now living with sight-threatening AMD in Europe, the USA, and Australia, respectively; this number is expected to increase by 50% by 2020 if preventive interventions are not developed [2]. AMD manifests tissue and cellular dysfunction in the forms of abnormal angiogenesis and proliferative neo-vascularization [3], excessive vascular permeability [4], immunoregulatory dysfunction [5], alterations in physiologic reduction-oxidation balance [6], and neuronal/retinal pigment epithelium (RPE) cell degeneration [4]. Lipid-based compounds, their precursors, cleavage and biosynthetic enzymes, and metabolites have the capacity to modulate processes and systems implicated in AMD pathogenesis [7–14]. A number of bioinformatic and analytic methods exist to guide investigations on joint actions of genes encoding elements of biologic pathways. These have been adapted to analysis of data from genome-wide association studies [15].

An emerging evidence base indicates a lower likelihood of advanced AMD among people reporting the highest levels of eicosapentaenoic acid (EPA, 20:5ω–3,), and docosahexaenoic acid (DHA, 22:6ω–3), EPA + DHA, or fish intake [12, 16–26]. DHA, a major dietary omega–3 (ω–3) long-chain polyunsaturated fatty acid (LCPUFA), is also a major structural lipid in sensory [27] and vascular [28, 29] retina. EPA is a major dietary ω–3 LCPUFA, the precursor to both DHA and a family of potent paracrine and autocine effectors with vaso- and immunoregulatory actions [30, 31]. While EPA is not detected in appreciable quantities within retinal phospholipids, it circulates in vascular tissue and is rapidly used for eicosanoid biosynthesis in various cellular and tissue compartments. The most efficient way to alter retinal DHA concentrations is through consumption of dietary DHA. Fish are the main dietary source of EPA and DHA [32–34]. Pioneering mechanistic studies informing inference on ω–3 LCPUFA-AMD relationships have been conducted over the past decade [7, 8, 10, 11, 14, 35–44], and breadth of findings from applied clinical research designs is now expanding.

Our central premise that *dietary and retinal fatty acids and their metabolites affect and are affected by metabolic and environmental factors and processes implicated in pathogenesis of neural and vascular retina* was developed from a number of extant reports and texts [13, 27, 45]. Elements of our conceptual framework exist in table 1. ω–3 LCPUFAs and their metabolites exhibit cytoprotective and reparative actions contributing to a number of anti-angiogenic [11] and neuroprotective [9, 46] mechanisms within the retina. AMD pathogenesis is associated with ischemia, chronic light exposure, oxidative stress, inflammation, cellular signaling mechanisms, and aging [3, 6]. ω–3 LCPUFAs operate within complex systems to impact production and activity of vaso- and immonoregulatory compounds classified as eicosanoids, angiogenic factors, matrix metalloproteinases, reactive oxygen species (ROS), cyclic nucleotides, neurotransmitters and neuromodulators, pro-inflammatory and immunoregulatory cytokines, and inflammatory phospholipids involved in these processes [reviewed in 13, 47]. Effects and actions of metabolic and environmental bioactivators and bioactive molecules include, but are not limited to, activation of phospholipase A_2 (PLA$_2$), cyclooxygenase (COX), and lipoxygenase (LOX), and fatty acid anhydrase. Balance and concentration of dietary ω–3 and ω–6 LCPUFA intake and tissue status impacts this enzyme system [34] to yield a pool of LCPUFAs and potent autocoids [8].

The sections that follow contain information on observed and putative relationships of ω–3 LCPUFAs with metabolic- and environment-based activators and bioactive compounds in the context of AMD pathogenesis models. We first present the body of evidence implicating LCPUFAs as key modulators of processes influencing AMD pathogenesis. We then apply empirical and inference-based methods for examining the relationship of genetic variation in LCPUFA -associated molecules with sight-threatening AMD. Our general conclusions are that: (1) there is consistent evidence to suggest that ω–3 LCPUFAs may act in protective roles for AMD; (2) whole-genome scanning technology may be applied to efficiently elucidate novel pathway and gene set-based associations with complex diseases like AMD, and (3) a knowledge-based approach to exposure ascertainment (in this case, identification and annotation of lipid-associated genes) is valuable in planning, implementation, analytic inference efforts to elucidate novel associations in complex systems.

Table 1. Central elements of our conceptual framework

Description and physiologic significance of LCPUFAs [reviewed in 45, 48–50]
- EPA has 20 carbons and 5 methylene-interrupted double bonds
- DHA has 22 carbons and 6 methylene-interrupted double bonds
- DHA, EPA are ω–3 LCPUFAs of physiologic significance; they act as constituents of lipid-protein complexes, substrates for bioactive autocoids and natural ligands to nuclear transcription factors

LCPUFA metabolism, intake, transport, and accretion [reviewed in 27, 45, 51]
- LCPUFAs may be of dietary or cellular origin
- Humans may not have capacity to meet retinal tissue needs for LCPUFA through biosynthesis
- Retinal LCPUFA tissue status is modifiable by and dependent on dietary intake
- The hepatocyte is the major site of LCPUFA biosynthesis
- LCPUFAs are esterified as components of triglycerides and phospholipids, integrated with chylomicrons or very low density lipoproteins before transport to the choriocapillaris
- LCPUFA-rich phospholipids are hydrolyzed and bind to a high affinity, receptor at the choroid-RPE interface. They are transported through the interphotoreceptor matrix to the photoreceptor inner segment. Esterified DHA-phospholipid compounds are then hydrolyzed, actively transferred to the inner segment cytosol and re-esterified into phospholipids, incorporated into photoreceptor disc membranes and transported to the outer segment. Discs migrate to the apical tip of the photoreceptor and are then shed and phagocytized by RPE cells. DHA is then stored within oil droplets in the RPE. DHA is efficiently recycled to the inner segment via a receptor-mediated process
- LCPUFAs may be biosynthesized on neural and vascular retinal endoplasmic reticulum and peroxisomes
- ω–3 LCPUFA-rich foods are based mainly in marine and lacrustine products [32, 33]
- DHA is accreted selectively and retained efficiently in photoreceptors [52]

LCPUFAs in retinal structure and function
- DHA is a major structural component of retinal membranes [27]
- DHA tissue status insufficiency is associated with altered visual processing capacity [53]
- DHA affects retinal cell signaling mechanisms in phototransduction [54–56]
- LCPUFAs influence gene expression [50, 57–59] and retinal cell differentiation, and survival [37–44, 60]

Impact of metabolic and environmental factors on LCPUFAs and implications for AMD pathogenesis [reviewed in 12, 13]
- PLA$_2$ cleaves LCPUFAs from their esterified form within membranes and lipoproteins to a free form capable of acting as a substrate for synthesis of potent autocrine and paracrine lipid mediators [7, 9–11, 14, 31, 46, 61]. PLA$_2$ is activated by light exposure, ischemia, oxidative stress, apoptosis, inflammation, cell-signaling molecules, and aging. Retinal diseases are associated with PLA$_2$ activity and with these metabolic and environmental factors
- COX and LOX catalyze conversion of LCPUFAs to eicosanoids. COX and LOX are activated by ischemia, oxidative stress, light exposure, apoptosis, inflammation, cell-signaling molecules, and aging. Retinal diseases of public health significance are associated both with COX/LOX activity and with these metabolic and environmental factors
- LCPUFAs demonstrate anti-angiogenic, anti-vasoproliferative, and neuroprotective actions on factors and processes implicated in the pathogenesis of vasoproliferative and neurodegenerative retinal diseases
- These actions affect eicosanoids, angiogenic factors, reactive oxygen species, matrix metalloproteinases, cyclic nucleotides, neurotransmitters and neuromodulators, pro-inflammatory and immunoregulatory cytokines, and inflammatory phospholipids

LCPUFAs and retinal diseases of public health significance [reviewed in 12, 13]
- LCPUFAs have the capacity to affect pathogenic processes implicated in retinal neovascularization
- LCPUFAs have the capacity to affect pathogenic processes implicated in retinal neural degeneration

The Nature of Essential Fatty Acids, LCPUFAs, and Their Distribution in Retina

Fatty acids are synthesized via condensation of malonyl coenzyme A (CoA) units by a fatty acid synthase complex. Two families of essential fatty acids (EFAs) exist, i.e. ω–3 and ω–6. Humans do not have capacity for de novo biosynthesis of EFAs (α-linolenic acid (ALA, 18:3ω–3) and linoleic acid (LA, 18:2ω–6), because of a natural absence of Δ15- and Δ12-desaturase enzymes. LCPUFAs may be obtained directly through the diet or formed from ALA (ω–3 LCPUFAs) or LA (ω–6 LCPUFAs).

ω–3 and ω–6 LCPUFAs contain a carboxyl head group and a carbon chain (≥18 carbons) with two or more methylene-interrupted double (unsaturated) bonds. EFAs and LCPUFAs are structurally classified by the number of carbons, double bonds, and proximity of the first double bond to the methyl (ω) terminal of the fatty acid acyl chain. Fatty acids of the ω–3 family contain a double bond at the third carbon and those of the ω–6 family contain a double bond at the sixth carbon. EPA contains 20 carbons, 5 double bonds, and has a molecular weight of 302.451. DHA has a carbon chain length of 22, 6 double bonds, and a molecular weight of 328.488. Arachidonic acid (AA, 20:4–ω6) is a major dietary ω–6 LCPUFA with 20 carbons, 4 double bonds, and a molecular weight of 304.467.

In humans, LCPUFA stores exist mainly as esterified complexes in the *sn-2* position of glycerophosphates (also known as glycerophospholipids or phospholipids) or trihydric glycerols (also known as triacylglycerols or triglycerides). Within the neural retina, phospholipids are the predominant LCPUFA-rich lipid class; these compounds act mainly as structural elements of membranes. Phosphatidylcholine (PC) represents 40–50% of retinal phospholipids and is localized mainly to the outer membrane leaflet. Phosphatidylethanolamine (PEA) and phosphatidylserine (PS) represent 30–35 and 5–10% of retinal phospholipids, respectively; both species tend to orient within the cytoplasmic leaflet. PEA and PS respectively represent 30–35 and 5–10% of retinal phospholipids; both tend to orient within the cytoplasmic leaflet. Phosphatidylinositol (PI) represents 3–6% of retinal phospholipid membrane domains [47].

Highest body concentrations of DHA per unit weight exist in phospholipids of retinal photoreceptor outer segments and the overall percent of DHA (30% of all retinal fatty acids) is 50 mol% greater than in the next most concentrated tissue [52]; DHA is also found in substantial amounts within retinal vascular tissue and glia. PEA and PS are the dominant retinal DHA-containing phospholipid species. AA is a major fatty acid of vascular and neural retinal tissue. The highest concentrations of AA are found in PC and PEA. EPA exists in vascular tissue and blood components, but does not accrue appreciable quantities to retinal tissue – it is quickly used in DHA or eicosanoid biosynthesis (reviewed in Nelson [62]).

The lipid composition of retinal photoreceptor outer segments is unique: 80–90% of structural lipids are phospholipids and 8–10% are neutral lipids [27, 63]. Neutral lipid species are mainly cholesterol, although free fatty acids can be detected as well. Retinal phospholipids are also unique because of their polyenoic nature. Polyenoic phospholipids contain PUFAs in the *sn-1* or *sn-2* positions of the molecule's glycerol backbone. Phospholipids in the outer segments are predominantly dipolyenoic [64–66]. Dipolyenoic species are known to increase rate of rhodopsin activation (metarhodopsin II formation) in model membrane systems [67]; this process is essential in phototransduction.

Fliesler and Anderson [27] provide a detailed review on chemistry and metabolism of lipids in the vertebrate retina. Vertebrate retinal phospholipid species include: (1) PEA as ~40% of outer segment lipids; (2) PS as ~12%, and (3) PC as ~10% of total outer segment lipids. PC, PE, PS, and PI respectively represent ~48, 32, 9, and 4% of retinal phospholipids. DHA exists as approximately 20% of the fatty acids for outer segment PC, and ~30% for each of PE and PS [27, 68]. Half of all PC fatty acids are saturated (~30% palmitic acid and ~20% stearic acid); in PE these values are ~10 and 36%, respectively. 30% of PS fatty acids are saturated, with the greatest proportion being stearic acid (~28%).

EPA, DHA, and AA are fatty acids of physiologic significance; they act as:

- *Key structural constituents of phospholipid membranes.* DHA and AA are major fatty acids of neural and vascular retinal tissue.
- *Ligands to transcription factors* for genes influencing: (a) cellular differentiation and growth; (b) lipid, protein, and carbohydrate metabolism. DHA and EPA affect gene expression through regulation of transcription factor activity and concentration within the nucleus. Transcription factors containing a LCPUFA-binding domain include peroxisome proliferator-activated receptors (PPARs), the retinoid X receptor (RXR), nuclear factor-κB (NF-κB), and sterol regulatory element-binding proteins (SREBPs). In some cases, metabolites of the EPA and DHA also act directly as ligands.
- *Effectors of signal transduction pathways regulating gene transcription.* These pathways include enzyme-based LOX, COX, protein kinase C (PKC), and sphingomyelinase. LCPUFAs may also regulate pathways affecting serine-threonine and tyrosine kinase-linked- and G-protein receptors.
- *Substrates for eicosanoid or endocannabinoids* of in inter- and intracellular signaling cascades influencing vascular, neural, and immune function.

EFA and LCPUFA Metabolism, Transport, and Accretion to the Retina
A detailed discussion of LCPUFA metabolism, transport, and accretion appears in Chow [45]. LCPUFAs are obtained through diet or derived from EFAs. EFAs may be desaturated (by insertion of double bonds) and elongated (by addition of 2-carbon units) to LCPUFAs on the hepatic or retinal endoplasmic reticulum (ER). ALA is the dietary precursor to EPA and DHA. LA is the dietary precursor to AA. Conversion from 24- to 22-carbon LCPUFAs requires β-oxidation in the peroxisome. Because ω−3 and ω−6 EFA families compete for the same desaturases and elongases, dietary lipid balance and composition will affect production and tissue accretion of these nutrients [33, 69, 70]. Although biosynthesis of LCPUFAs from EFAs is possible, the

efficiency of tissue accretion is highest when they are ingested in the preformed state [71]. Photoreceptors are constrained in their capacity to synthesize DHA [72, 73]. RPE [73], retinal endothelium [74], and brain astrocytes [75] are able to synthesize DHA.

Gordon and Bazan [47] and Rodriguez deTurco et al. [76] present pathways through which LCPUFAs enter the retina. Within foods, EFAs and LCPUFAs exist mainly in esterified forms as triacylglycerols (TGs). During early phases of absorption, free fatty acids are hydrolyzed within the intestine from the *sn-1* and *sn-3* positions of TGs by pancreatic lipase. DHA is most likely to occupy the *sn-2* position of the resulting 2-monoglyceride. EPA exists mainly at the *sn-3*, and to a lesser extent, the *sn-1* position [32]. Free LCPUFAs and LCPUFA-monoacylglycerol complexes are subsequently re-esterified to phospholipids and TGs within enterocytes of the intestinal epithelium. TGs and phospholipids are next integrated to chylomicrons and very low density lipoproteins (VLDL), secreted into the lymphatic system, and circulated to the liver from the thoracic duct via blood. The bulk of DHA biosynthesis from ALA occurs in liver [77]. ALA enters the hepatocyte through a receptor-mediated process and is activated by CoA. The fatty acid complex subsequently enters the smooth ER where it is elongated and desaturated to DHA-CoA. DHA-CoA enters the rough ER and is esterified to phospholipids and then complexes with apoproteins. The complex arrives to the Golgi bodies in vesicular form where they are assembled into lipoproteins and secreted [78]. DHA of cellular and dietary origin is transported via VLDL lipoproteins to the choriocapillaris. Lipoprotein lipase hydrolyzes chylomicrons remnants and VLDL within the choriocapillaris. The great majority of lymph-borne esterified LCPUFAs are transported in TGs of the chylomicron and VLDL fractions; they exist to a lesser extent as free fatty acids and within PC, cholesterol ester, monoglyceride, and diglyceride pools. DHA is accreted mainly to phospholipids species composing membranes (PEA, PC, PS) in the retina. Within the circulation, LCPUFAs on chylomicron-bound TGs are hydrolyzed to their free forms by capillary-endothelial-cell-derived lipoprotein lipase. These free fatty acids may subsequently form non-covalent bonds with albumin in blood plasma for delivery to tissues.

Retinal biosynthesis of DHA is slow and may be insufficient to sustain the needs of photoreceptors [72, 73]. In addition to photoreceptors, cellular sources of DHA exist in RPE [73], retinal endothelium [74], and brain astrocytes [75]. Scott and Bazan [77] and Li et al. [79] present evidence that the liver is a key site for LCPUFA biosynthesis. Hepatic biosynthesis determines availability and distribution of LCPUFAs in plasma lipids and lipoproteins, lipoprotein assembly, and tissue uptake [47].

DHA transport via the choriocapillaris to the RPE and inner segments is likely to be mediated by a high affinity receptor-mediated uptake. Hepatectomized rats exhibit rapid accretion of LCPUFAs in neural tissue [80], suggesting that transport systems and specific binding proteins for these compounds operate effectively within the mammalian nervous system. DHA travels from the choriocapillaris via the RPE cells and interphotoreceptor matrix (an extracellular region between the RPE and outer limiting membrane). The hydrophobic nature of fatty acids requires specific cytoplasmic transport mechanisms, binding proteins, and receptors to transport LCPUFAs to the photoreceptors. As there is no direct contact between choroidal circulation and photoreceptors, adjacent cell types including RPE cells, astrocytes, and Müller cells must aid in the process.

LCPUFA Delivery to Subcellular Membrane Systems in the Photoreceptor. LCPUFA-containing phospholipids enter the RPE and photoreceptor inner segment via a receptor-mediated transport process involving a high affinity fatty acid-binding protein with a lipoprotein lipase [47]. LCPUFAs enter the photoreceptor inner segment in a smooth ER-dense area adjacent to the base of the outer segment. After enzymatic degradation of the DHA-containing triglyceride in the inner segment, activation of fatty acid co-enzyme A initiates esterification of DHA to phosphatidic acid. De novo phospholipid, di- and triglyceride biosynthesis occurs following this process. DHA-containing phospholipids are subsequently integrated as structural constituents of photoreceptor disc membranes and are retained in proximity to rhodopsin molecules across the lifespan of the photoreceptor disc. Efficient mechanisms of repair for oxidized DHA exist and this condition allows the molecule to remain intact within photoreceptor discs. Properties of DHA retention and repair are unique among photoreceptor lipids. As discs migrate to the outer segment-RPE interface, are shed, and phagocytized the photoreceptor, the DHA content is not altered appreciably. Phagosomes are degraded in the RPE to form oil droplets containing DHA-rich triglycerides. These triglycerides are then transported back to the myoid of the inner segment for re-uptake. RPE cytosol remains virtually free of DHA-containing lipid and lipoprotein species and this condition may have important consequences for AMD prevention.

LCPUFAs in the Vascular Retina. Lecompte et al. [29] reported on fatty acid composition of isolated bovine retinal microvessels. DHA and AA each represent approximately 10% of total fatty acids in purified intact vessels. In primary cultures (confluent endothelial cell/pericyte monolayers) the value for DHA was reduced to approximately 2%; the value for AA did not change. DHA levels were restored in the cell culture with 10 μM supplementation of unesterified DHA. In endothelial cells, AA concentration was unchanged; in the case of pericytes, AA concentration was reduced. Levels of EPA in both systems were more than 10 times less than those of DHA and AA. While substantial variation existed across model systems, the mol% of EPA in retinal microvessels was 5-fold higher than that in non-vascular retina (0.5 vs. 0.1%). This is an important issue, as retroconversion of DHA to EPA is estimated at 9–11% [81, 82] in human serum [81, 82]. Also, endothelial cultures from bovine macrovascular networks (aorta) exhibit considerable retroconversion. In the Lecompte et al. [29] report, retroconversion was negligible, demonstrating specificity of fatty acid metabolism that is based on the origin of vascular tissue.

Delton-Vandenbroucke et al. [74] reported that cultured bovine retinal endothelial cells are capable of biosythesizing DHA via desaturation of docosapentaenoic acid (DPA, 22:5) of the ω–3 family. Although EPA was the major metabolite of DPA ω–3 desaturation, DPA has been shown to represent 2 mol% of isolated and purified bovine microvessels [29].

EFA and LCPUFA Intake and Supplementation

Hibbeln et al. [33] provide estimates of ω–3 and ω–6 fatty acid intake across more than 30 countries. US residents typically consume approximately 1.6 g/day (approximately 0.7% of total energy intake) of ω–3 fatty acids [83]. The bulk of this is ALA. EPA and DHA usually represent 6–12% of total ω–3 intake (0.1–0.2 g/day). The main sources of ALA are vegetable oils. Linseed, canola, and soybean oils contain the highest levels. EPA and DHA are concentrated in fatty fish and this is the main source in the Western diet. Roughly 10% of DHA is typically derived from eggs. Products fortified with DHA and EPA are now entering the US consumer market. These products usually contain <75 mg/serving. ω–3 LCPUFAs are available as dietary supplements. Capsules typically contain 120 mg DHA and 180 mg EPA [84]. In these products EPA is usually provided from fish oil. DHA may be derived from single-celled organisms or fish oil. A list of commercially available supplements containing DHA and/or EPA, the nutrient composition of these supplements, and the supplement manufacturers exists at The Natural Medicines Comprehensive Database (http://www.naturaldatabase.com). Data from the 2003–2004 National Health and Nutrition Survey indicate that approximately 1 in 20 US residents aged ≥20 years is now taking a supplement containing ω–3 LCPUFAs.

The American Heart Association statement on ω–3 fatty acids and cardiovascular disease reviews safety of ω–3 fatty acids and fish [84] and cites dietary intake recommendations of 0.3–0.5 g/day of EPA + DHA from the World Health Organization, North Atlantic Treaty Organization, and National Health Ministries of Australia, Canada, Japan, Sweden, and the United Kingdom. Gebauer et al. [85] provide a history of recommendations. The US Food and Drug Administration (FDA) [86] stated that consumption of up to 3 g/day of marine-based ω–3 fatty acids is generally regarded as safe (GRAS). The FDA [87] has also approved a health claim for DHA and EPA in supplement form. Governmental regulatory bodies have issued statements concerning the potential for hemorrhagic risk with intake of ω–3 LCPUFAs >3 g/day [87; discussed in 84]. The antithrombotic and antihemostatic effects of ω–3 LCPUFAs operate within physiologic limits at intakes between 1.0 and 3.0 g/day [88–92]; at these levels, hemorrhagic risk is not considered a major issue, and most studies using higher amounts, up to 6 g/day, have not reported any adverse effects.

DHA Is an Essential Structural Component of Retinal Membranes

Biophysical and biochemical properties of DHA affect membrane function by altering permeability, fluidity, thickness, lipid phase properties, and the activation of membrane-bound proteins [93, 94]. DHA-rich membranes impart properties to outer segments that impact the dynamic of cellular communication processes [67, 95–99]. The stereochemical structure of DHA allows efficient conformational change of the transmembrane protein rhodopsin, in response to the capture of light that initiates visual sensation. LCPUFA-rich membranes exhibit less rigid global properties than those concentrated in cholesterol or saturated fatty acids, since multiple unsaturated bonds and long carbon chains in LCPUFAs do not permit dense packing of the hydrophobic fatty acid components. A more fluid membrane enables faster response to light stimulation. For DHA, the position of the first unsaturated bond at the ω–3 (between Δ20 and Δ19) carbon yields gains in efficiency for membrane dynamics over those observed in an otherwise structurally identical fatty acid with the first double bond at the ω–6 carbon [100].

Biochemical characteristics of DHA provide biologic credibility of its concentration in the metabolically active retinal outer segment. The highly unsaturated nature of DHA makes it highly susceptible to oxidation in the metabolically active photoreceptor. The evolutionary significance of concentrating DHA in the photoreceptor may be that membrane-bound DHA is a primary source of lipid-derived signaling molecules that modulate intercellular communication and autocrine signaling from the plasma membrane. These processes have the capacity to influence the nuclear control of gene expression [101–105]. While esterified AA is more efficiently released from membrane stores than DHA [54], retinal astrocytes can provide a readily mobilized source of DHA for such purposes [106].

DHA Tissue Status Is Associated with Alterations in Retinal and Visual Function
Litman et al. [67, 96, 98] investigated mechanisms by which membrane fatty acid composition may affect phototransduction. Phototransduction is the process through which the retina processes light energy and converts it to a cellular signal. In a dark-adapted state, retinal photoreceptors maintain a depolarizing 'dark current' that is mediated by the effect of high cytosolic concentrations of 3′,5′-cyclic guanosine monophosphate (cGMP) that open Na^+/Ca^{2+} channels. Phototransduction starts with the capture of a photon by rhodopsin. Rhodopsin is subsequently transformed to metarhodopsin II (M(II)). M(II) binds to and activates the α-subunit of the trimeric G-protein transducin. The M(II)-transducin complex binds to and activates tetrameric cGMP phosphodiesterase (PDE) through extraction of one of inhibitory γ-subunit. Activated PDE hydrolyzes cGMP to GMP, which produces a hyperpolarized membrane due to dissociation of cGMP from Na^+/Ca^{2+} ion channels. The hyperpolarized state of the photoreceptor yields a graded decrease of glutamate release on horizontal and bipolar cells. Bipolar cells form synapses with retinal ganglion cells; axons of the retinal ganglion cells form the optic nerve that connects to brain centers that work in visual sensation and perception. The process is stopped when rhodopsin is phosphorylated by rhodopsin kinase and then bound with visual arrestin; this process inhibits formation of the M(II)-transducin complex.

Litman and Mitchell [67] demonstrated that M(II) formation to an activated membrane-bound receptor state was higher in DHA-containing model membrane systems than in those containing AA and cholesterol. DHA enhances production of M(II) and activation of the M(II)-transducin complex is more than 2-fold greater in DHA-containing systems than it is in those concentrated with saturated and mono-unsaturated fatty acid species [54]. These findings support the concept that interaction in M(II)-transducin coupling is enhanced (essentially rendered more efficient) in DHA-rich membranes. Similar relationships were observed for PDE activity [96].

Actions and Associations of ω–3 LCPUFAs on Processes Implicated in AMD Pathogenesis

A number of metabolic and environmental factors and processes activate molecules associated with abnormal angiogenesis, proliferative neovascularization, excessive vascular endothelial permeability, immunoregulatory dysfunction, alterations in physiologic redox balance, and neuronal/RPE cell degeneration observed in AMD. As mentioned above, key factors and processes associated with AMD pathogeneis include ischemia, light exposure, oxidative stress, apoptosis, inflammation, neuroactive cell signaling molecules, and age-related developmental processes. These factors and processes operate in a complex system, share common modulators, and yield common outcomes. It is essential to note that in addition to affecting molecules associated with the pathogenesis of retinal disease, AMD-associated factors and processes are capable of activating: (1) PLA_2, leading to release of unesterified LCPUFAs from phospholipid membranes, and (2) COXs and LOXs that drive eicosanoid synthesis. As the concentration and composition of ω–3 LCPUFAs stored in phospholipid membranes is modifiable by and dependent upon dietary intake, the balance of free LCPUFAs and their metabolites is thus affected after activation of PLA_2, COX, and LOX. It is also essential to consider the role of factors capable of altering the concentrations of free LCPUFAs and the activity of key fatty acid cleavage and biosynthetic enzymes when investigating potential actions of ω–3 LCPUFAs in the retina. As such, we first review basic concepts related to PLA_2, COX, and LOX in the context of AMD-associated metabolic and environmental exposures. Table 2 contains references to the evidence base on the relationship of these AMD-associated factors and PLA_2, COX, and LOX.

PLA_2 in LCPUFA Hydrolysis. PLA_2s catalyze hydrolysis of fatty acids from the ester bond at the *sn-2* position of phospholipids. Hydrolysis yields free LCPUFAs and lysophospholipids. Approximately 20 groups of PLA_2s have been identified; PLA_2s are generally classified into cytosolic ($cPLA_2$), secretory ($sPLA_2$), and calcium-independent ($iPLA_2$) isoforms [111]. $cPLA_2$s are high molecular weight and cleave AA preferentially; Ca^{2+}-dependent and -independent forms exist. Intracellular $sPLA_2$s are low molecular weight; these enzymes do not show specificity for particular fatty acids. $cPLA_2\alpha$ has an *N*-terminal calcium-dependent phospholipid domain that may permit post-translational regulation by Ca^{2+} or phosphorylation via mitogen-activated protein kinase (MAPK) and PKC [129–133]. Extracellular signal-regulated kinases (ERKs) act in communication between $cPLA_2\alpha$ and $sPLA_2$s [134, 135]. DHA has been

Table 2. AMD-associated processes usually increase enzyme expression or activity of PLA$_2$, COX, and LOX

Disease-associated factor	Enzyme		
	PLA$_2$	COX	LOX
Ischemia [3]	↑ PLA$_2$ activity [107, 108]	↑ COX activity [109, 110]	↑ LOX activity [111]
Light exposure [112]	↑20:4ω–6 release [113]	↑ COX-2 production [114]	↑ LTB$_4$ production [115]
Redox balance [6]	ROS ↑ PLA$_2$ activity [116]	ROS ↑ COX-2 mRNA [117, 118]	ROS ↑ 5-LOX activity [119]
Cell cycle [3]	↑ [116]	Necrosis ↑ COX-2 mRNA [120]	
Inflammation [121]	↑ PLA$_2$ activity [122]	PAF ↑ COX-2 mRNA [123–125]	5-LOX ↓ with Rx [126]
Aging [2]	↑ [127]	↑COX-2 in senescent cells [128]	

PLA$_2$ = Phospholipase A$_2$, COX = cyclooxygenase, LOX = lipoxygenase, Redox = oxidation-reduction; ROS = reactive oxygen species; PAF = platelet-activating factor; ↑ = increases; ↓ = decreases.

shown to decrease PLA$_2$ activity in nerve growth cones of nerve growth factor-differentiated PC12 cells, with a predominant effect on sPLA$_2$ in calcium-independent pathways [136].

COX in Eicosanoid Biosynthesis. COX (prostaglandin endoperoxide synthase) is a protein complex that converts 20-carbon LCPUFA substrates from ω–6 (AA) and ω–3 (EPA) families to G-prostaglandin endoperoxides. Figure 1 presents a basic structure of eicosanoid metabolism. This process involves hydrogen subtraction (at carbon 11) and subsequent addition of 2 molecules of oxygen. A hydroperoxidase subsequently uses glutathione to convert the G-prostaglandins to H-prostaglandins. FitzGerald [137] reviews basic aspects of COX production, structure, and actions of COX metabolites. The constitutive form of COX (COX-1) exists mainly in the gastric mucosa, kidney and platelets, and operates primarily in the role of hemostatic regulation. The inducible form (COX-2) is expressed constitutively in the central nervous system, is activated by cytokines and mitogens, and acts in formation of prostaglandins in inflammatory response. Ringbom et al. [138] have demonstrated that DHA and EPA are effective in inhibiting COX-1- and COX-2-catalyzed prostaglandin biosynthesis with an in vitro assay. COX-2 showed higher potency. Corey et al. [139] discuss potential for DHA to operate as a competitive inhibitor of COX. COXs are activated in response to PLA$_2$ activation and free LCPUFA concentration.

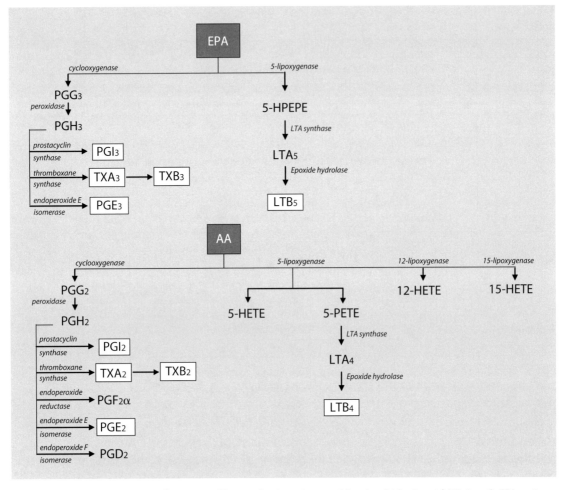

Fig. 1. Overview of eicosanoid biosynthetic pathways. AA = Arachidonic acid (20:4ω–6); EPA = eicosapentaenoic acid (20:5ω–3); HETE = hydroxyeicosatetraenoic acid; HPETE = hydroperoxyeicosatetraenoic acid; LT = leukotriene; PG = prostaglandin; TX = thromboxane.

LOX in Eicosanoid Biosynthesis. 5-LOX converts AA or EPA to hydroperoxides (hydroperoxyeicosatetraenoic acids, HPETE); this process involves removal of hydrogen at carbon 7 and insertion of molecular oxygen at carbon 5. HPETE is essential for leukotriene biosynthesis; it may also be reduced to hydroxyeicosatetraenoic acid (HETE). Activation of 5-LOX is modulated by Ca^{2+}, ATP, and 5-LOX-activating protein. 5-LOX metabolites act in immunoregulation within the inflammatory response [reviewed in 140]. LOXs are activated in response to PLA_2 activation and free LCPUFA concentration. 12- and 15-LOX are other LOX enzymes that catalyze conversion of EPA and AA to other potent compounds of physiological significance.

Ischemia, O_2 Delivery, and Hemodynamics in AMD. Retinal ischemia and concomitant hemodynamic change is associated with AMD [141, 142]. Lipid-based modulators of retinal ischemia operate as paracrine and autocrine effectors within blood and on vascular membranes to alter blood flow and O_2 regulation. LCPUFAs are precursors to vasoregulatory thromboxanes (TX) and prostaglandins (PG) affecting blood flow [143], vasomotility, platelet activity, and platelet aggregation [88–91]. As precursors to lipid mediators and endogenous ligands to nuclear transcription factors, ω–3 LCPUFAs are associated with beneficial or non-damaging cellular response in vascular systems subjected to physiologic stresses that alter blood flow, oxygen delivery [70, 143–148] and lipoprotein metabolism [50, 149, 150].

Chronic Light Exposure and AMD. Under normal physiological conditions, retinal photic damage is unlikely to occur, despite the high density of photosensitive compounds (chromophores) and the chronic nature of light exposure. Findings on sunlight exposure and AMD are equivocal [151], however photic damage is difficult to measure in free-living humans. Boulton et al. [112] review plausible processes that may operate in retinal diseases associated with an overstimulation of photoreceptors; in some cases, models of chronic light exposure may offer important insight to relationships between photoreceptor activity and AMD. Cellular response to chronic light exposure (light adaptation) alters rhodopsin and membrane fatty acid concentration. As a result of this regulation the healthy retina exhibits a stable capacity for photon capture that is independent of stimulus intensity. In this way cells maintain sensitive response to light without sustaining injury from high metabolic demand. DHA may impact this process, as IRBP, a key transport protein involved in photopigment regeneration, contains a high-affinity DHA-binding site [152, 153]. Light exposure leads to transformation of 11-*cis*-retinaldehyde to all-*trans*-retinaldehyde (a chromophore with a peak absorption spectrum in the range of high-energy short-wavelength light associated with photic damage) and all-*trans*-retinol (a by-product of phototransduction with membranolytic characteristics) [112]. The cycle of rhodopsin regeneration from all-*trans*-retinaldehyde to 11-*cis*-retinaldehyde and reduction of all-*trans*-retinol is implicated in photoreceptor survival. IRBP transports regenerated 11-*cis*-retinaldehyde from the RPE to the photoreceptor. Chen et al. [152] reported that DHA rapidly and specifically displaced 11-*cis*-retinaldehyde from IRBP of bovine samples and suggest that the gradient of DHA between RPE (3.5% of total lipids as DHA) and photoreceptor cells (20% of total lipids as DHA) would enable a swap of 11-*cis*-retinaldehyde for DHA as IRBP approaches the RPE. All-*trans*-retinol exhibits a high affinity to IRBP. As the protein comes in contact with the DHA-rich photoreceptor, the 11-*cis*-retinoid may be released, allowing DHA to bind in its place. All-*trans*-retinol also exhibits a high affinity to the receptor in and may thus bind to the complex as it approaches the outer segments in transit to the RPE.

In the healthy retina, light adaptation is related to reduction of oxidative stress, as it leads to a decrease in photoreceptor oxygen consumption [142]. Organisciak et al. [154] provide evidence to suggest that light damage and photopigment concentration affect oxidative processes since heme oxygenase, an oxygen-sensitive stress protein, is upregulated by retinal photic injury and rhodopsin loss.

Retinal Energy Production, Regulation, Metabolism, Reduction-Oxidation Balance and AMD. Beatty et al. [6] discuss how natural characteristics of the retina affect cellular oxidation-reduction (redox) balance to favor oxidation. These are: the volume of O_2 consumption required to support the metabolic needs of the photoreceptors, the high concentration of photosensitizing compounds in the photoreceptors and RPE, the high concentration of PUFAs in photoreceptors, and active phagocytosis of photoreceptor outer segments by the RPE. The metabolically active neural retina supports energy requirements with ATP produced from oxygen and nutrient-based substrates (fatty acids and glucose, pyruvate, and lactate) within photoreceptor inner segment mitochondria. As a means of supporting the metabolic needs of the cell, photoreceptor inner segments are densely packed with these with organelles.

Mitochondria are the major site of ROS generation and gains in energy processing efficiency are believed to lower production rates and volume of these compounds. ROS can damage bases in nucleic acids, amino acid side chains in proteins, and unsaturated bonds in fatty acids. Mitochondria are the main site for superoxide anion ($O_2^{-\bullet}$) generation; because it is highly reactive, superoxide is unlikely to exist far from mitochondria-dense cytosolic regions. The superoxide anion is produced via addition of an electron to molecular oxygen; it may react with nitric oxide (NO) to form peroxynitrate ($ONOO^-$). Superoxide may also be converted to hydrogen peroxide. Hydrogen peroxide has a long enough half-life to allow it to travel to the nuclear domain; hydrogen peroxide oxidizes –SH groups of resident proteins and reacts with divalent metal catalysts (released from injury of hemolysis), and via single electron transfer, yields highly reactive hydroxyl radicals. The hydroxyl radical is the most ROS in the body. The half-life of the hydroxyl radical is short ($\sim 10^{-8}$ s), but it has a relatively high oxidation potential. The hydroxyl radical can be formed in the nucleus and produce covalent cross-linking of nucleic acid bases. The hydroxyl radical reacts with esterified membrane lipids to yield lipid radicals. Lipid radicals combine with oxygen to yield highly reactive lipid peroxyl and –hydroperoxyl radicals. Lipid peroxyl and –hydroperoxyl radicals exist mainly in biological membranes rich in PUFA. Phospholipid bilayers of cell membranes, when concentrated with PUFAs, are rich sources of electrons used to reduce ROS. Balazy and Nigam [127] review the multiple aspects of lipid peroxidation. Free radicals extract hydrogen from unsaturated bonds of membrane lipids, yielding lipid peroxyl radicals and lipid peroxides. Adjacent fatty acids are subsequently oxidized in the attempt to reduce the peroxyl radical to a stable compound.

DHA may be important as a structural or signaling molecule (or precursor for a molecule) in mitochondrial function. DHA-supplemented primary photoreceptor cultures exhibit no change in proportion of cells maintaining mitochondrial membrane potential after exposure to oxidative stress from paraquat (a superoxide anion generator), while 50% of cells in unsupplemented cultures cannot sustain function [41]. A 20% higher proportion of cells with functional mitochondria are observed in the same model system when comparing DHA- and DHA-free cultures exposed to ambient air [42]. Brenna and Diau [155] report that brain DHA concentration increases directly as a function metabolic of rate in vervet monkeys and suggest that DHA may act as an essential structural element in bioenergetic processes.

A number of model systems have demonstrated increased efficiency of ATP production and energy use within mitochondrial membranes of cardiac tissue in animals with higher levels of phospholipid ω–3 LCPUFAs [156]. After ischemic challenge, recovery of cardiac mitochondrial function in rats fed a fish oil diet was better than that observed in a group consuming an ω–3 LCPUFA-free diet [157]. These results suggest that ω–3 LCPUFAs enhance processes of energy metabolism with minimal cost of energy substrate expenditure. It is currently unknown whether ω–3 LCPUFAs may influence efficiency of energy production within the retina.

Age-Related Developmental Processes and Chronic Environmental Exposures in AMD. Structure and metabolic efficiency of the retina changes across developmental periods. These events may be driven by systemic development processes or exposures and we offer information in this context. Pieri [158] notes the kinetics of aging are impacted by multiple causes and presents biochemical evidence to support the free radical theory of aging. This theory evolved from its original form (oxygen is a causal factor of aging) to the oxidative stress theory (age-related injury in cellular systems may result from an insufficient antioxidant potential and excessive oxidative stress that coexists with insufficient damage repair and detoxification activity). Yu and Yang [159] provide elements of the oxidative stress theory: (1) there is a diverse physiological origin of reactive species (oxygen, glucose, protein, DNA, NO, aldehyde); (2) there is value in assessing the balance of oxidants to antioxidant defense systems – defense processes and factors include cellular compartmentalization, DNA repair, antioxidant enzymes, antioxidant vitamins, other compounds with antioxidant properties, and (3) there are various types of reactions between ROS and other bioactive molecules – these include damage, damage repair, detoxification. Beatty et al. [6] suggest changes in oxidant load, elastin, collagen, and mitochondrial and nuclear DNA as putative pathogenic factors associated with age-related oxidative retinal damage. These authors observe that exogenous and endogenous retinal defense systems are compromised with advancing age.

Mitochondrial structure and function are affected with age [160]; these changes may lead to increased production of ROS. In addition to the potential effects of age-related cumulative oxygen load, there is a concomitant alteration in tissue status of aqueous and lipid-soluble vitamins with antioxidant properties [reviewed in 112]. Mitochondrial aging involves membrane composition and fluidity alterations that are purported to negatively affect biophysical response in bioenergetics. Study of this topic is germane to issues discussed throughout this work because the bulk of free radicals in retina are derived from mitochondrial respiration. Aging membranes become less fluid and fluidity is determined largely in part by membrane lipid concentration and composition (phospholipid species, fatty acid acyl chain length, number of double bonds, position of the first double bond from the methyl terminal, phospholipids-to-cholesterol ratio). Mitochondria produce ROS that target membrane lipids. The role of mitochondria in AMD is discussed in the section above and has been a central focus in our research.

The biochemical nature of DHA and AA and the selective tissue distribution of these compounds to metabolically active retinal tissue are paradoxical, as it would appear to facilitate formation of lipid radicals, lipid peroxyl radicals, and lipid peroxides. The importance of LCPUFAs in the retina is indicated by the efficient conservation and use of these 'easily oxidized' lipids in areas highly susceptible to oxidative stress and under conditions that facilitate production of ROS [47]. There is evidence to suggest that foveal regions exposed to highest intensity light have lower concentration of LCPUFAs [161]; in age-related (chronic) retinal disease the fovea is often spared until late stages of disease.

In vitro studies generally report reactive LCPUFA peroxidation in response to energy or oxygen exposure, implicating these compounds as 'suicide antioxidants.' In contrast, most in vivo studies have reported relationships in the direction of benefit. Muggli [162] reviews studies reporting relationships of ω–3 LCPUFA or fish intake with ROS-mediated events, effects on ROS biomarkers, and effects on antioxidant defense systems. Free radical-induced hemolysis [163] and in vitro LDL oxidation [164] were both reduced in samples from people on fish oil diets. Urinary F2-isoprostanes are in vivo markers of lipid peroxidation and oxidant stress. Non-smoking, treated-hypertensive, type 2 diabetic subjects consuming 4 g/day of purified EPA and DHA had lower levels of this biomarker than a matched comparison group consuming an olive oil supplement [165]. Fish oil exposure is also associated with reduction in superoxide anion generation in human samples [166, 167]. In some cases, in vivo oxidation of LDL was not altered as a function of LCPUFA intake [168–170]; in others it was decreased [171]. In elderly subjects, ω–3 LCPUFA intake at low doses (180 mg/day) was associated with decreases in oxidative stress within platelets [88]. At higher doses (50 μmol/l) DHA operated as a pro-oxidant [172].

An in vitro study on human cells reported an age- and area-related susceptibility to peroxidation, with higher posterior pole oxidation within tissue from the oldest subjects [173]. The oxidative damage of peripheral retina did not vary with age. Rotstein et al. [40] applied an in vitro model of oxidative stress on pure rat retina neurons to elucidate a mechanism by which DHA may operate as a neuroprotective factor. After primary retinal cells were exposed to an environmental oxidant that generates the superoxide anion, they were observed to die by apoptosis; loss of mitochondrial membrane integrity was seen as a key factor in this event. Addition of DHA to the cultures protected photoreceptors from oxidative stress-induced apoptosis. Authors speculate that DHA operates to preserve mitochondrial membrane structure and function by reducing Bax and increasing Bcl-2 expression. In rats, lower DHA tissue status is associated with lower susceptibility to light damage from acute exposure of 700–800 lx followed by 90 min of darkness [174]. After exposure to intense green light using intermittent or hyperthermic light treatments, rats fed a depleted ω–3 diet exhibited better structural outcomes than rats fed a linolenic acid-enriched diet from flaxseed [175]. A series of intriguing studies on the role of CYP450 EPA-derived epoxides in regulation of vascular systems is now emerging to suggest that oxygenated ω–3 LCPUFAs may have positive physiologic significance [176].

Cellular Differentiation and Survival. DHA acts as a trophic molecule in photoreceptor development, differentiation, and growth. It works in part by increasing opsin expression and apical process differentiation [37, 38, 177]. The proportion DHA-fed cells expressing opsin was significantly higher than in those from a DHA-free culture. Opsin combines with 11-*cis*-retinal to form rhodopsin; the relevance of this issue for retinal health is that expression of the opsin gene may be required for assembly of photoreceptor disc membranes [178]. Although DHA may not act in determination of photoreceptor fate, it was shown to enhance differentiation in cone-rod homeobox (Crx)-expressing cells [43]. Crx in photoreceptor progenitors is necessary for expression of transcripts associated with photoreceptor maturation.

DHA or its metabolities prolong retinal cell survival and prevent apoptosis in model systems of photoreceptors [37–40, 177] and RPE cells [7, 9, 10, 14, 46]. The proportion photoreceptors supplemented with DHA that survived for 11 days in vitro was approximately twice that observed from cultures existing on DHA-free media. Measures of apoptosis (fragmented photoreceptor nuclei) suggested a protective effect of DHA at post-plating days 7 and 11. In primary cultures of rat neural retina cells, DHA acted as a protective agent against oxidant- and ceramide-induced cell death by upregulating expression of the anti-apoptotic factor, Bcl-2 [179]. Ceramide is a lipid-based mediator of apoptosis; DHA acts via ceramide glycosylation to limit endogenous levels of this molecule [179]. In photoreceptor cultures DHA was also shown to act on the ERK/MAPK pathway to prevent apoptosis [42]. DHA-derived neuroprotectin 1 acts as a potent cytokine- and oxidant-induced factor preventing apoptosis in RPE cell cultures [8]. In these systems NPD1 decreased proapoptotic proteins Bax and Bad, upregulated the anti-apoptotic Bcl-2 and Bcl-x(L) expression, inhibited oxidative-stress-induced caspase-3 activation [7, 14]. Detailed coverage on the role of NPD1 in the retina and its relationship with neurotrophins exists elsewhere in this issue of *WRND*.

Inflammation and Lipid-Based Molecules. Calder et al. [61, 180, 181] provide a number of excellent reviews on the modulatory role of ω–3 LCPUFAs in immune and inflammatory processes. We have reviewed the putative relationship of LCPUFAs with retinal inflammation in detail elsewhere [13]. Inflammation, the immediate biologic response to injury or infection, is the result of increased capillary permeability and blood flow. Increased capillary permeability enables regulatory proteins (antibodies, complement, and cytokines) and leukocytes (monocytes, macrophages, natural killer (NK) lymphocytes, and granulocytes) to pass from the bloodstream across the vascular endothelial wall. Integration of this innate immune response with an acquired one subsequently occurs as activated macrophages and monocytes present antigen to cytotoxic (CD8+) and helper (CD4+) T lymphocytes.

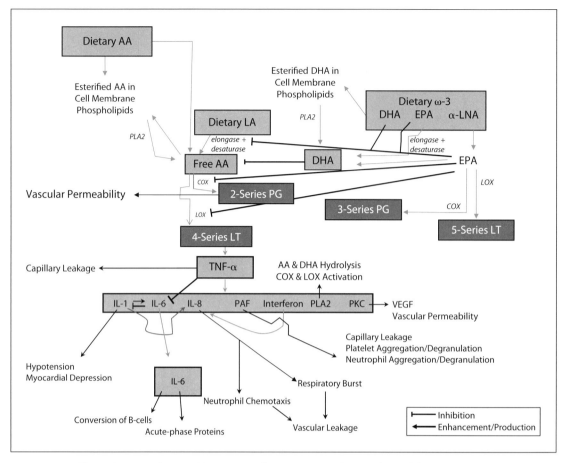

Fig. 2. Impact of ω–3 LCPUFAs on inflammatory mediators derived from arachidonic acid. AA = Arachidonic acid (20:4ω–6); COX = cyclooxygenase; DHA = docosahexaenoic acid (22:6ω–3); EPA = eicosapentaenoic acid (20:5ω–3); HETE = hydroxyeicosatetraenoic acid; HPETE = hydroperoxyeicosatetraenoic acid; IFN = interferon; Ig = immunoglobulin; IL = interleukin; LOX = lipoxygenase; LT = leukotriene; PAF = platelet-activating factor; PKC = protein kinase C; PLA$_2$ = phospholipase A$_2$; PG = prostaglandin; TX = thromboxane.

Helper T lymphocytes express CD4+ receptors that recognize peptide fragments on cell surfaces that are bound in the class II major histocompatibility complex (MHCII). These peptides are derived from extracellular pathogens that have been phagocytosed by macrophages or endocytosed by antigen-presenting cells (macrophages, dendritic cells, B lymphocytes). Inflammation activates PLA$_2$, COX, and LOX. An emerging evidence base suggests that inflammatory processes [121] as well as genes affecting and affected by such processes [5] are implicated processes and factors in AMD pathogenesis, and ROP. ω–3 LCPUFAs act as the precursors to a number of bioactive lipid-based immuno- and inflammatory eicosanoids, resolvins, and neuroprotectins [7–10, 14, 182]. Metabolic pathways of eicosanoid biosynthesis are presented in figure 1.

ω–3 LCPUFAs modulate production of AA-derived eicosanoids and this is important for a number of reasons. First, LTB_4 is associated with TNF-α production [183]. TNF-α mediates production of a number of potent pro-inflammatory and immunoregulatory cytokines [180]. Also, ω–3 LCPUFA-derived eicosanoids may operate directly on factors in the immune system or via a number soluble mediators, the inflammatory phospholipids platelet-activating factor (PAF), NO, and tyrosine and serine/threonine kinases. While AA-derived eicosanoids play different roles in the inflammatory process, they are all associated with vascular leakage. PGE_2 decreases T-cell proliferation, lymphocyte migration, and secretion of IL-1 and IL-2. PGI_2 blocks leukocyte aggregation, T-cell proliferation, and lymphocyte migration and secretion of IL-1 and IL-2. TXA_2 increases lymphocyte proliferation. LTB_4 increases leukocyte chemotaxis and aggregation, T-cell proliferation, and the release of TNF-α, IFN-γ, IL-1, and IL-2. Figure 2 presents one scenario on the putative effect of ω–3 LCPUFAs and their metabolites on AA metabolites (and associated compounds) implicated in inflammatory processes.

AA-based COX and LOX metabolites are extremely potent at low concentrations and act as autocoids through G-protein-mediated signaling pathways to increase cAMP levels at the site of biosynthesis. PGE_2, PGI_2, TXA_2, and LTB_4 are the most potent AA-derived angiogenic eicosanoids. PGE_2 increases vasodilation and enhances vasodilatory effects of bradykinin and histamine. PGI_2 induces vasodilation and cAMP production and inhibits leukocyte and platelet aggregation – thus the tissue system in which this molecule acts is an important consideration when speculating about its role in health and disease. TXA_2 induces platelet aggregation and vasoconstriction and LTB_4 induces vascular permeability. As capillary integrity is broached, vascular leakage and recruitment of immune system cells occurs.

The immune system cells are capable of producing pathogenic inflammatory mediators and angiogenic growth factors. The existing instability of the capillary basement membrane then permits out-migration of activated vascular endothelial cells seen in abnormal angiogenesis. AA metabolites of the COX pathway induce vascular endothelial cell migration and tube formation [184]. The AA-derived LOX product 12-HETE promotes tumor angiogenesis through induction of mitogenic activity and migration in microvascular endothelial cells [185, 186]. 12-HETE also induces cell surface integrin $α_vβ_3$ expression [187, 188] in cell cultures from rodent models [187, 188]. AA-derived leukotrienes affect the production of TNF-α [189], a potent cytokine activating numerous cascades that modulate systemic inflammation and apoptosis. ω–3 LCPUFAs alter both substrate and enzymes involved in the production of immuno- and vasoregulatory eicosanoids.

Calder [61, 180] proposes mechanisms by which ω–3 LCPUFAs may reduce the effect of AA-derived angiogenic eicosanoids – these are: (1) ω–6-based eicosanoid precursor (AA) displacement. This action alters AA availability for catalysis in membrane phospholipids. (2) PLA_2 inhibition. PLA_2 is the enzyme necessary to release the precursor for metabolism. (3) Biosynthetic eicosanoid synthase and peroxidase quenching. These enzymes are used for series-2 prostanoid and series-4 leukotriene production. (4) Decreased 3-series (PG and TX) and the 5-series (LT) eicosanoid production. ω–3 LCPUFAs act as the precursors to these molecules. 3- and 5-series eicosanoids are in most cases less potent than AA-based eicosanoids of the 2- and 4-series. In many cases the ω–3 LCPUFA metabolites have been linked to protective actions in model cell systems.

AA-derived LTB_4 affects the production of TNF-α [189]. TNF-α is detectable in retinal vascular tissue and extracellular matrix of fibrovascular tissue in people with vasoproliferative diabetic retinopathy (PDR) [190]. A TNF-α gene polymorphism in the MCH of people with non-insulin-dependent diabetes mellitus (NIDDM) is associated with PDR and vitreous levels of soluble TNF-α receptors were higher in eyes with PDR than in eyes of healthy people without diabetes [191]; these results were interpreted to represent a form of genetic susceptibility [192]. People with insulin-dependent diabetes mellitus (IDDM) and PDR have higher concentrations of soluble TNF-α receptors than both (1) people with IDDM who are PDR-free, and (2) healthy controls [193]. TNF-α production and expression are also modified in a rodent model ischemia-induced retinopathy affecting retinal vasculature [194] – while ischemia may play less of a part in AMD pathogenesis than in that of PDR, it is reasonable to suspect that the shared neovascular component may be modulated by similar factors and processes.

A large body of evidence implicates ω–3 LCPUFAs in alteration of the innate and acquired immune systems and the inflammatory response within neural and vasucular tissue. Model studies on human cell lines incubated with ω–3 LCPUFAs demonstrated decreased: (1) monocyte cell surface antigen presentation [195] and TNF-α and IL-1β expression [196]; (2) neutrophil superoxide presentation [167]; (3) NK lymphocyte activation [197, 198], and (4) lymphocyte proliferation [197, 199–204], antigen expression [205], and IL-2 production [197, 199]. De Caterina et al. [206] have added DHA to adult saphenous vein endothelial cell cultures activated by cytokines to observe reduced expression of IL-6 and IL-8.

Animal feeding studies demonstrate differences in immune system function in comparison of animals receiving ω–3 LCPUFA-rich diets to those consuming ω–3 LCPUFA-free diets; in these studies animals on ω–3 LCPUFA-rich diets show decreased: (a) macrophage-based ROS production [207–210], cell surface antigen presentation [211, 212], TNF-α expression [183, 213–215], IL-1β expression [183, 213–215], IL-6 expression [183, 213–215], and IFN-γ receptor expression [216]; (b) monocyte IL-1β and TNF-α expression [217]; (c) NK cell activation [218–221]; (d) cytotoxic T-lymphocyte activation [222], and (e) lymphocyte proliferation [218, 222–232] and production of IL-2 and IFN-γ [233].

Human feeding studies demonstrate similar results at high doses of ω–3 LCPUFAs. Human studies also emphasize the importance of considering the balance of ω–3/ω–6 LCPUFAs. Three [234–236] of four studies demonstrate reduced monocyte chemotaxis in populations consuming ω–3 LCPUFA-rich diets. Subjects in the study that did not demonstrate a difference between dietary groups [237] consumed a relatively lower amount of ω–3 LCPUFAs. Monocyte surface antigen expression, NK lymphocyte activation [238] and lymphocyte proliferation [239, 240] decreased in people consuming high levels of ω–3 LCPUFAs. The relationship between intake of ω–3 LCPUFAs and production of pro-inflammatory cytokines is not clear from studies in human populations. Approximately half [236, 239, 241, 242] of the existing studies [237, 240, 243–245] show an inhibitory effect of ω–3 LCPUFA feeding on TNF-α expression. Four [202, 236, 239, 241, 242] feeding studies demonstrated an inhibitory effect on IL-1β expression while others did not [237, 240, 243–246]. An inhibitory effect on IL-6 expression was reported from two [239, 247] of four [237, 244] studies. All feeding studies examining the effect of ω–3 LCPUFAs on IL-2 production and IFN-γ production demonstrated an inhibitory effect in people consuming ω–3 LCPUFAs [239, 242].

In addition to their effects on AA-eicosanoid metabolism, ω–3 LCPUFAs may influence vascular function and inflammatory response via modulation of intracellular signaling pathways and transcription factor activation [102, 103]. DHA and EPA act as natural ligands to a number of nuclear hormone receptors that affect transcriptional activities. Among these are PPAR [105] and RXR [104]. The activated PPAR-γ/RXR heterodimer regulates genes modulating induction of inflammatory signaling pathways (NF-κB, MAP kinase pathways, IL-2 secretion). DHA binds to specific DNA motifs on *cis*-regulatory elements in promoter regions of target genes. DHA binding impacts activation of the PPAR and RXR receptors that subsequently operate as transcription factors [248]. α, β, and γ isoforms of PPAR receptors are affected by DHA [248–250]. DHA can act directly in transcription, as it is concentrated in PS, a negatively charged aminophospholipid known to activate protein kinases involved in gene expression [54]. DHA may also operate at the posttranscriptional level to induce changes of phosphorylation events in native mRNA processing, mRNA transport and stabilization, and mRNA degradation rates [178]. These pathways modulate production of inflammatory mediators. The activated PPAR-γ/RXR complex also leads to cell proliferation, production of adhesion molecules (VCAM-1, ICAM-1, E- and P-selectins) and modulation of endothelial-leukocyte adhesion pathways in vascular tissue [251]. Jump [252] and De Caterina and Madonna [57] provide review of the role and actions of dietary PUFAs in regulation of gene transcription.

Increased levels of inflammatory mediators are associated with AMD [121]. How may proliferative retinopathies be affected by inflammation? A number of retinal diseases characterized partially by an inflammatory component involve leukocyte migration and adhesion within the retinal vasculature; this is preceded by induction of inflammatory (TNF-α, VCAM-1) and redox-sensitive genes (NF-κB). TNF-α plays a dominant role in modulating endothelial adhesion molecules. Ischemia- and inflammation-induced activation of COX-2 regulates the production of VEGF. Both VEGF and TNF-α upregulate ICAM-1 via NF-κB and serine/threonine kinase Akt-PI3 kinase-eNOS signaling pathways [253]. PKC may be an important factor in

Table 3. Vasoregulatory or vasotrophic factors affected by LCPUFAs, eicosanoids, COX, or LOX

Molecule		Reference
Angiogenin	Angiogenin $\rightarrow$ PLA$_2$	262
Angiopoietin (Ang)-2	DHA $\downarrow$ Ang-2	263
Angiotensin II	EPA and DHA $\uparrow$ response to Ang II in diabetes	264
Fibroblast growth factors: acidic/basic	EPA $\uparrow$ cell migration in response to bFGF	265 (no effect), 266
Follistatin	PGE$_2$ $\uparrow$ follistatin-related gene (FLRG) mRNA	267
Granulocyte colony-stimulating factor (G-CSF)	COX-2 inhibitor $\downarrow$ G-CSF mRNA	268
Interleukin-8 (IL-8)	DHA $\downarrow$ endothelial IL-8 expression	206
Leptin	EPA and DHA $\downarrow$ leptin secretion	269, 270
Platelet-derived growth factor-BB	EPA $\dashv$ PDGF-induced mitogenesis	271–273
Transforming growth factor-β	EPA $\uparrow$ TGF-β secretion	272, 274
Tumor necrosis factor-α	EPA and DHA $\downarrow$ TNF-α mRNA	275–278
Vascular endothelial growth factor	EPA $\downarrow$ VEGF and $\dashv$ VEGF receptor expression	265, 279–284

$\rightarrow$ = Activates; $\uparrow$ increases; $\dashv$ = suppresses; $\downarrow$ decreases.

retinal vascular pathology; PKC activates PLA$_2$ [254]. Recall that PLA$_2$ is responsible for releasing esterified AA as a substrate for COX- and LOX-based eicosanoid production. These processes are associated with blood-retinal barrier degradation and manifested in increased vascular permeability. Extant data from model systems suggests relationships between angiogenesis and enzymes synthesizing eicosanoids from LCPUFAs. Nude mice with human breast cancer xenografts and fed ω–3 LCPUFA-rich diets showed displacement of AA from tumor cell membranes, a reduction in PGE$_2$ and 12-HETE [255, 256], loss of COX-2 mRNA expression [257], and reduction in COX-2- and COX-1-immunoreactive protein [258]. Both EPA and DHA inhibit COX-2 and COX-1 induction of PG biosynthesis [138]. There may be a link between this pathway, growth factor expression, and angiogenesis as the selective COX-2 inhibitor celecoxib (SC-58635) is capable of regulating production of VEGF and VEGF receptors in animal models of retinal neovascularization [259, 260]. This agent is also effective in suppressing FGF-2-induced corneal angiogenesis in rats [261].

Inflammation, Vascular Pathology, and Proteins Impacting and Impacted by Lipid-Based Molecules. A number of immunoregulatory cytokines, angiogenic growth factors, and their signaling pathways are affected by and affect LCPUFAs, eicosanoids, and PLA_2, COX, and LOX activities (table 3). We review VEGF, TGF-β, TNF-α, angiogenin, angiopoietin-1, FGF, follistatin, G-CSF, IL-8, leptin, and PDGF-BB. Cytokines are regulatory proteins that function as chemical messengers between natural and acquired immune systems and within the acquired immune system. Cytokines are also ligands for cell surface receptors that induce cellular growth, development, and activity related to vascular remodeling. They can potently induce capillary leakage and leukocyte migration. The LOX-5-catalyzed AA-metabolite (LTB_4) directly increases the production of the pro-inflammatory cytokine TNF-α [189]. Through its effect on this factor, LTB_4 indirectly enhances production other pro-inflammatory cytokines (IL-1, IL-2, IL-8, IL-6, IFN-γ) and the inflammatory lysophospholipid PAF. Figure 2 illustrates these relationships.

Angiogenic growth factors operate directly or indirectly on endothelial cells. Direct activity occurs via endothelial cell-surface receptors and induces endothelial cell migration and proliferation. Macrophage- and mast cell-derived polypeptide growth factors such as vascular endothelial growth factor (VEGF) and basic fibroblast growth factor (bFGF) operate as such. Indirect mechanisms act via chemotactic induction in macrophages that subsequently secrete VEGF and bFGF. This is the case of the eicosanoids reviewed above.

VEGF is a 45-kDa glycoprotein produced in the neural retina by astrocytes. It has specificity to several tyrosine kinase receptors (Flk-1, Flt-1) and has been identified as a central factor involved in retinal vasoproliferation [285]. VEGF is a key molecule in induction of: endothelial cell migration and proliferation, microvascular permeability, endothelial cell release of metalloproteinases and interstitial collagenases, and endothelial cell tube formation [286]. VEGF stimulates capillary meshwork formation in vivo [283] and has thus been implicated as a proangiogenic factor in ischemia-induced proliferative retinopathies [287–289]. Insulin-like growth factor (IGF-1) modulates VEGF-induced activation of MAPK. MAPK is involved in endothelial cell proliferation. Low levels of IGF-1 inhibit VEGF-induced activation of protein kinase B (Akt). The Akt/PI-3 kinase system modulates processes controlling vascular endothelial cell activation and survival, as well as leukocyte migration and adhesion.

In some cases, LCPUFAs affect activation and expression of VEGF-specific tyrosine kinase receptors. EPA affected VEGF-induced proliferation of bovine carotid artery endothelial (BAE) cells by inhibition of the fetal liver tyrosine kinase 1 (Flk-1) receptor, a factor essential for endothelial cell differentiation and proliferation. Neither DHA nor AA affected this system. The *fms*-like tyrosine kinase receptor (Flt-1), a factor involved in vessel construction [283], was not affected by EPA, DHA, or AA. bFGF-induced endothelial cell proliferation was not inhibited by EPA, DHA, or AA. However, EPA inhibited VEGF-induced activation of

MAPK. EPA downregulated Flk-1 receptor expression in a dose-dependent manner and upregulated Flt-1 receptor expression [283]. It also inhibited endothelial cell tube formation in vitro [290]. EPA-treated endothelial cells had low MAPK activity relative to cells that were not incubated with EPA. The mechanism of VEGF receptor downregulation may occur at the tyrosine kinase NF-κB site as EPA treatment caused suppression of NF-κB activation. NF-κB is a nuclear transcription factor that upregulates COX-2 expression, NO synthase, and intracellular adhesion molecule (ICAM) [291].

ω–3 LCPUFAs may also influence activation of IGF-1 pathways necessary to mediate effects of VEGF. In a study on burn patients (burns reduce IGF-1 levels) applying a nutritional intervention with a 15% fat diet with fish oil (50% of total dietary lipids from fish oil vs. 15 and 30% fat without fish oil), subjects returned to normal serum IGF-1 concentrations by 30 days post-intervention. Subjects in the no fish oil groups were consistently lower on IGF-1 and did not approach normal values within the first month of the study [292]. IGF-1 and VEGF interact in retinal neovascularization via the Akt/PI-3 kinase signaling pathway, a serine/threonine kinase activated system. DHA-enriched Neuro 2A cells survived a staurosporine-induced apoptotic signal through inhibition of normally observed decreases in Akt phosphorylation and activity [293]. Akt activity is essential for vascular endothelial cell survival [294].

Role of LCPUFAs in Structure and Function of Vascular Retina
The evidence base reviewed until this point suggests that ω–3 LCPUFAs have the capacity to modulate production and activities of a number of factors and processes implicated in retinal neovascularization, inflammation of retinal vasculature, and alterations in retinal capillary ultrastructure. Vascular pathology in AMD is localized predominantly within the choriocapillaris. Increased microvascular density is usually accompanied by alterations in the integrity of the capillary walls. Choroidal permeability may lead to abnormal vascular remodeling, capillary leakage, inflammation, and thrombosis. These processes are manifested in vitreous hemorrhage, fibrovascular scarring, mechanical stress, and subsequent retinal detachment. Table 4 contains an overview of potential points in a neovascular cascade at which ω–3 LCPUFAs may exert a meaningful impact. Table 5 contains similar information in the context of a number of etiologic factors for AMD.

The following section contains an application of knowledge base discussed above within the framework of a genome-wide association study on functionally relevant gene sets and pathways. We started with a general approach to inquiry on the role of lipid-associated compounds in AMD for the purpose of conducting an unbiased descriptive analysis that was optimized for discovery of novel relationships. Evidence converged to allow inference on a number of biologically credible explanations of our findings. It is our hope that this work will be extended in replicate samples.

Relationships of Advanced AMD with Lipid-Associated Gene Variants in the Age-Related Eye Disease Study

The Age-Related Eye Disease Study (AREDS) was a US-based, multi-center, 12-year prospective project examining the clinical course of AMD and age-related cataract. Analyses of AREDS data on dietary ω–3 LCPUFA-AMD relationships yielded inverse (protective) associations of reported intake with prevalent neovascular AMD [12] and progression to geographic atrophy [26] (a neurodegenerative form of the disease). AREDS genetic samples were used in one of the first successful applications of microarray technology to identify susceptibility variants in a complex disease [318].

The single marker elucidated in our original genome-wide association study has led to a set of important findings on inflammatory and immunoregulatory processes in AMD pathogenesis. The polygenic nature of AMD and the variable expressivity in the disease also warrants study on joint action of functionally-related genes encoding elements of metabolic or signaling pathways. In the context of our ω–3 LCPUFA-AMD relationships, we felt that it would be informative to examine the putative impact of sequence variants in genes encoding structures affecting and affected by lipid-based molecules as they relate to AMD. We used data from 508 AREDS participants examined in a genome-wide association study with a 100K microarray. Joint action models predicted a 99-fold increased susceptibility of advanced AMD from 11 variants of 11 inositol-related genes (odds ratio = 99.2, $p \leq 1.0 \times 10^{-17}$). Comparison of these findings against p value distributions from 1,500 analyses on randomly selected sets of single nucleotide polymorphisms (SNPs) (obtained from our complete panel of 96,774) indicated that these results were not likely due to random sampling error; in no instance did any of the 1,500 test models yield a p value $<1.2 \times 10^{-9}$. These novel results may provide meaningful insight into the role of molecular genetics in modifying nutrient-AMD relationships.

Methods

Study Population
All data in this work are from elderly self-identified white, non-Hispanic US residents participating in the AREDS. Details on the design and sample demographics of the study exist in extant publications [319]. Our final experimental population contained 368 people with advanced AMD and 141 people who had no clinical signs of AMD across the entire course of the study.

Outcomes
Masked professional graders at the University of Wisconsin Fundus Photography Reading Center ascertained phenotype annually across a 12-year period from stereoscopic color fundus images using a standardized and validated protocol. All photographs were taken with a standardized method by certified photographers. AREDS

Table 4. Potential influence of ω–3 LCPUFAs at key points in the neovascular progression

Step in neovascular cascade	Putative action of ω–3 LCPUFAs
Growth factors bind on endothelial cells	VEGF Flk-1 expression inhibited in EPA-treated bovine carotid artery endothelial (BAE) cells. Flk-1 expression increased [283]
Activated endothelial cells send signals to the nucleus for production of signaling molecules and enzymes	EPA selectively inhibits VEGF-induced, but not bFGF-induced activation of MAPK [283]. Members of the ERK-MAPK family respond to proliferative and mitogenic stimuli, regulate changes in transcription, and are associated with cellular differentiation and proliferation. c-Jun amino-terminal kinase (JNK) and p38 MAPK pathways may be activated by exposures associated with retinal disease; these include hypoxia, ultraviolet light, inflammatory cytokines, osmotic shock, or environmental stress [295]. MAPKs are important mediators in endothelial barrier function [296]
Enzymatic BM digestion	Incubation of human vascular ECs with EPA protects against gap junctional intercellular communication injury after hypoxia/reperfusion challenge. Effect mediated by inhibition of tyrosine kinase activation [297]. EPA inhibits urokinase-type plasminogen (uPA) activator activity [298]. uPA catalyzes conversion of plasminogen to plasmin. Plasmin is a serine proteinase involved in conversion of fibrin to soluble forms. uPA implicated in retinal neovascularization and may affect cell associated proteolytic activity [299]
EC division and migration through BM	ω–3 LCPUFAs prevent serotonin-induced EC proliferation [300]. Bovine aortic endothelial cells, treated with 0–5 µg/ml EPA for 48 h, displayed dose-dependent suppression to VEGF-induced proliferation [283]. EPA inhibited cell growth in a dose-dependent manner in bovine carotid ECs cultured between collagen gels [290]. Prostacyclin (PGI$_2$) is the main prostanoid in most vascular systems. PGI$_2$ regulates vascular EC proliferation. DHA and EPA incubation led to changes in fatty acid composition of membrane phospholipids of human umbilical vein endothelial cells (HUVEC) co-incubated with allogeneic peripheral blood lymphocytes and resulted in reduced basal PGI$_2$ production [302]
Adhesion molecules or integrins (α$_v$β$_3$, α$_v$β$_5$) pull blood vessel sprouts forward.	Incubation of human adult saphenous vein endothelial cell cultures with DHA reduced endothelial expression of VCAM-1, E-selectin, ICAM-1, IL-6 and IL-8 after challenge with IL-1, IL-4, TNF-α, or bacterial endotoxin [206]. Primary HUVECs activated with IL-1β produce ICAM-1, E-selectin and VCAM-1 transcripts. Both EPA and DHA attenuate induction of these adhesion molecules after challenge with IL-1β [303]
Matrix metalloproteinases (MMP) dissolve tissue in front of the sprouting vessel tip. As the vessel extends, the tissue is remolded around it	MMPs are a family of neutral zinc endopeptidases secreted as pro-enzymes in extracellular areas. MMPs modulate aspects of angiogenesis, inflammation, and affect tissue remodeling through: degradation of specific extracellular matrix components; destruction of proteinase inhibitors, cell surface proteins, cytokines; and activation or release of signaling molecules and proteinases. Expression of MMPs is induced by cytokines, growth factors, and reactive oxygen species. Endogenous

Table 4. Continued

Step in neovascular cascade	Putative action of ω−3 LCPUFAs
	tissue inhibitors of metalloproteinases (TIMPs) bind non-covalently to zinc-dependent active site of MMPs to regulate their activity. MMP-2 (Gelatinase A) and MMP-9 (Gelatinase B) operate against type IV collagens and laminins in vascular endothelial basement membranes. MMP-2 binds on vascular EC surfaces to $\alpha_v\beta_3$ integrin during capillary tube formation. MMP-9 is constitutively produced in the retinal ganglion cell layer. These MMPs exist in the interphotoreceptor matrix and are implicated in pathogenesis of retinopathy of prematurity and proliferative diabetic retinopathy [304]
	MMP-2 and MMP-9 expression was elevated in C557Bl/J6 mice with ischemia-induced retinal neovascularization, relative to animals reared under normal conditions [305]. TIMP-1 (MMP-9 inhibitor) and TIMP-2 (MMP-2 inhibitor) were decreased within the same animals, indicating that these extracellular proteinases are important in retinal angiogenesis. The mechanism by which MMPs are expressed occurs via soluble mediators TNF-α and VEGF (not via the hypoxic insult introduced in the ischemic challenge) [306]. Serum MMP-2 and -9 activity decreased in female CD-VAF rats fed DHA-containing diets with various compositions of EFAs and LCPUFAs, relative to a comparison group fed DHA-free diets [307]. CDF_1 and BALB/c mice receiving diets enriched in DHA had lower MMP-9 activity in tumor tissue extract than animals fed an LCPUFA-free diet. MMP-9 activities were also significantly lower in animals consuming DHA + oleic acid and DHA + LA, relative to controls fed a DHA-free diet. Gelatinolytic (MMP-2 and -9) activities were not different between controls and animals consuming oleic acid, LA, EPA, and EPA + DHA enriched diets [308]. EPA treatment in nude mice prevented development of lung metastases from MDA-MB-435 human breast cancer cell mammary fat pad solid tumors. Incubation with yielded in a dose-related inhibition of cultured MDA-MB-435 cell 92-kDa type IV collagenase (MMP-9) mRNA expression [309]
ECs sprout from tubes	Bovine carotid artery ECs treated for 2 days with EPA showed dose-dependent inhibition of tube formation. AA increased tube formation, and docosahexaenoic acid had no effect [290]. DPA (22:5ω−3) suppressed tube-forming activity in endothelial cells induced by vascular endothelial growth factor [279]. ECs cultured in collagen gel and treated with EPA displayed a dose-dependent suppression of tube formation, VEGF-induced proliferation, and activation of p42/p44 MAP kinase [265]

BM = Basement membrane, EC = endothelial cell, PDR = proliferative diabetic retinopathy, ROP = retinopathy of prematurity.

Table 5. Etiologic factors for AMD and putative actions of ω–3 LCPUFAs

Factor/process	Putative pathogenic mode of action	Putative action of ω–3 LCPUFAs
Neovascularization		
VEGF	VEGF → vascular endothelial cell proliferation VEGF → vascular endothelial cell migration VEGF → vascular endothelial cell survival VEGF → vascular endothelial cell permeability VEGF → uPA + tPA → ECM degradation VEGF → MMP → ECM degradation VEGF ↔ NO → vascular hyperpermeability VEGF → ICAM-1	EPA ⊣ VEGF KDR [265] ω–3 LCPUFA ⊣ VEGF KDR [279] EPA ⊣ VEGF Flk-1 [283] EPA ⊣ urokinase activity [298] DHA ⊣ MMP-2 [307] DHA ⊣ ICAM-1 [206] DHA ⊣ VCAM [206]
Angiopoietins	Ang1 → pericyte recruitment → vascular integrity Ang2 ⊣ Ang1 Ang2 + VEGF → neovascularization	DHA ⊣ Ang-2 [310]
Nitric oxide	NO → integrin $α_vβ_3$ → endothelial cell migration NO → integrin $α_vβ_3$ → endothelial cell different VEGF ↔ NO → vascular hyperpermeability VEGF → eNOS → NO → VEGF eNOS → vaso-obliteration eNOS → vitreous neovascularization iNOS ⊣ VEGF receptor expression	DHA → iNOS [311,312]
Extracellular matrix	Integrins + ECM proteins → endothelial migration TNF-α → $α_vβ_3$ → endothelial cell migration MMP → ECM degradation TIMP-3 ⊣ VEGF-ind. endothelial cell migration	DHA ⊣ TNF-α [196] DHA ⊣ MMP-2 [307] ω–3 LCPUFA → TIMP [313]
Oxidative stress		
Reactive O_2 intermediates	Membrane lipid peroxidation Mitochondrial DNA damage H_2O_2 → p53/p21 → apoptosis H_2O_2 ⊣ Bcl-2 ⊣ apoptosis tBHP → caspase → mito. damage → apoptosis H_2O_2 → VEGF in RPE → apoptosis	Fish oil → mitochondrial function [157] Fish oil → ATP metabolism [314] DHA → Bcl-2 [40] DHA ⊣ caspase-3 [315] DHA → Akt/PI3 pathway [293]
Hypoxia	Hypoxia → VEGF in RPE Hypoxia → Ang2	See VEGF and Ang sections of table
Lipofuscin/A2E	Short wavelength light-induced RPE apoptosis A2E ⊣ photoreceptor lysosomal degradation Physical disruption of RPE cytoarchitecture	DHA → IRBP [152]

Table 5. Continued

Factor/process	Putative pathogenic mode of action	Putative action of ω–3 LCPUFAs
AGE/RAGE	AGE → RPE aging genes AGE → VEGF in RPE	ω–3 LCPUFA ⊣ AGE [316]
Hemo-hydrodynamic Δ		
Bruch's membrane	Thickening ⊣ diffusion ⊣ choroidal perfusion	DHA → IRBP [152] DHA ⊣collagen aggregation [147]
Choriocapillaris	↓ diameter ⊣ choroidal perfusion → transport ↓ density ⊣choroidal perfusion → RPE transport	DHA → vascular compliance [143]
Neutral fat deposits	Modification of diffusion characteristics of BM	DHA → IRBP [152]
RPE senescence		
Age	AGE ⊣ gene expression lysosomal enzymes AGE shortened chromosomal telomeres	ω–3 LCPUFA ⊣ AGE [316]
β-Galactosidase	↓ proteolytic activity → RPE deposits	ω–3 LCPUFA → galactosidase [317]

The conceptual structure of this table was partially adapted from Ambati et al. [3]. AGE = Advanced glycation end products; Ang = angiopoietin; bFGF = basic fibroblast growth factor; BM = Bruch's membrane; eNOS = endothelial nitric oxide synthase; ECM = extracellular matrix; H_2O_2 = hydrogen peroxide; iNOS = inducible nitric oxide synthase; ICAM = intracellular adhesion molecule; IRBP = interphotoreceptor-binding protein; KDR = VEGF receptor-2, kinase insert domain-containing receptor; MMP = matrix metalloproteinase; mitochond. fct = mitochondrial function; NO = nitric oxide; PEDF = pigment epithelium derived factor; ROI = reactive O_2 intermediates; RAGE = receptor for advanced glycation end products; RPE = retinal pigment epithelium; SWL = near-UV light; TIMP = tissue inhibitor of matrix metalloproteinase; tPA = tissue-type plasminogen activator; uPA = urokinase-type plasminogen activator; VEGF = vascular endothelial growth factor; Δ = change; ↓ = reduction; ⊣ = decreased expression, inhibition or deactivation; → = factor or process leads to outcome.

Report 1 [319] contains details on the process of outcome ascertainment. Advanced AMD cases meet the following criteria: (1) presence in either eye of geographic atrophy or neovascular AMD defined as photocoagulation or other treatment for choroidal neovascularization (based on clinical center reports), or (2) photographic documentation of any of the following: non-drusenoid retinal pigment epithelial detachment, serous or hemorrhagic retinal detachment, hemorrhage under the retina or RPE, and/or subretinal fibrosis either at baseline or during the course of the study.

Our AMD-free group had good vision in both eyes and no existing eye disease. Controls were selected to be the oldest AREDS participants with DNA available who had a drusen area of <5 small drusen (<63 μm diameter) and no pigmentary abnormalities in both eyes at all visits for which fundus photographs were gradable. Both eyes had visual acuity of 20/32 or better measured by a standard protocol, ocular media was clear enough for good quality fundus photographs, and there was absence of any ocular disorder that might obscure assessment of either AMD or lens opacities. The AMD-free group has three distinguishing characteristics that make it a robust and appropriate comparison group: (1) phenotype was determined annually over a 12-year period with a standardized protocol by multiple professional graders who were masked to phenotypic information from previous years – adjudication with a standardized protocol occurred when discrepancies emerged; (2) criteria for AMD-free classification (≤5 drusen of ≤63 μm in both eyes for the entire 12-year period) is stringent relative to those applied in previous association studies for AMD; (3) the age of the AREDS AMD-free group is in the range that AMD prevalence increases ~3 times (from ~4% in those aged 74–79 years to ~12% in those aged ≥80 years) in population-based studies.

The mean age (±SE) of controls in was 76.9 ± 0.38 years; the value for the advanced AMD group was 79.7 ± 0.26 years. Half of those in the AMD-free group were women, while the corresponding value for the advanced AMD group was 58%. 5% of people in the AMD-free group were current smokers; the value for the advanced AMD group was 11%.

Bioinformatics and Statistical Modeling

Our bioinformatic and statistical approach is described in figure 3. In phase 1 we employed an empirical process to identify candidate gene sets and pathways associated with advanced AMD (steps 1–6). The first issue was to apply a valid definition of the lipid-associated genes from which we would interrogate relevant variants (step 1). The Lipid Metabolites and Pathways (LIPIDMAPS) Research Group maintains a proteomic database of 2,919 human transcripts related to lipid-associated enzymatic activity, metabolic processes, and signaling pathways described in the Kyoto Encyclopedia of Genes and Genomes (www.genome.ad.jp/kegg) and Gene Ontology (www.geneontology.org). We used transcript identifiers to extract information on the nature and positional coordinates of genes encoding these structures (step 2). Positional coordinates of gene regions in the range of ±10,000 base pairs from current gene boundaries were searched with utilities at The National Center for Biotechnology Information (NCBI) and Ensembl to define the universe of known variants from genes encoding LIPIDMAPS structures (step 3). We applied this information filter to microarray data from our 12-year natural history on AMD to extract SNPs for relationship with AMD (step 4). These variants were tested for association with advanced AMD in age-, sex-, and smoking-adjusted logistic regression models using a log-additive coding scheme (step 5). Results of these analyses were used to make inferences on candidate pathways and gene sets in the context of evidence on: (a) molecular genetics of AMD and (b) extant findings on processes both impacted by ω–3 LCPUFAs and implicated in health and disease of neural or vascular retina (step 6). Multiple single markers were associated with of inositol-based metabolic or signaling pathways.

In phase 2 we applied a knowledge-based approach to evaluate the predictive utility of our gene set in determining the likelihood of having advanced AMD (steps

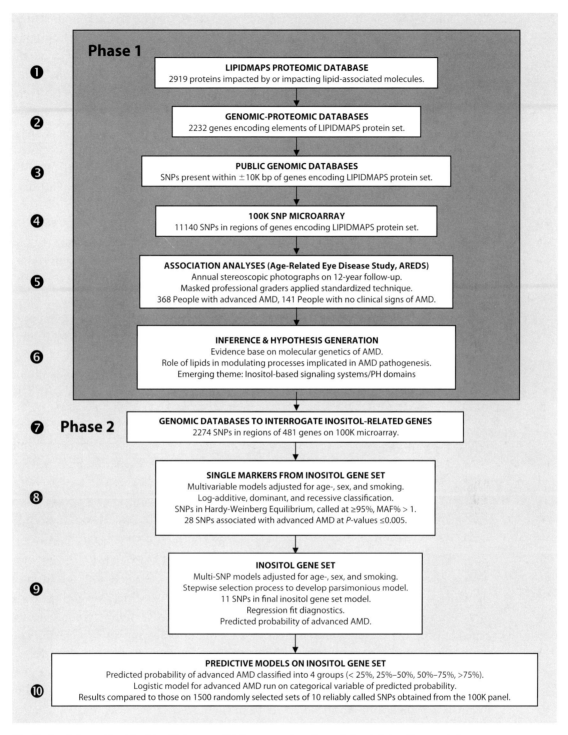

Fig. 3. Analytic method for identifying candidate gene set and specifying joint-action models.

7–10). Our analytic methods are based on those developed by Lesnick et al. [15] to examine joint actions of common gene variations within biologic pathways as predictors of disposition to complex disease. We used the NCBI search engine to obtain lists of all catalogued human genes associated with inositol (step 7). Positional coordinates of these genes ± 10,000 base pairs were obtained and used to filter SNPs in from our 100K microarray. Distributions of inositol-related SNPs in Hardy-Weinberg equilibrium, called reliably at ≥95%, and present in at least 1% of the total sample, were examined for log-additive, dominant, and recessive associations with advanced AMD in age-, sex-, and smoking-adjusted logistic regression models (step 8). We specified a candidate inositol gene set with single markers containing complete data for all participants and attaining two-sided p values ≤0.005. We then ran age-, sex-, and smoking-adjusted joint action logistic regression models with members of this set. A stepwise selection process was applied to develop parsimonious models and regression diagnostics with the Hosmer and Lemershow lackfit method were run to determine whether variance of the final model violated assumptions necessary for valid inference (step 9). Eleven SNPs persisted in the final model. We modeled these variants simultaneously on occurrence of advanced AMD to derive the predicted probability of having AMD for each participant (values may range naturally from 0 to 1) and classified these values into groups by increments of 0.25 (<0.25, 0.25–0.50, 0.50–0.75, and 0.75–1.00). These probability categories represented the primary independent variable of likelihood estimates in final predictive models of advanced AMD occurrence (step 10). The distribution of p *values* from 1,500 randomly selected sets of variants drawn from our total panel (96,774 SNPs) was used to evaluate significance of our findings.

Results

At the time of publication the LIPIDMAPS database contained 2,919 proteins. We identified 2,232 genes encoding elements of these structures. Our 100K microarray contains 11,140 variants in gene regions associated with the LIPIDMAPS constructs. After examining results from this set, a number of AMD-associated variants with diverse positions across the genome emerged for genes associated with the inositol signaling pathway. There were 2,274 variants in a NCBI-specified inositol gene set present on our microarray; of these, 28 that were in Hardy-Weinberg equilibrium, called reliably at ≥95%, and present in at least 1% of the total sample also yielded p values ≤0.005 (fig. 4). This candidate inositol gene set was used in joint action models.

Eleven common variants with complete data from 11 inositol-related genes persisted in the final model (table 6). This set yielded predictive probabilities that distinguished people with advanced AMD from their AMD-free peers (fig. 5). Relative to people with a predicted probability of advanced AMD <0.25 from our final model, the likelihood of having AMD among people with probabilities of >0.75 was increased 99-fold (p = 1.0×10^{-17}, Model 1, table 7). The overall p value of the model is 3.1×10^{-21}. For each 25% increase in predicted probability there was a 3.5-fold increased

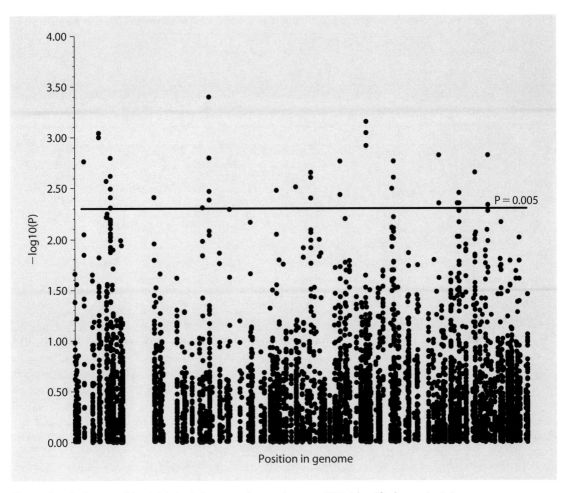

Fig. 4. Results from multivariable logistic regression analyses on SNPs identified as variants in genes encoding elements of inositol signaling pathways.

likelihood of having advanced AMD (odds ratio = 3.5, 95% confidence interval = 2.8–4.7). Comparison of our findings to those derived from p value distributions of 1,500 analyses on randomly selected sets of SNPs from our complete array panel indicated that results were not likely due to random sampling error. None of the 1,500 test models yielded a p value <1.2×10^{-9}. In addition to analyses on variants with complete data, we applied our approach to a set with less than 10% missing data for single markers. The final analysis in this model contained 19 SNPs that were present in 339 people with advanced AMD and 128 AMD-free people (Model 2, table 7). Results did not change appreciably from the original model.

Discussion
These novel findings implicate molecular events driven by elements of inositol metabolism and signaling pathways in AMD pathogenesis. Our primary intent was

Table 6. Variants included in the final predictive model for inositol-related factors and processes

Variant	Gene		MAF%		
	HGNC symbol	Prox. exon (~bp)	no AMD	adv. AMD	p value
rs4146894[R]	PLEKHA1	<2,100	45.4	37.5	0.0001
rs2270960[R]	ITPR2	<50	46.5	37.4	0.0009
rs2038490[A]	PIGH	<100	28.0	17.3	0.0013
rs2575876[A]	ABCA1	<200	31.2	21.3	0.0022
rs1759752[R]	PPAP2B	<3,000	48.9	55.6	0.0028
rs2816955[A]	NR5A2	>5,000	40.4	49.7	0.0040
rs1424166[D]	CDH13	<2,000	49.3	55.8	0.0040
rs3784789[A]	CSK	>5,000	40.8	32.6	0.0055
rs3795451[R]	CDC42BPA	3' UTR	46.8	44.4	0.0087
rs697852[A]	ITPKB	>5,000	23.0	16.2	0.0095
rs766366[D]	DGKB	>5,000	46.5	37.9	0.0110
rs1529819[A]	DEPDC2	<300	44.3	36.5	0.0116

The 'no AMD' (n = 141) group consisted of people who were AMD-free across the study. People in the advanced (Adv.) AMD group (n = 368) have neovascular AMD and/or geographic atrophy. p values are two-sided and from multivariable models including age at last photograph used to ascertain outcome, sex, and smoking (never, past, current). Superscripts in the 'Variant' column represent form of the variable applied in the final model: A = additive, D = dominant, R = recessive. Prox. exon = proximity to exon. ~bp = approximate number of base pairs. MAF = Minor allele frequency, PLEKHA1 = pleckstrin homology domain containing, family A (phosphoinositide-binding specific) member 1; ITPR2 = inositol 1,4,5-triphosphate receptor, type 2; PIGH = phosphatidylinositol glycan anchor biosynthesis, class H; ABCA1 = ATP-binding cassette, subfamily A (ABC1), member 1; PPAP2B = phosphatidic acid phosphatase type 2B; NR5A2 = nuclear receptor subfamily 5, group A, member 2; CDH13 = cadherin 13, H-cadherin; CSK = c-src tyrosine kinase; CDC42BPA = CDC42 binding protein kinase α (DMPK-like); ITPKB = inositol 1,4,5-trisphosphate 3-kinase B; DGKB = diacylglycerol kinase, β; DEPDC2 = DEP domain containing 2.

to determine whether the *joint action* of common gene variations within members a systematically identified lipid-associated gene set could predict predisposition to advanced AMD. It is important to emphasize that inferences are most appropriately applied to the inositol-associated *gene set* (and not the individual variants used for predictive modeling) since our microarray panel did not have complete coverage of all genes, and in some cases did not contain variants in (or in linkage disequilibrium with those in) coding regions. The magnitude of effect in the joint action model exceeded that of any single marker. In the absence of mechanistic validation studies we cannot yet make conclusive inferences; however, extant work on molecular genetics of AMD provides essential guidance in assessing the value of our findings.

We thus consider our results in the context of two biologically credible and related lines of evidence. The first is related to pleckstrin homology (PH) domain-containing

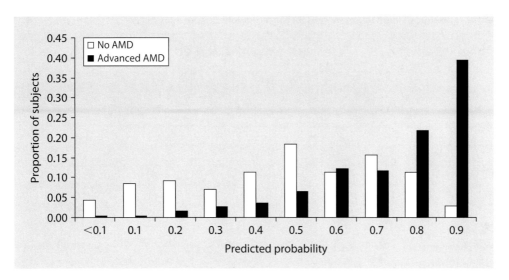

Fig. 5. Predicted probabilities of advanced AMD based upon the final joint action model of variants in inositol-related genes (cf. table 6). The explanatory value of the final model is strongest for the advanced AMD group, as approximately 7 in 10 people with AMD have at least a 70% predicted probability of having advanced AMD with the current set of variants (~40% of people with AMD have probability scores ≥0.90). In most instances, people in the no AMD group have lower probabilities than those with AMD. Within probability categories there is usually a clear separation between groups. Fit of the model may be improved (~20% of controls have predicted probabilities between 0.70 and 0.90) with data on additional SNPs.

effectors. A strong and often replicated susceptibility locus for advanced AMD exists on chromosome 10q26 [320–322]. PH domain-containing, family A (phosphoinositide binding-specific) member 1 (PLEKHA1) occupies this region and represents 1 of the 3 genes most strongly associated with AMD worldwide. The other two genes (LOC387715/age-related maculopathy susceptibility 2 (ARMS2) and HtrA serine peptidase 1 gene (HTRA1)) are proximally positioned on 10q26 and in linkage disequilibrium with PLEKHA1 [322]. Pleckstrin is a PKC substrate containing two PH domains that bind *phosphoinositides*; it is involved in plasma membrane-based signaling systems [323]. PH domains represent approximately 1 in 10 of all domain structures in the human proteome [324] and exist on a number of protein kinases, GTPases/GTP regulators, adaptors, and phospholipases central to physiologic function [324, 325]. Figure 6 includes examples of molecules containing PH domains along with phosphoinositide-binding specificity. The key points are that PH domains bind phosphoinositides and act in recruitment and translocation of host proteins to the plasma membrane so that macromolecules of PI3K, GTP, and Ras signaling systems may be assembled.

DHA modulates Akt signaling in neuronal survival by influencing events at the PH domain. DHA acts as an effect modifier in the process of PH-mediated membrane translocation for the Akt system in a model system of neuronal cell survival [326].

Table 7. Results of joint action models for inositol-related genes

Inositol-related genes	Comparison (probability group)			OR (95% CI)	p value
	A	vs.	B		
Model 1					
Full data set	linear model	–		3.5 (2.8–4.7)	3.1×10^{-21}
11 markers	<0.25		0.25–0.50	10.5 (2.3–48.5)	0.64
	<0.25		0.50–0.75	19.8 (4.5–87.0)	0.04
	<0.25		0.75–1.00	99.2 (22.3–440.9)	1.0×10^{-17}
Model 2					
95% complete data	linear model	–		4.3 (3.3–5.7)	2.0×10^{-25}
19 markers	<0.25		0.25–0.50	7.8 (2.4–25.1)	0.26
	<0.25		0.50–0.75	13.4 (4.5–40.6)	0.26
	<0.25		0.75–1.00	114.9 (37.4–353.0)	5.5×10^{-25}

Odds ratios (OR) represent the increased likelihood of having advanced AMD relative to a one-step change in the scale of predicted probabilities ('linear model', e.g. moving from <0.25 to 0.25–0.50 or 0.25–0.50 to 0.50–0.75) or each predicted probability category relative to the <0.25 group (A vs. B). All p values are two-sided. Model 1 was run on SNPs with 100% base calls for all participants (listed in table 6: 'No AMD' group, n = 141; AMD group, n = 368). Model 2 was run on SNPs from Model 1 and others with ≥90% call frequency. Results for Model 2 are based on 128 people without AMD and 339 people with AMD.

This action has been linked to DHA enrichment of PS, a phospholipid present in appreciable quantities within the neural retina. Increases in PS concentration facilitate interaction of Akt's PH domain with the plasma membrane and thus allow a more efficient phosphorylation of the Akt. Akt activation in this system inhibits a key step in the apoptotic cascade and thereby promotes cell survival. How do these results relate to our own? PLEKHA1 binds specifically and with high affinity within the plasma membrane to phosphatidylinositol 3,4-bisphosphate (PtdIns(3,4)P2), a bioactive lipid and the dephosphorylation product of phosphatidylinositol-3,4,5-trisphosphate (PtdIns(3,4,5)P3). PtdIns(3,4,5)P3 is produced from a phosphatidylinositol-4,5-bisphosphate (PtdIns(4,5)P2) substrate after class IB phosphoinositide 3-kinase (PI3Kγ) activation. PI3Kγ ligands have been associated with atrophic and vasoproliferative retinal pathology in model systems; these ligands include chemokines (IL-8, RANTES, macrophage inflammatory protein (MIP)-1a, MIP-2, MCP-1, Gro-α), pro-inflammatory lipids (PAF), leukotrienes (LTB$_4$), angiotensin II, and complement component C5. PtdIns(3,4)P2- and PtdIns(3,4,5)P3-pleckstrin complexes work within the PI3K pathway to regulate innate and adaptive immune cells, vascular smooth muscle cells,

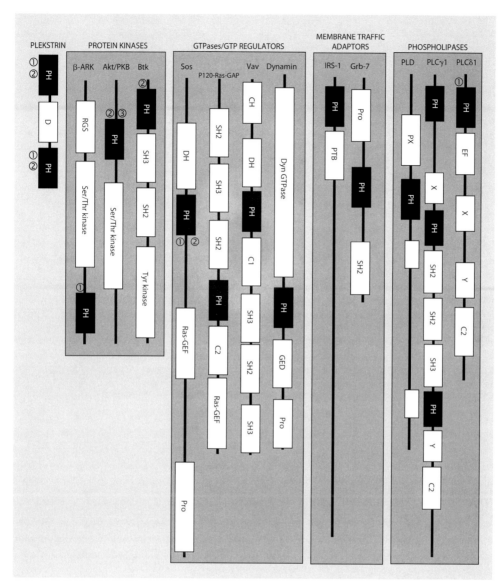

Fig. 6. Pleckstrin homology domains and phosphoinositide-binding sites adapted from Itoh and Takenawa [323]. Non-specific binding to PH domains from PtdIns3P and PtdIns4P. Specific binding according to the following symbols: ① = PtdIns(4,5)P2, ② = PtdIns(3,4,5)P3, ③ = PtdIns(3,4)P2. PH = Pleckstrin homology domain; D = disheveled, Egl-10, and pleckstrin; DH = Dbl homology; Dyn = dynamin; GEF = guanine nucleotide exchanging factor; GAP = GTPase-activating protein; CH = calponin homology; C1 = protein kinase C conserved region 1; C2 = protein kinase C conserved region 2; GED = GTPase effector domain; X = phospholipase C catalytic domain X; Y = phospholipase C catalytic domain Y; EF = EF hand; RGS = regulator of G-protein signaling; PL = phospholipase; Pro = proline-rich; PTB = phosphotyrosine binding; SH2 = Src homology 2; SH3 = Src homology 3; b-ARK = β-adhesion-related kinase; Btk = Bruton's tyrosine kinase; Sos = guanine nucleotide-exchange factor Son of sevenless; Vav = guanine-nucleotide exchange factor Vav.

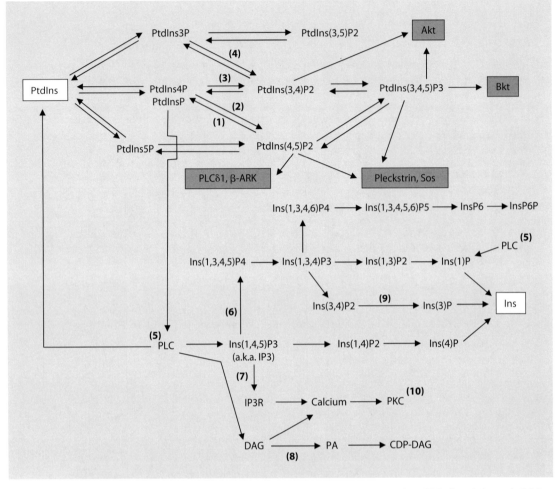

Fig. 7. Pathways are adapted from KEGG Pathway 04070. CPD-DAG = CDP-diacylglycerol; DAG = diacylglycerol; PA = phosphatidic acid; PtdIns = phosphatidylinositol; Ins = inositol. Numerals are used to represent roles of genes in this signaling pathway that contain variants associated with advanced age-related macular degeneration at p values ≤0.05 in age-, sex-, and smoking-adjusted logistic regression models. The HGNC symbols for genes containing AMD-associated variants are as follows: (1) INPP5E, SYNJ2; (2) PIP4K2A, PIP4K2B, PIP5K1A, PIP5K1C; (3) PIK3C2G; (4) INPP4B; (5) PLCB2, PLCE1, PLCG2; (6) ITPKB; (7) ITPR1, ITPR2; (8) DGKA, DGKB, DGKH, DGKI; (9) INPP4B; (10) PRKCA, PRKCB1. INPP5E = Inositol polyphosphate-5-phosphatase; SYNJ2 = synaptojanin 2, inositol phosphate 5′-phosphatase-2; PIP4K2A = phosphatidylinositol-5-phosphate 4-kinase, type II, α; PIP4K2B phosphatidylinositol-5-phosphate 4-kinase, type II, β; PIP5K1A = phosphatidylinositol-4-phosphate 5-kinase, type I, α; PIP5K1C = phosphatidylinositol-4-phosphate 5-kinase, type I, γ; PIK3C2G = phosphoinositide-3-kinase, class 2, γ polypeptide; INPP4B = inositol polyphosphate-4-phosphatase, type II; PLCB2 = phospholipase C, β 2; PLCE1 = phospholipase C, ε 1; PLCG2 = phospholipase C, γ 2 (phosphatidylinositol-specific); ITPKB = inositol 1,4,5-trisphosphate 3-kinase B; ITPR1 = inositol 1,4,5-triphosphate receptor, type 1; ITPR2 = inositol 1,4,5-triphosphate receptor, type 2; DGKA = diacylglycerol kinase, α; DGKB = diacylglycerol kinase, β; DGKH = diacylglycerol kinase, η; DGKI = diacylglycerol kinase, ι; INPP4B = inositol polyphosphate-4-phosphatase, type II; PRKCA = protein kinase C, α; PRKCB1 = protein kinase C, β 1.

and platelets partially through their interaction with PH domains on serine/threonine kinases in the protein kinase B (Akt) signaling pathway. Figure 7 plots information on gene variants associated with AMD within the framework of the PI signaling system (genes containing sequence variants associated with advanced AMD at p values ≤0.05 are represented in the diagram). The PH domains for Akt and pleckstrin share a specific affinity to PtdIns(3,4,5)P3. There are a number of points in figure 7, particularly (3) and (4), at which variants present in greater frequency among people with AMD may impact production of the precursor pool for the specific plekstrin ligand. These findings are intriguing as a number of research groups have emphasized the difficulty of making inferences about the independent effects of PLEKHA1, LOC387715/ARMS2, and HTRA1 because of the tendency for shared inheritance of haplotypes. Our findings support the importance of PLEKHA1 as part of an inositol-based system as there was a great diversity in the position of inositol-related genes specified in the final joint action model. The variant from our final model within the PLEKHA1 gene region yielded the strongest relationship of all 11 SNPs in the final model; but it is important to note, omitting this variable led to negligible change in the results. Table 8 contains annotations for the 20 genes represented in figure 7. These genes exist on 14 chromosomes. It is intriguing to observe genes with similar functions existing on different chromosomes were associated with our outcomes (diacylglycerol kinases on chromosomes 7 and 12, PKC isoforms on chromosomes 16 and 17, and phospholipase C isoforms on chromosomes 10, 15, and 16).

A second line of evidence supported by our findings involves the relationship of dietary lipids, phosphoinositides, and genetics with calcium signaling. Szado et al. [327] demonstrated that phosphorylation of inositol triphosphate (IP_3) receptors by the Akt system, prevented programmed cell death in a model cell system through inhibition of calcium release. This point is germane to our work, as ω–3 LCPUFAs have been shown to influence calcium homeostasis [328, 329]. Points (7) and (10) in figure 7 highlight the potential for disrupted inositol-modulated calcium signaling in people with advanced AMD.

Summary and Future Directions

Our general conclusions are that: (1) there is consistent evidence to suggest that ω–3 LCPUFAs may act in protective roles for AMD; (2) genome-wide association studies may be applied to efficiently elucidate novel pathway- and gene set-based associations with complex diseases like AMD, and (3) a knowledge-based approach to exposure ascertainment (in this case, identification and annotation of lipid-associated genes) is valuable in planning, implementation efforts necessary to make valid inference about complex systems. The essential need for replication of findings in an independent sample is now being planned.

Table 8. Annotations and positional coordinates of genes represented in the inositol-signaling system (cf. fig. 7)

Figure 7 group	Chr	Start bp	HGNC ID	Symbol	Gene name
(6)	1	224886016	6179	ITPKB	inositol 1,4,5-trisphosphate 3-kinase B
(2)	1	149437696	8994	PIP5K1A	phosphatidylinositol-4-phosphate 5-kinase, type I, α
(7)	3	4510136	6180	ITPR1	inositol 1,4,5-triphosphate receptor, type 1
(4) and (9)	4	143168636	6075	INPP4B	inositol polyphosphate-4-phosphatase, type II
(1)	6	158322907	11504	SYNJ2	synaptojanin, synaptic inositol 1,4,5-triphosphate 5 phosphatase, inositol phosphate 5′-phosphatase 2
(8)	7	14153770	2850	DGKB	diacylglycerol kinase, β
(8)	7	136724925	2855	DGKI	diacylglycerol kinase, ι
(1)	9	138442896	21474	INPP5E	inositol polyphosphate-5-phosphatase
(2)	10	22865829	8997	PIP4K2A	phosphatidylinositol 5 phosphate 4 kinase type 2 α
(5)	10	95743736	17175	PLCE1	phospholipase C, epsilon 1
(8)	12	54611213	2849	DGKA	diacylglycerol kinase, α
(7)	12	26379552	6181	ITPR2	inositol 1,4,5-triphosphate receptor, type 2
(3)	12	18305741	8973	PIK3C2G	phosphoinositide-3-kinase, class 2, γ polypeptide
(8)	13	41520889	2854	DGKH	diacylglycerol kinase, η
(5)	15	38367392	9055	PLCB2	phospholipase C, β 2 1 phosphatidylinositol 4,5-bisphosphate phosphodiesterase β
(5)	16	80370408	9066	PLCG2	phospholipase C, γ 2 (phosphatidylinositol-specific) 1-phosphatidylinositol 4,5-bisphosphate phosphodiesterase γ 1
(10)	16	23754823	9395	PRKCB1	protein kinase C, β 1
(2)	17	34175470	8998	PIP4K2B	phosphatidylinositol-5-phosphate 4-kinase, type II, β
(10)	17	61729216	9393	PRKCA	protein kinase C, α
(2)	19	3581182	8996	PIP5K1C	phosphatidylinositol-4-phosphate 5-kinase, type I, γ

Figure 7 contains labels in the far left column of this table to represent positions in the inositol pathway. Chr = Chromosome; bp = base pair.

New and emerging concepts related to the content of the work we present should focus on the interrelationship of LCPUFAs with genetic factors impacting neural and vascular structure and function. Dietary LCPUFAs operate as key structural and signaling molecules. They affect and are affected by key compounds with known vaso-, neuro-, and immunomodulatory actions. We have applied bioinformatic and statistical genetic techniques in an effort to examine lipid-dependent metabolism and signaling mechanisms as a step forward in guiding researchers in discovery of key pathways driving retinal response to developmental, demographic, environmental, and metabolic factors. To the extent that retinal tissue status of DHA is dependent upon and modifiable by diet, we may eventually arrive at some reasonable understanding of whether alterations in dietary or cellular lipid composition or modulation of lipid precursors, cleavage and biosynthetic enzymes, or metabolites will serve as an effective preventive intervention for retinal diseases.

Acknowledgements

The datasets used for the analyses described in this work were obtained from the Age-Related Eye Disease Study (AREDS) Database found at http://www.ncbi.nlm.nih.gov/sites/entrez?db = gap through dbGaP accession number phs000001.v1.p1. The authors would like to thank the AREDS participants, the AREDS Research Group, the AREDS Coordinating Center Staff at the EMMES Corporation, and the AREDS Project Office for their valuable contribution to this project. AREDS was funded by contracts from the National Eye Institute, National Institutes of Health, Department of Health and Human Services, Bethesda, Md., USA. The authors would like to acknowledge the contributions of Elvira Argrón (NEI) for her help in programming the data simulations and Emily Chew (NEI), Traci Clemons (EMMES Corp.), and Alice Henning (EMMES Corp.) for their technical advice on classification of AREDS participants.

References

1 Congdon N, O'Colmain B, Klaver CC, Klein R, Munoz B, Friedman DS, Kempen J, Taylor HR, Mitchell P: Causes and prevalence of visual impairment among adults in the United States. Arch Ophthalmol 2004;122:477–485.

2 Friedman DS, O'Colmain BJ, Munoz B, Tomany SC, McCarty C, de Jong PT, Nemesure B, Mitchell P, Kempen J: Prevalence of age-related macular degeneration in the United States. Arch Ophthalmol 2004; 122:564–572.

3 Ambati J, Ambati BK, Yoo SH, Ianchulev S, Adamis AP: Age-related macular degeneration: etiology, pathogenesis, and therapeutic strategies. Surv Ophthalmol 2003;48:257–293.

4 Holz FG, Pauleikhoff D, Klein R, Bird AC: Pathogenesis of lesions in late age-related macular disease. Am J Ophthalmol 2004;137:504–510.

5 Moshfeghi DM, Blumenkranz MS: Role of genetic factors and inflammation in age-related macular degeneration. Retina 2007;27:269–275.

6 Beatty S, Koh H, Phil M, Henson D, Boulton M: The role of oxidative stress in the pathogenesis of age-related macular degeneration. Surv Ophthalmol 2000; 45:115–134.

7 Mukherjee PK, Chawla A, Loayza MS, Bazan NG: Docosanoids are multifunctional regulators of neural cell integrity and fate: significance in aging and disease. Prostaglandins Leukot Essent Fatty Acids 2007;77:233–238.

8 Bazan NG: Homeostatic regulation of photoreceptor cell integrity: significance of the potent mediator neuroprotectin D1 biosynthesized from docosahexaenoic acid: the proctor lecture. Invest Ophthalmol Vis Sci 2007;48:4864–4881.

9 Mukherjee PK, Marcheselli VL, Barreiro S, Hu J, Bok D, Bazan NG: Neurotrophins enhance retinal pigment epithelial cell survival through neuroprotectin D1 signaling. Proc Natl Acad Sci USA 2007; 104:13152–13157.

10 Mukherjee PK, Marcheselli VL, de Rivero Vaccari JC, Gordon WC, Jackson FE, Bazan NG: Photoreceptor outer segment phagocytosis attenuates oxidative stress-induced apoptosis with concomitant neuroprotectin D1 synthesis. Proc Natl Acad Sci USA 2007;104:13158–13163.

11 Connor KM, SanGiovanni JP, Lofqvist C, Aderman CM, Chen J, Higuchi A, Hong S, Pravda EA, Majchrzak S, Carper D, Hellstrom A, Kang JX, Chew EY, Salem N Jr, Serhan CN, Smith LE: Increased dietary intake of omega–3-polyunsaturated fatty acids reduces pathological retinal angiogenesis. Nat Med 2007;13:868–873.

12 SanGiovanni JP, Chew EY, Clemons TE, Davis MD, Ferris FL 3rd, Gensler GR, Kurinij N, Lindblad AS, Milton RC, Seddon JM, Sperduto RD: The relationship of dietary lipid intake and age-related macular degeneration in a case-control study: AREDS Report No 20. Arch Ophthalmol 2007;125:671–679.

13 SanGiovanni JP, Chew EY: The role of omega–3 long-chain polyunsaturated fatty acids in health and disease of the retina. Prog Retin Eye Res 2005;24:87–138.

14 Mukherjee PK, Marcheselli VL, Serhan CN, Bazan NG: Neuroprotectin D1: a docosahexaenoic acid-derived docosatriene protects human retinal pigment epithelial cells from oxidative stress. Proc Natl Acad Sci USA 2004;101:8491–8496.

15 Lesnick TG, Papapetropoulos S, Mash DC, Ffrench-Mullen J, Shehadeh L, de Andrade M, Henley JR, Rocca WA, Ahlskog JE, Maraganore DM: A genomic pathway approach to a complex disease: axon guidance and Parkinson disease. PLoS Genet 2007;3:e98.

16 Seddon JM, Cote J, Rosner B: Progression of age-related macular degeneration: association with dietary fat, transunsaturated fat, nuts, and fish intake. Arch Ophthalmol 2003;121:1728–1737.

17 Seddon JM, Rosner B, Sperduto RD, Yannuzzi L, Haller JA, Blair NP, Willett W: Dietary fat and risk for advanced age-related macular degeneration. Arch Ophthalmol 2001;119:1191–1199.

18 Smith W, Mitchell P, Leeder SR: Dietary fat and fish intake and age-related maculopathy. Arch Ophthalmol 2000;118:401–404.

19 Mares-Perlman JA, Brady WE, Klein R, Vanden-Langenberg GM, Klein BE, Palta M: Dietary fat and age-related maculopathy. Arch Ophthalmol 1995;113:743–748.

20 Heuberger RA, Mares-Perlman JA, Klein R, Klein BE, Millen AE, Palta M: Relationship of dietary fat to age-related maculopathy in the third national health and nutrition examination survey. Arch Ophthalmol 2001;119:1833–1838.

21 Cho E, Hung S, Willett WC, Spiegelman D, Rimm EB, Seddon JM, Colditz GA, Hankinson SE: Prospective study of dietary fat and the risk of age-related macular degeneration. Am J Clin Nutr 2001;73:209–218.

22 Seddon JM, George S, Rosner B: Cigarette smoking, fish consumption, omega–3 fatty acid intake, and associations with age-related macular degeneration: the US Twin Study of Age-Related Macular Degeneration. Arch Ophthalmol 2006;124:995–1001.

23 Tan JS, Mitchell P, Kifley A, Flood V, Smith W, Wang JJ: Smoking and the long-term incidence of age-related macular degeneration: The Blue Mountains Eye Study. Arch Ophthalmol 2007;125:1089–1095.

24 Arnarsson A, Sverrisson T, Stefansson E, Sigurdsson H, Sasaki H, Sasaki K, Jonasson F: Risk factors for five-year incident age-related macular degeneration: The Reykjavik Eye Study. Am J Ophthalmol 2006; 142:419–428.

25 Delcourt C, Carriere I, Cristol JP, Lacroux A, Gerber M: Dietary fat and the risk of age-related maculopathy: The Polanut Study. Eur J Clin Nutr 2007;61: 1341–1344.

26 SanGiovanni JP, Chew E, Agrón E, Clemons TE, Davis MD, Ferris FL 3rd, Gensler GR, Kurinij N, Lindblad AS, Milton RC, Seddon JM, Klein R, Sperduto RD, AREDS Research Group: The relationship of dietary lipid intake with incident age-related macular degeneration: a prospective study in the Age-Related Eye Disease Study. AREDS Report No 23. Arch Ophthalmol 2008;126:1274–1279.

27 Fliesler SJ, Anderson RE: Chemistry and metabolism of lipids in the vertebrate retina. Prog Lipid Res 1983;22:79–131.

28 Kulkarni P, Cai J, Hurst HE: Lipids and nitric oxide in porcine retinal and choroidal blood vessels. J Ocul Pharmacol Ther 2002;18:265–275.

29 Lecomte M, Paget C, Ruggiero D, Wiernsperger N, Lagarde M: Docosahexaenoic acid is a major n–3 polyunsaturated fatty acid in bovine retinal microvessels. J Neurochem 1996;66:2160–2167.

30 Serhan CN, Chiang N: Endogenous pro-resolving and anti-inflammatory lipid mediators: a new pharmacologic genus. Br J Pharmacol 2008;153(suppl 1): S200–S215.

31 Bazan NG: The metabolism of omega–3 polyunsaturated fatty acids in the eye: the possible role of docosahexaenoic acid and docosanoids in retinal physiology and ocular pathology. Prog Clin Biol Res 1989;312:95–112.

32 Nettleton JA: Omega–3 Fatty Acids and Health. New York, Chapman & Hall, 1995.

33 Hibbeln JR, Nieminen LR, Blasbalg TL, Riggs JA, Lands WE: Healthy intakes of n–3 and n–6 fatty acids: estimations considering worldwide diversity. Am J Clin Nutr 2006;83:1483S–1493S.

34 Simopoulos AP: Essential fatty acids in health and chronic disease. Am J Clin Nutr 1999;70:560S–569S.

35 Leung IY, Sandstrom MM, Zucker CL, Neuringer M, Max Snodderly D: Nutritional manipulation of primate retinas. IV. Effects of n–3 fatty acids, lutein, and zeaxanthin on S-cones and rods in the foveal region. Exp Eye Res 2005;81:513–529.

36 Leung IY, Sandstrom MM, Zucker CL, Neuringer M, Snodderly DM: Nutritional manipulation of primate retinas. II. Effects of age, n–3 fatty acids, lutein, and zeaxanthin on retinal pigment epithelium. Invest Ophthalmol Vis Sci 2004;45:3244–3256.

37 Rotstein NP, Aveldano MI, Barrantes FJ, Roccamo AM, Politi LE: Apoptosis of retinal photoreceptors during development in vitro: protective effect of docosahexaenoic acid. J Neurochem 1997;69:504–513.

38 Rotstein NP, Politi LE, Aveldano MI: Docosahexaenoic acid promotes differentiation of developing photoreceptors in culture. Invest Ophthalmol Vis Sci 1998;39:2750–2758.

39 Rotstein NP, Aveldano MI, Barrantes FJ, Politi LE: Docosahexaenoic acid is required for the survival of rat retinal photoreceptors in vitro. J Neurochem 1996;66:1851–1859.

40 Rotstein NP, Politi LE, German OL, Girotti R: Protective effect of docosahexaenoic acid on oxidative stress-induced apoptosis of retina photoreceptors. Invest Ophthalmol Vis Sci 2003;44:2252–2259.

41 Chucair AJ, Rotstein NP, Sangiovanni JP, During A, Chew EY, Politi LE: Lutein and zeaxanthin protect photoreceptors from apoptosis induced by oxidative stress: relation with docosahexaenoic acid. Invest Ophthalmol Vis Sci 2007;48:5168–5177.

42 German OL, Insua MF, Gentili C, Rotstein NP, Politi LE: Docosahexaenoic acid prevents apoptosis of retina photoreceptors by activating the ERK/MAPK pathway. J Neurochem 2006;98:1507–1520.

43 Garelli A, Rotstein NP, Politi LE: Docosahexaenoic acid promotes photoreceptor differentiation without altering CRX expression. Invest Ophthalmol Vis Sci 2006;47:3017–3027.

44 Insua MF, Garelli A, Rotstein NP, German OL, Arias A, Politi LE: Cell cycle regulation in retinal progenitors by glia-derived neurotrophic factor and docosahexaenoic acid. Invest Ophthalmol Vis Sci 2003; 44:2235–2244.

45 Chow KC: Fatty Acids in Foods and Their Health Implications, ed 2. New York, Dekker, 2000.

46 Bazan NG: Cell survival matters: docosahexaenoic acid signaling, neuroprotection and photoreceptors. Trends Neurosci 2006;29:263–271.

47 Gordon WC, Bazan NG: Retina; in Harding JJ (ed): Biochemistry of the Eye. London, Chapman & Hall, 1997, pp 144–275.

48 Uauy R, Mena P, Rojas C: Essential fatty acids in early life: structural and functional role. Proc Nutr Soc 2000;59:3–15.

49 Simopoulos AP: Omega–3 fatty acids in health and disease and in growth and development. Am J Clin Nutr 1991;54:438–463.

50 Simopoulos AP: The role of fatty acids in gene expression: health implications. Ann Nutr Metab 1996;40:303–311.

51 Simopoulos AP, Leaf A, Salem N Jr: Workshop statement on the essentiality of and recommended dietary intakes for omega–6 and omega–3 fatty acids. Prostaglandins Leukot Essent Fatty Acids 2000;63:119–121.

52 Neuringer M: The relationship of fatty acid composition to function in the retina and visual system; in Dobbing J (ed): Lipids, Learning, and the Brain: Fats in Infant Formulas. 103rd Ross Conference on Pediatric Research. Adelaide, South Australia, Ross Laboratories, 1993, pp 134–158.

53 Martinez M, Vazquez E, Garcia-Silva MT, Manzanares J, Bertran JM, Castello F, Mougan I: Therapeutic effects of docosahexaenoic acid ethyl ester in patients with generalized peroxisomal disorders. Am J Clin Nutr 2000;71:376S–385S.

54 Salem N Jr, Litman B, Kim HY, Gawrisch K: Mechanisms of action of docosahexaenoic acid in the nervous system. Lipids 2001;36:945–959.

55 Niu SL, Mitchell DC, Lim SY, Wen ZM, Kim HY, Salem N Jr, Litman BJ: Reduced G-protein-coupled signaling efficiency in retinal rod outer segments in response to n–3 fatty acid deficiency. J Biol Chem 2004;279:31098–31104.

56 Neuringer M, Jeffrey BG: Visual development: neural basis and new assessment methods. J Pediatr 2003;143:S87–S95.

57 De Caterina R, Madonna R: Nutrients and gene expression. World Rev Nutr Diet. Basel, Karger, 2004, vol 93, pp 99–133.

58 De Caterina R, Madonna R: Role of nutrients and physical activity in gene expression. World Rev Nutr Diet. Basel, Karger, 2005, vol 94, pp 107–119.

59 De Urquiza AM, Liu S, Sjoberg M, Zetterstrom RH, Griffiths W, Sjovall J, Perlmann T: Docosahexaenoic acid, a ligand for the retinoid X receptor in mouse brain. Science 2000;290:2140–2144.

60 Politi L, Rotstein N, Carri N: Effects of docosahexaenoic acid on retinal development: cellular and molecular aspects. Lipids 2001;36:927–935.

61 Calder PC: Omega–3 polyunsaturated fatty acids, inflammation and immunity. World Rev Nutr Diet. Basel, Karger, 2001;88:109–116.

62 Nelson GJ: Effects of dietary fatty acids on lipid metabolism; in Chow KC (ed): Fatty Acids in Foods and Their Health Implications. New York, Dekker, 2000, pp 481–516.

63 Daemen FJ: Vertebrate rod outer segment membranes. Biochim Biophys Acta 1973;300:255–288.

64 Choe HG, Anderson RE: Unique molecular species composition of glycerolipids of frog rod outer segments. Exp Eye Res 1990;51:159–165.

65 Wiegand RD, Koutz CA, Stinson AM, Anderson RE: Conservation of docosahexaenoic acid in rod outer segments of rat retina during n–3 and n–6 fatty acid deficiency. J Neurochem 1991;57:1690–1699.

66 Aveldano MI, Sprecher H: Very long chain (C24 to C36) polyenoic fatty acids of the n–3 and n–6 series in dipolyunsaturated phosphatidylcholines from bovine retina. J Biol Chem 1987;262:1180–1186.

67 Litman BJ, Mitchell DC: A role for phospholipid polyunsaturation in modulating membrane protein function. Lipids 1996;31(suppl):S193–S197.

68 Anderson RE: Lipids of ocular tissues. IV. A comparison of the phospholipids from the retina of six mammalian species. Exp Eye Res 1970;10:339–344.

69 Lands WE: Impact of daily food choices on health promotion and disease prevention. World Rev Nutr Diet. Basel, Karger, 2001, vol 88, pp 1–5.

70 Simopoulos AP: Evolutionary aspects of diet, the omega–6/omega–3 ratio and genetic variation: nutritional implications for chronic diseases. Biomed Pharmacother 2006;60:502–507.

71 Su HM, Bernardo L, Mirmiran M, Ma XH, Corso TN, Nathanielsz PW, Brenna JT: Bioequivalence of dietary α-linolenic and docosahexaenoic acids as sources of docosahexaenoate accretion in brain and associated organs of neonatal baboons. Pediatr Res 1999;45:87–93.

72 Wetzel MG, Li J, Alvarez RA, Anderson RE, O'Brien PJ: Metabolism of linolenic acid and docosahexaenoic acid in rat retinas and rod outer segments. Exp Eye Res 1991;53:437–446.

73 Wang N, Anderson RE: Synthesis of docosahexaenoic acid by retina and retinal pigment epithelium. Biochemistry 1993;32:13703–13709.

74 Delton-Vandenbroucke I, Grammas P, Anderson RE: Polyunsaturated fatty acid metabolism in retinal and cerebral microvascular endothelial cells. J Lipid Res 1997;38:147–159.

75 Moore SA: Polyunsaturated fatty acid synthesis and release by brain-derived cells in vitro. J Mol Neurosci 2001;16:195–201.

76 Rodriguez de Turco EB, Parkins N, Ershov AV, Bazan NG: Selective retinal pigment epithelial cell lipid metabolism and remodeling conserves photoreceptor docosahexaenoic acid following phagocytosis. J Neurosci Res 1999;57:479–486.

77 Scott BL, Bazan NG: Membrane docosahexaenoate is supplied to the developing brain and retina by the liver. Proc Natl Acad Sci USA 1989;86:2903–2907.

78 Bazan NG: Supply of n–3 polyunsaturated fatty acids and their significance in the central nervous system; in Wurtman RJ, Wurtman JJ (eds): Nutrition and the Brain. New York, Raven Press, 1990, vol 8, pp 1–24.

79 Li F, Chen H, Anderson RE: Biosynthesis of docosahexaenoate-containing glycerolipid molecular species in the retina. J Mol Neurosci 2001;16:205–221.

80 Anderson GJ, Connor WE: Uptake of fatty acids by the developing rat brain. Lipids 1988;23:286–290.

81 Conquer JA, Holub BJ: Supplementation with an algae source of docosahexaenoic acid increases (n–3) fatty acid status and alters selected risk factors for heart disease in vegetarian subjects. J Nutr 1996;126:3032–3039.

82 Conquer JA, Holub BJ: Dietary docosahexaenoic acid as a source of eicosapentaenoic acid in vegetarians and omnivores. Lipids 1997;32:341–345.

83 Kris-Etherton PM, Taylor DS, Yu-Poth S, Huth P, Moriarty K, Fishell V, Hargrove RL, Zhao G, Etherton TD: Polyunsaturated fatty acids in the food chain in the United States. Am J Clin Nutr 2000;71:179S–188S.

84 Kris-Etherton PM, Harris WS, Appel LJ: Fish consumption, fish oil, omega–3 fatty acids, and cardiovascular disease. Circulation 2002;106:2747–2757.

85 Gebauer SK, Psota TL, Harris WS, Kris-Etherton PM: n–3 fatty acid dietary recommendations and food sources to achieve essentiality and cardiovascular benefits. Am J Clin Nutr 2006;83:1526S–1535S.

86 DHHS/FDA: Department of Health and Human Services, US Food and Drug Administration: Substances affirmed as generally recognized as safe: menhaden oil. Federal Register. June 5, 1997. Vol 62, No 108, pp 30751–30757. 21 cfr part 184. Docket No. 86g-0289. 1997. 2003.

87 DHHS/FDA: Office of Nutritional Products, Labeling, and Dietary Supplements, Center for Food Safety and Applied Nutrition, US Food and Drug Administration: Letter responding to a request to reconsider the qualified claim for a dietary supplement health claim for omega–3 fatty acids and coronary heart disease. Docket No. 91n-0103. February 8, 2002. 2002.

88 Vericel E, Calzada C, Chapuy P, Lagarde M: The influence of low intake of n–3 fatty acids on platelets in elderly people. Atherosclerosis 1999;147:187–192.

89 Dyerberg J, Bang HO: Lipid metabolism, atherogenesis, and haemostasis in Eskimos: the role of the prostaglandin-3 family. Haemostasis 1979;8:227–233.

90 Von Schacky C, Fischer S, Weber PC: Long-term effects of dietary marine omega–3 fatty acids upon plasma and cellular lipids, platelet function, and eicosanoid formation in humans. J Clin Invest 1985;76:1626–1631.

91 Levine PH, Fisher M, Schneider PB, Whitten RH, Weiner BH, Ockene IS, Johnson BF, Johnson MH, Doyle EM, Riendeau PA, et al: Dietary supplementation with omega–3 fatty acids prolongs platelet survival in hyperlipidemic patients with atherosclerosis. Arch Intern Med 1989;149:1113–1116.

92 Li XL, Steiner M: Dose response of dietary fish oil supplementations on platelet adhesion. Arterioscler Thromb 1991;11:39–46.

93 Jumpsen J, Clandinin MT: Brain Development: Relationship to Dietary Lipid and Lipid Metabolism. Champaign/IL, AOCS Press, 1997.

94 Clandinin MT, Jumpsen J, Suh M: Relationship between fatty acid accretion, membrane composition, and biologic functions. J Pediatr 1994;125:S25–S32.

95 Treen M, Uauy RD, Jameson DM, Thomas VL, Hoffman DR: Effect of docosahexaenoic acid on membrane fluidity and function in intact cultured y-79 retinoblastoma cells. Arch Biochem Biophys 1992;294:564–570.

96 Litman BJ, Niu SL, Polozova A, Mitchell DC: The role of docosahexaenoic acid containing phospholipids in modulating G protein-coupled signaling pathways: visual transduction. J Mol Neurosci 2001;16:237–242, 279–284.

97 Niu SL, Mitchell DC, Litman BJ: Manipulation of cholesterol levels in rod disk membranes by methyl-β-cyclodextrin: effects on receptor activation. J Biol Chem 2002;277:20139–20145.

98 Niu SL, Mitchell DC, Litman BJ: Optimization of receptor-G protein coupling by bilayer lipid composition. II. Formation of metarhodopsin ii-transducin complex. J Biol Chem 2001;276:42807–42811.

99 Mitchell DC, Niu SL, Litman BJ: Optimization of receptor-G protein coupling by bilayer lipid composition. I. Kinetics of rhodopsin-transducin binding. J Biol Chem 2001;276:42801–42806.

100 Mitchell DC, Niu SL, Litman BJ: Enhancement of G-protein-coupled signaling by DHA phospholipids. Lipids 2003;38:437–443.

101 Doucet JP, Squinto SP, Bazan NG: Fos-jun and the primary genomic response in the nervous system. Possible physiological role and pathophysiological significance. Mol Neurobiol 1990;4:27–55.

102 Yaqoob P: Lipids and the immune response. Curr Opin Clin Nutr Metab Care 1998;1:153–161.

103 Miles EA, Calder PC: Modulation of immune function by dietary fatty acids. Proc Nutr Soc 1998;57:277–292.

104 De Urquiza AM, Liu S, Sjoberg M, Zetterstrom RH, Griffiths W, Sjovall J, Perlmann T: Docosahexaenoic acid, a ligand for the retinoid X receptor in mouse brain. Science 2000;290:2140–2144.

105 Lin Q, Ruuska SE, Shaw NS, Dong D, Noy N: Ligand selectivity of the peroxisome proliferator-activated receptor α. Biochemistry 1999;38:185–190.

106 Kim HY, Edsall L: The role of docosahexaenoic acid (22:6n–3) in neuronal signaling. Lipids 1999;34(suppl):S249–S250.

107 Kolko M, de Turco EB, Diemer NH, Bazan NG: Secretory phospholipase A_2-mediated neuronal cell death involves glutamate ionotropic receptors. Neuroreport 2002;13:1963–1966.

108 Phillis JW, O'Regan MH: A potentially critical role of phospholipases in central nervous system ischemic, traumatic, and neurodegenerative disorders. Brain Res Brain Res Rev 2004;44:13–47.

109 Ju W-K, Kim K-Y, Neufeld AH: Increased activity of cyclooxygenase-2 signals early neurodegenerative events in the rat retina following transient ischemia. Exp Eye Res 2003;77:137–145.

110 Candelario-Jalil E, Gonzalez-Falcon A, Garcia-Cabrera M, Alvarez D, Al-Dalain S, Martinez G, Leon OS, Springer JE: Assessment of the relative contribution of COX-1 and COX-2 isoforms to ischemia-induced oxidative damage and neurodegeneration following transient global cerebral ischemia. J Neurochem 2003;86:545–555.

111 Phillis JW, O'Regan MH: The role of phospholipases, cyclooxygenases, and lipoxygenases in cerebral ischemic/traumatic injuries. Crit Rev Neurobiol 2003;15:61–90.

112 Boulton M, Rózanowska M, Rózanowski B: Retinal photodamage. J Photochem Photobiol B 2001;64:144–161.

113 Jung H, Reme C: Light-evoked arachidonic acid release in the retina: illuminance/duration dependence and the effects of quinacrine, mellitin and lithium. Light-evoked arachidonic acid release. Graefes Arch Clin Exp Ophthalmol 1994;232:167–175.

114 Hendrickx N, Volanti C, Moens U, Seternes OM, de Witte P, Vandenheede JR, Piette J, Agostinis P: Upregulation of cyclooxygenase-2 and apoptosis resistance by p38 MAPK in hypericin-mediated photodynamic therapy of human cancer cells. J Biol Chem 2003;278:52231–52239

115 Naveh N, Weissman C, Marshall J: Lipoxygenase metabolism following laser induced retinal injury in rabbits. Curr Eye Res 2000;21:554–559.

116 Goldman R, Moshonov S, Chen X, Berchansky A, Furstenberger G, Zor U: Crosstalk between elevation of $[Ca^{2+}]_i$, reactive oxygen species generation and phospholipase A_2 stimulation in a human keratinocyte cell line. Adv Exp Med Biol 1997;433:41–45.

117 Feng L, Xia Y, Garcia GE, Hwang D, Wilson CB: Involvement of reactive oxygen intermediates in cyclooxygenase-2 expression induced by interleukin-1, tumor necrosis factor-α, and lipopolysaccharide. J Clin Invest 1995;95:1669–1675.

118 Kiritoshi S, Nishikawa T, Sonoda K, Kukidome D, Senokuchi T, Matsuo T, Matsumura T, Tokunaga H, Brownlee M, Araki E: Reactive oxygen species from mitochondria induce cyclooxygenase-2 gene expression in human mesangial cells: potential role in diabetic nephropathy. Diabetes 2003;52:2570–2577.

119 Werz O, Szellas D, Steinhilber D: Reactive oxygen species released from granulocytes stimulate 5-lipoxygenase activity in a B-lymphocytic cell line. Eur J Biochem 2000;267:1263–1269.

120 Bizik J, Kankuri E, Ristimaki A, Taieb A, Vapaatalo H, Lubitz W, Vaheri A: Cell-cell contacts trigger programmed necrosis and induce cyclooxygenase-2 expression. Cell Death Differ 2004;11:183–195.

121 Penfold PL, Madigan MC, Gillies MC, Provis JM: Immunological and aetiological aspects of macular degeneration. Prog Retin Eye Res 2001;20:385–414.

122 Bazan NG, Colangelo V, Lukiw WJ: Prostaglandins and other lipid mediators in Alzheimer's disease. Prostaglandins Other Lipid Mediat 2002;68–69: 197–210.

123 Sennlaub F, Valamanesh F, Vazquez-Tello A, El-Asrar AM, Checchin D, Brault S, Gobeil F, Beauchamp MH, Mwaikambo B, Courtois Y, Geboes K, Varma DR, Lachapelle P, Ong H, Behar-Cohen F, Chemtob S: Cyclooxygenase-2 in human and experimental ischemic proliferative retinopathy. Circulation 2003;108:198–204.

124 Bazan HE, Tao Y, DeCoster MA, Bazan NG: Platelet-activating factor induces cyclooxygenase-2 gene expression in corneal epithelium. Requirement of calcium in the signal transduction pathway. Invest Ophthalmol Vis Sci 1997;38:2492–2501.

125 Dubois RN, Abramson SB, Crofford L, Gupta RA, Simon LS, Van De Putte LB, Lipsky PE: Cyclooxygenase in biology and disease. FASEB J 1998;12:1063–1073.

126 Flamand N, Surette ME, Picard S, Bourgoin S, Borgeat P: Cyclic AMP-mediated inhibition of 5-lipoxygenase translocation and leukotriene biosynthesis in human neutrophils. Mol Pharmacol 2002;62:250–256.

127 Balazy M, Nigam S: Aging, lipid modifications and phospholipases – new concepts. Ageing Res Rev 2003;2:191–209.

128 Han JH, Roh MS, Park CH, Park KC, Cho KH, Kim KH, Eun HC, Chung JH: Selective COX-2 inhibitor, NS-398, inhibits the replicative senescence of cultured dermal fibroblasts. Mech Ageing Dev 2004; 125:359–366.

129 Nemenoff R, Winitz S, Qian N, Van Putten V, Johnson G, Heasley L: Phosphorylation and activation of a high molecular weight form of phospholipase A_2 by p42 microtubule-associated protein 2 kinase and protein kinase C. J Biol Chem 1993;268:1960–1964.

130 Qiu Z, Leslie C: Protein kinase C-dependent and -independent pathways of mitogen- activated protein kinase activation in macrophages by stimuli that activate phospholipase A_2. J Biol Chem 1994; 269:19480–19487.

131 Lin LL, Wartmann M, Lin AY, Knopf JL, Seth A, Davis RJ: cPLA2 is phosphorylated and activated by MAP kinase. Cell 1993;72:269–278.

132 Kramer RM, Roberts EF, Um SL, Borsch-Haubold AG, Watson SP, Fisher MJ, Jakubowski JA: P38 mitogen-activated protein kinase phosphorylates cytosolic phospholipase A_2 (cPLA$_2$) in thrombin-stimulated platelets. Evidence that proline-directed phosphorylation is not required for mobilization of arachidonic acid by cPLA$_2$. J Biol Chem 1996;271: 27723–27729.

133 Geijsen N, Dijkers PF, Lammers JJ, Koenderman L, Coffer PJ: Cytokine-mediated cPLA$_2$ phosphorylation is regulated by multiple MAPK family members. FEBS Lett 2000;471:83–88.

134 Balsinde J, Dennis EA: Distinct roles in signal transduction for each of the phospholipase A_2 enzymes present in P388D1 macrophages. J Biol Chem 1996; 271:6758–6765.

135 Hernandez M, Burillo SL, Crespo MS, Nieto ML: Secretory phospholipase A_2 activates the cascade of mitogen-activated protein kinases and cytosolic phospholipase A_2 in the human astrocytoma cell line 1321N1. J Biol Chem 1998;273:606–612.

136 Martin RE: Docosahexaenoic acid decreases phospholipase A_2 activity in the neurites/nerve growth cones of PC12 cells. J Neurosci Res 1998;54:805–813.

137 FitzGerald GA: COX-2 and beyond: approaches to prostaglandin inhibition in human disease. Nat Rev Drug Discov 2003;2:879–890.

138 Ringbom T, Huss U, Stenholm A, Flock S, Skattebol L, Perera P, Bohlin L: COX-2 inhibitory effects of naturally occurring and modified fatty acids. J Nat Prod 2001;64:745–749.

139 Corey EJ, Shih C, Cashman JR: Docosahexaenoic acid is a strong inhibitor of prostaglandin but not leukotriene biosynthesis. Proc Natl Acad Sci USA 1983;80:3581–3584.

140 Romano M, Claria J: Cyclooxygenase-2 and 5-lipoxygenase converging functions on cell proliferation and tumor angiogenesis: Implications for cancer therapy. FASEB J 2003;17:1986–1995.

141 Osborne NN, Casson RJ, Wood JP, Chidlow G, Graham M, Melena J: Retinal ischemia: mechanisms of damage and potential therapeutic strategies. Prog Retin Eye Res 2004;23:91–147.

142 Wangsa-Wirawan ND, Linsenmeier RA: Retinal oxygen: fundamental and clinical aspects. Arch Ophthalmol 2003;121:547–557.

143 Knapp HR: Dietary fatty acids in human thrombosis and hemostasis. Am J Clin Nutr 1997;65: 1687S–1698S.

144 Mori A, Saito M, Sakamoto K, Nakahara T, Ishii K: Intravenously administered vasodilatory prostaglandins increase retinal and choroidal blood flow in rats. J Pharmacol Sci 2007;103:103–112.

145 Appel LJ, Miller ER 3rd, Seidler AJ, Whelton PK: Does supplementation of diet with 'fish oil' reduce blood pressure? A meta-analysis of controlled clinical trials. Arch Intern Med 1993;153:1429–1438.

146 Morris MC, Sacks F, Rosner B: Does fish oil lower blood pressure? A meta-analysis of controlled trials. Circulation 1993;88:523–533.

147 Agren JJ, Vaisanen S, Hanninen O, Muller AD, Hornstra G: Hemostatic factors and platelet aggregation after a fish-enriched diet or fish oil or docosahexaenoic acid supplementation. Prostaglandins Leukot Essent Fatty Acids 1997;57:419–421.

148 Mori TA, Beilin LJ, Burke V, Morris J, Ritchie J: Interactions between dietary fat, fish, and fish oils and their effects on platelet function in men at risk of cardiovascular disease. Arterioscler Thromb Vasc Biol 1997;17:279–286.

149 Harris WS: n–3 fatty acids and serum lipoproteins: human studies. Am J Clin Nutr 1997;65:1645S– 1654S.

150 Jump DB: Dietary polyunsaturated fatty acids and regulation of gene transcription. Curr Opin Lipidol 2002;13:155–164.

151 Khan JC, Shahid H, Thurlby DA, Bradley M, Clayton DG, Moore AT, Bird AC, Yates JR: Age-related macular degeneration and sun exposure, iris colour, and skin sensitivity to sunlight. Br J Ophthalmol 2006;90:29–32.

152 Chen Y, Houghton LA, Brenna JT, Noy N: Docosahexaenoic acid modulates the interactions of the interphotoreceptor retinoid-binding protein with 11-cis-retinal. J Biol Chem 1996;271:20507–20515.

153 Chen Y, Saari JC, Noy N: Interactions of all-trans-retinol and long-chain fatty acids with interphotoreceptor retinoid-binding protein. Biochemistry 1993;32:11311–11318.

154 Organisciak DT, Darrow RM, Barsalou L, Darrow RA, Kutty RK, Kutty G, Wiggert B: Light history and age-related changes in retinal light damage. Invest Ophthalmol Vis Sci 1998;39:1107–1116.

155 Brenna JT, Diau GY: The influence of dietary docosahexaenoic acid and arachidonic acid on central nervous system polyunsaturated fatty acid composition. Prostaglandins Leukot Essent Fatty Acids 2007;77:247–250.

156 Grynberg A, Demaison L: Fatty acid oxidation in the heart. J Cardiovasc Pharmacol 1996;28:S11–S17.

157 Demaison L, Sergiel JP, Moreau D, Grynberg A: Influence of the phospholipid n–6/n–3 polyunsaturated fatty acid ratio on the mitochondrial oxidative metabolism before and after myocardial ischemia. Biochim Biophys Acta 1994;1227:53–59.

158 Pieri C: Fatty acids and aging; in Chow KC (ed): Fatty Acids in Foods and Their Health Implications. New York, Dekker, 2000, pp 763–776.

159 Yu BP, Yang R: Critical evaluation of the free radical theory of aging. A proposal for the oxidative stress hypothesis. Ann NY Acad Sci 1996;786:1–11.

160 Feher J, Kovacs B, Kovacs I, Schveoller M, Papale A, Balacco Gabrieli C: Improvement of visual functions and fundus alterations in early age-related macular degeneration treated with a combination of acetyl-L-carnitine, n–3 fatty acids, and coenzyme q10. Ophthalmologica 2005;219:154–166.

161 Van Kuijk FJ, Buck P: Fatty acid composition of the human macula and peripheral retina. Invest Ophthalmol Vis Sci 1992;33:3493–3496.

162 Muggli R: n–3 long-chain polyunsaturated fatty acids and vitamin E in cardiovascular disease prevention: epiphenomenon or causal dependency? In Huang YS, Lin SJ, Huang PC (eds): Essential Fatty acids and Eicosanoids – Invited Papers from the Fifth International Congress. Champaign/IL, AOCS Press, 2003, pp 65–70.

163 Mabile L, Piolot A, Boulet L, Fortin LJ, Doyle N, Rodriguez C, Davignon J, Blache D, Lussier-Cacan S: Moderate intake of n–3 fatty acids is associated with stable erythrocyte resistance to oxidative stress in hypertriglyceridemic subjects. Am J Clin Nutr 2001;74:449–456.

164 Wander RC, Du SH, Thomas DR: Influence of long-chain polyunsaturated fatty acids on oxidation of low density lipoprotein. Prostaglandins Leukot Essent Fatty Acids 1998;59:143–151.

165 Mori TA, Puddey IB, Burke V, Croft KD, Dunstan DW, Rivera JH, Beilin LJ: Effect of omega–3 fatty acids on oxidative stress in humans: GC-MS measurement of urinary F2-isoprostane excretion. Redox Rep 2000;5:45–46.

166 Luostarinen R, Saldeen T: Dietary fish oil decreases superoxide generation by human neutrophils: relation to cyclooxygenase pathway and lysosomal enzyme release. Prostaglandins Leukot Essent Fatty Acids 1996;55:167–172.

167 Chen LY, Lawson DL, Mehta JL: Reduction in human neutrophil superoxide anion generation by n–3 polyunsaturated fatty acids: role of cyclooxygenase products and endothelium-derived relaxing factor. Thromb Res 1994;76:317–322.

168 Higgins S, Carroll YL, McCarthy SN, Corridan BM, Roche HM, Wallace JM, O'Brien NM, Morrissey PA: Susceptibility of LDL to oxidative modification in healthy volunteers supplemented with low doses of n–3 polyunsaturated fatty acids. Br J Nutr 2001; 85:23–31.

169 Brude IR, Drevon CA, Hjermann I, Seljeflot I, Lund-Katz S, Saarem K, Sandstad B, Solvoll K, Halvorsen B, Arnesen H, Nenseter MS: Peroxidation of LDL from combined-hyperlipidemic male smokers supplied with omega–3 fatty acids and antioxidants. Arterioscler Thromb Vasc Biol 1997;17:2576–2588.

170 Bonanome A, Biasia F, De Luca M, Munaretto G, Biffanti S, Pradella M, Pagnan A: n–3 fatty acids do not enhance LDL susceptibility to oxidation in hypertriacylglycerolemic hemodialyzed subjects. Am J Clin Nutr 1996;63:261–266.

171 Ando M, Sanaka T, Nihei H: Eicosapentanoic acid reduces plasma levels of remnant lipoproteins and prevents in vivo peroxidation of LDL in dialysis patients. J Am Soc Nephrol 1999;10:2177–2184.

172 Vericel E, Polette A, Bacot S, Calzada C, Lagarde M: Pro- and antioxidant activities of docosahexaenoic acid on human blood platelets. J Thromb Haemost 2003;1:566–572.

173 De La Paz M, Anderson RE: Region and age-dependent variation in susceptibility of the human retina to lipid peroxidation. Invest Ophthalmol Vis Sci 1992;33:3497–3499.

174 Bush RA, Reme CE, Malnoe A: Light damage in the rat retina: the effect of dietary deprivation of n–3 fatty acids on acute structural alterations. Exp Eye Res 1991;53:741–752.

175 Organisciak DT, Darrow RM, Jiang YL, Blanks JC: Retinal light damage in rats with altered levels of rod outer segment docosahexaenoate. Invest Ophthalmol Vis Sci 1996;37:2243–2257.

176 Barbosa-Sicard E, Markovic M, Honeck H, Christ B, Muller DN, Schunck WH: Eicosapentaenoic acid metabolism by cytochrome P450 enzymes of the CYP2C subfamily. Biochem Biophys Res Commun 2005;329:1275–1281.

177 Politi LE, Rotstein NP, Carri NG: Effect of GDNF on neuroblast proliferation and photoreceptor survival: additive protection with docosahexaenoic acid. Invest Ophthalmol Vis Sci 2001;42:3008–3015.

178 Uauy R, Hoffman DR, Peirano P, Birch DG, Birch EE: Essential fatty acids in visual and brain development. Lipids 2001;36:885–895.

179 German OL, Miranda GE, Abrahan CE, Rotstein NP: Ceramide is a mediator of apoptosis in retina photoreceptors. Invest Ophthalmol Vis Sci 2006;47:1658–1668.

180 Calder PC: Polyunsaturated fatty acids, inflammation, and immunity. Lipids 2001;36:1007–1024.

181 Sijben JW, Calder PC: Differential immunomodulation with long-chain n–3 PUFA in health and chronic disease. Proc Nutr Soc 2007;66:237–259.

182 Serhan CN: Resolution phase of inflammation: novel endogenous anti-inflammatory and prore-solving lipid mediators and pathways. Annu Rev Immunol 2007;25:101–137.

183 Wallace FA, Miles EA, Calder PC: Activation state alters the effect of dietary fatty acids on pro-inflammatory mediator production by murine macrophages. Cytokine 2000;12:1374–1379.

184 Rose DP, Connolly JM: Regulation of tumor angiogenesis by dietary fatty acids and eicosanoids. Nutr Cancer 2000;37:119–127.

185 Nie D, Hillman GG, Geddes T, Tang K, Pierson C, Grignon DJ, Honn KV: Platelet-type 12-lipoxygenase in a human prostate carcinoma stimulates angiogenesis and tumor growth. Cancer Res 1998;58:4047–4051.

186 Tang DG, Renaud C, Stojakovic S, Diglio CA, Porter A, Honn KV: 12(S)-HETE is a mitogenic factor for microvascular endothelial cells: its potential role in angiogenesis. Biochem Biophys Res Commun 1995; 211:462–468.

187 Tang DG, Diglio CA, Bazaz R, Honn KV: Transcriptional activation of endothelial cell integrin alpha v by protein kinase C activator 12(S)-HETE. J Cell Sci 1995;108:2629–2644.

188 Liu B, Timar J, Howlett J, Diglio CA, Honn KV: Lipoxygenase metabolites of arachidonic and linoleic acids modulate the adhesion of tumor cells to endothelium via regulation of protein kinase C. Cell Regul 1991;2:1045–1055.

189 Talvani A, Machado FS, Santana GC, Klein A, Barcelos L, Silva JS, Teixeira MM: Leukotriene B_4 induces nitric oxide synthesis in *Trypanosoma cruzi*-infected murine macrophages and mediates resistance to infection. Infect Immun 2002;70:4247–4253.

190 Limb GA, Chignell AH, Green W, LeRoy F, Dumonde DC: Distribution of TNF-α and its reactive vascular adhesion molecules in fibrovascular membranes of proliferative diabetic retinopathy. Br J Ophthalmol 1996;80:168–173.

191 Limb GA, Hollifield RD, Webster L, Charteris DG, Chignell AH: Soluble TNF receptors in vitreoretinal proliferative disease. Invest Ophthalmol Vis Sci 2001;42:1586–1591.

192 Hawrami K, Hitman GA, Rema M, Snehalatha C, Viswanathan M, Ramachandran A, Mohan V: An association in non-insulin-dependent diabetes mellitus subjects between susceptibility to retinopathy and tumor necrosis factor polymorphism. Hum Immunol 1996;46:49–54.

193 Limb GA, Soomro H, Janikoun S, Hollifield RD, Shilling J: Evidence for control of tumour necrosis factor-α (TNF-α) activity by TNF receptors in patients with proliferative diabetic retinopathy. Clin Exp Immunol 1999;115:409–414.

194 Yossuck P, Yan Y, Tadesse M, Higgins RD: Dexamethasone alters TNF-α expression in retinopathy. Mol Genet Metab 2001;72:164–167.

195 Hughes DA, Southon S, Pinder AC: n–3 polyunsaturated fatty acids modulate the expression of functionally associated molecules on human monocytes in vitro. J Nutr 1996;126:603–610.

196 Baldie G, Kaimakamis D, Rotondo D: Fatty acid modulation of cytokine release from human monocytic cells. Biochim Biophys Acta 1993;1179:125–133.

197 Purasiri P, McKechnie A, Heys SD, Eremin O: Modulation in vitro of human natural cytotoxicity, lymphocyte proliferative response to mitogens and cytokine production by essential fatty acids. Immunology 1997;92:166–172.

198 Yamashita N, Yokoyama A, Hamazaki T, Yano S: Inhibition of natural killer cell activity of human lymphocytes by eicosapentaenoic acid. Biochem Biophys Res Commun 1986;138:1058–1067.

199 Calder PC, Newsholme EA: Polyunsaturated fatty acids suppress human peripheral blood lymphocyte proliferation and interleukin-2 production. Clin Sci (Lond) 1992;82:695–700.

200 Santoli D, Phillips PD, Colt TL, Zurier RB: Suppression of interleukin-2-dependent human T-cell growth in vitro by prostaglandin E (PGE) and their precursor fatty acids. Evidence for a PGE-independent mechanism of inhibition by the fatty acids. J Clin Invest 1990;85:424–432.

201 Calder PC, Bevan SJ, Newsholme EA: The inhibition of T-lymphocyte proliferation by fatty acids is via an eicosanoid-independent mechanism. Immunology 1992;75:108–115.

202 Virella G, Fourspring K, Hyman B, Haskill-Stroud R, Long L, Virella I, La Via M, Gross AJ, Lopes-Virella M: Immunosuppressive effects of fish oil in normal human volunteers: correlation with the in vitro effects of eicosapentanoic acid on human lymphocytes. Clin Immunol Immunopathol 1991;61: 161–176.

203 Khalfoun B, Thibault G, Lacord M, Gruel Y, Bardos P, Lebranchu Y: Docosahexaenoic and eicosapentaenoic acids inhibit human lymphoproliferative responses in vitro but not the expression of T-cell surface activation markers. Scand J Immunol 1996; 43:248–256.

204 Brouard C, Pascaud M: Modulation of rat and human lymphocyte function by n–6 and n–3 polyunsaturated fatty acids and acetylsalicylic acid. Ann Nutr Metab 1993;37:146–159.

205 Tappia PS, Man WJ, Grimble RF: Influence of unsaturated fatty acids on the production of tumour necrosis factor and interleukin-6 by rat peritoneal macrophages. Mol Cell Biochem 1995;143:89–98.

206 De Caterina R, Liao JK, Libby P: Fatty acid modulation of endothelial activation. Am J Clin Nutr 2000;71:213S–223S.

207 Eicher SD, McVey DS: Dietary modulation of Kupffer cell and splenocyte function during a *Salmonella typhimurium* challenge in mice. J Leukoc Biol 1995;58:32–39.

208 D'Ambola JB, Aeberhard EE, Trang N, Gaffar S, Barrett CT, Sherman MP: Effect of dietary n-3 and n-6 fatty acids on in vivo pulmonary bacterial clearance by neonatal rabbits. J Nutr 1991;121:1262–1269.

209 Joe B, Lokesh BR: Role of capsaicin, curcumin and dietary n–3 fatty acids in lowering the generation of reactive oxygen species in rat peritoneal macrophages. Biochim Biophys Acta 1994;1224:255–263.

210 Hubbard NE, Somers SD, Erickson KL: Effect of dietary fish oil on development and selected functions of murine inflammatory macrophages. J Leukoc Biol 1991;49:592–598.

211 Huang SC, Misfeldt ML, Fritsche KL: Dietary fat influences Ia antigen expression and immune cell populations in the murine peritoneum and spleen. J Nutr 1992;122:1219–1231.

212 Sanderson P, MacPherson GG, Jenkins CH, Calder PC: Dietary fish oil diminishes the antigen presentation activity of rat dendritic cells. J Leukoc Biol 1997;62:771–777.

213 Yaqoob P, Calder P: Effects of dietary lipid manipulation upon inflammatory mediator production by murine macrophages. Cell Immunol 1995;163:120–128.

214 Billiar TR, Bankey PE, Svingen BA, Curran RD, West MA, Holman RT, Simmons RL, Cerra FB: Fatty acid intake and Kupffer cell function: fish oil alters eicosanoid and monokine production to endotoxin stimulation. Surgery 1988;104:343–349.

215 Renier G, Skamene E, DeSanctis J, Radzioch D: Dietary n–3 polyunsaturated fatty acids prevent the development of atherosclerotic lesions in mice. Modulation of macrophage secretory activities. Arterioscler Thromb 1993;13:1515–1524.

216 Feng C, Keisler DH, Fritsche KL: Dietary omega–3 polyunsaturated fatty acids reduce IFN-γ receptor expression in mice. J Interferon Cytokine Res 1999; 19:41–48.

217 Grimm H, Tibell A, Norrlind B, Blecher C, Wilker S, Schwemmle K: Immunoregulation by parenteral lipids: impact of the n–3 to n–6 fatty acid ratio. JPEN J Parenter Enteral Nutr 1994;18:417–421.

218 Peterson LD, Jeffery NM, Thies F, Sanderson P, Newsholme EA, Calder PC: Eicosapentaenoic and docosahexaenoic acids alter rat spleen leukocyte fatty acid composition and prostaglandin E_2 production but have different effects on lymphocyte functions and cell-mediated immunity. Lipids 1998; 33:171–180.

219 Meydani SN, Yogeeswaran G, Liu S, Baskar S, Meydani M: Fish oil and tocopherol-induced changes in natural killer cell-mediated cytotoxicity and PGE_2 synthesis in young and old mice. J Nutr 1988;118: 1245–1252.

220 Yaqoob P, Newsholme EA, Calder PC: Inhibition of natural killer cell activity by dietary lipids. Immunol Lett 1994;41:241–247.

221 Sanderson P, Yaqoob P, Calder PC: Dietary lipid modulation of cell-mediated immunity in the rat. Biochem Soc Trans 1995;23:273S.

222 Fritsche KL, Cassity NA: Dietary n–3 fatty acids reduce antibody-dependent cell cytotoxicity and alter eicosanoid release by chicken immune cells. Poult Sci 1992;71:1646–1657.

223 Jolly CA, Jiang YH, Chapkin RS, McMurray DN: Dietary n–3 polyunsaturated fatty acids suppress murine lymphoproliferation, interleukin-2 secretion, and the formation of diacylglycerol and ceramide. J Nutr 1997;127:37–43.

224 Sanderson P, Thies F, Calder PC: Extracellular release of free fatty acids by rat T lymphocytes is stimulus-dependent and is affected by dietary lipid manipulation. Cell Biochem Funct 2000;18:47–58.

225 Yaqoob P, Newsholme EA, Calder PC: Fatty acid oxidation by lymphocytes. Biochem Soc Trans 1994; 22:116S.

226 Yaqoob P, Newsholme EA, Calder PC: The effect of dietary lipid manipulation on rat lymphocyte subsets and proliferation. Immunology 1994;82:603–610.

227 Yaqoob P, Calder PC: The effects of dietary lipid manipulation on the production of murine T-cell-derived cytokines. Cytokine 1995;7:548–553.

228 Alexander NJ, Smythe NL: Dietary fat modulation of in vitro lymphocyte function. Ann Nutr Metab 1988;32:192–199.

229 Kelley DS, Nelson GJ, Serrato CM, Schmidt PC, Branch LB: Effects of type of dietary fat on indices of immune status of rabbits. J Nutr 1988;118:1376–1384.

230 Fritsche KL, Cassity NA, Huang SC: Effect of dietary fat source on antibody production and lymphocyte proliferation in chickens. Poult Sci 1991;70:611–617.

231 Kuratko CN: Proliferation of colonic lymphocytes in response to inflammatory cytokines is lower in mice fed fish oil than in mice fed corn oil. Cancer Lett 2000;148:27–32.

232 Wallace FA, Miles EA, Evans C, Stock TE, Yaqoob P, Calder PC: Dietary fatty acids influence the production of Th1- but not Th2-type cytokines. J Leukoc Biol 2001;69:449–457.

233 Wallace FA: Dietary fatty acids influence the production of Th1- but not Th2-type cytokines. J Leukoc Biol 2001;69:449–457.

234 Schmidt EB, Pedersen JO, Ekelund S, Grunnet N, Jersild C, Dyerberg J: Cod liver oil inhibits neutrophil and monocyte chemotaxis in healthy males. Atherosclerosis 1989;77:53–57.

235 Schmidt EB, Varming K, Pedersen JO, Lervang HH, Grunnet N, Jersild C, Dyerberg J: Long-term supplementation with n–3 fatty acids. II. Effect on neutrophil and monocyte chemotaxis. Scand J Clin Lab Invest 1992;52:229–236.

236 Endres S, Ghorbani R, Kelley VE, Georgilis K, Lonnemann G, van der Meer JW, Cannon JG, Rogers TS, Klempner MS, Weber PC, et al: The effect of dietary supplementation with n–3 polyunsaturated fatty acids on the synthesis of interleukin-1 and tumor necrosis factor by mononuclear cells. N Engl J Med 1989;320:265–271.

237 Schmidt EB, Varming K, Moller JM, Bulow Pedersen I, Madsen P, Dyerberg J: No effect of a very low dose of n–3 fatty acids on monocyte function in healthy humans. Scand J Clin Lab Invest 1996;56:87–92.

238 Thies F, Nebe-von-Caron G, Powell JR, Yaqoob P, Newsholme EA, Calder PC: Dietary supplementation with eicosapentaenoic acid, but not with other long-chain n–3 or n–6 polyunsaturated fatty acids, decreases natural killer cell activity in healthy subjects aged >55 years. Am J Clin Nutr 2001;73:539–548.

239 Meydani SN, Endres S, Woods MM, Goldin BR, Soo C, Morrill-Labrode A, Dinarello CA, Gorbach SL: Oral n-3 fatty acid supplementation suppresses cytokine production and lymphocyte proliferation: comparison between young and older women. J Nutr 1991;121:547–555.

240 Molvig J, Pociot F, Worsaae H, Wogensen LD, Baek L, Christensen P, Mandrup-Poulsen T, Andersen K, Madsen P, Dyerberg J, et al: Dietary supplementation with omega–3-polyunsaturated fatty acids decreases mononuclear cell proliferation and interleukin-1β content but not monokine secretion in healthy and insulin-dependent diabetic individuals. Scand J Immunol 1991;34:399–410.

241 Caughey GE, Mantzioris E, Gibson RA, Cleland LG, James MJ: The effect on human tumor necrosis factor-α and interleukin 1β production of diets enriched in n–3 fatty acids from vegetable oil or fish oil. Am J Clin Nutr 1996;63:116–122.

242 Gallai V, Sarchielli P, Trequattrini A, Franceschini M, Floridi A, Firenze C, Alberti A, Di Benedetto D, Stragliotto E: Cytokine secretion and eicosanoid production in the peripheral blood mononuclear cells of ms patients undergoing dietary supplementation with n–3 polyunsaturated fatty acids. J Neuroimmunol 1995;56:143–153.

243 Yaqoob P, Pala HS, Cortina-Borja M, Newsholme EA, Calder PC: Encapsulated fish oil enriched in α-tocopherol alters plasma phospholipid and mononuclear cell fatty acid compositions but not mononuclear cell functions. Eur J Clin Invest 2000;30:260–274.

244 Cooper AL, Gibbons L, Horan MA, Little RA, Rothwell NJ: Effect of dietary fish oil supplementation on fever and cytokine production in human volunteers. Clin Nutr 1993;12:321–328.

245 Blok WL, Deslypere JP, Demacker PN, van der Ven-Jongekrijg J, Hectors MP, van der Meer JW, Katan MB: Pro- and anti-inflammatory cytokines in healthy volunteers fed various doses of fish oil for 1 year. Eur J Clin Invest 1997;27:1003–1008.

246 Cannon JG, Fiatarone MA, Meydani M, Gong J, Scott L, Blumberg JB, Evans WJ: Aging and dietary modulation of elastase and interleukin-1β secretion. Am J Physiol 1995;268:R208–R213.

247 Meydani SN, Lichtenstein AH, Cornwall S, Meydani M, Goldin BR, Rasmussen H, Dinarello CA, Schaefer EJ: Immunologic effects of national cholesterol education panel step-2 diets with and without fish-derived n–3 fatty acid enrichment. J Clin Invest 1993;92:105–113.

248 Gottlicher M, Demoz A, Svensson D, Tollet P, Berge RK, Gustafsson JA: Structural and metabolic requirements for activators of the peroxisome proliferator-activated receptor. Biochem Pharmacol 1993;46:2177–2184.

249 Dreyer C, Keller H, Mahfoudi A, Laudet V, Krey G, Wahli W: Positive regulation of the peroxisomal β-oxidation pathway by fatty acids through activation of peroxisome proliferator-activated receptors. Biol Cell 1993;77:67–76.

250 Yu K, Bayona W, Kallen CB, Harding HP, Ravera CP, McMahon G, Brown M, Lazar MA: Differential activation of peroxisome proliferator-activated receptors by eicosanoids. J Biol Chem 1995;270:23975–23983.

251 Dubuquoy L, Dharancy S, Nutten S, Pettersson S, Auwerx J, Desreumaux P: Role of peroxisome proliferator-activated receptor γ and retinoid X receptor heterodimer in hepatogastroenterological diseases. Lancet 2002;360:1410–1418.

252 Jump DB: Fatty acid regulation of gene transcription. Crit Rev Clin Lab Sci 2004;41:41–78.

253 Joussen AM, Poulaki V, Mitsiades N, Kirchhof B, Koizumi K, Dohmen S, Adamis AP: Nonsteroidal anti-inflammatory drugs prevent early diabetic retinopathy via TNF-α suppression. FASEB J 2002;16:438–440.

254 Williams B, Schrier RW: Glucose-induced protein kinase C activity regulates arachidonic acid release and eicosanoid production by cultured glomerular mesangial cells. J Clin Invest 1993;92:2889–2896.

255 Rose DP, Connolly JM, Rayburn J, Coleman M: Influence of diets containing eicosapentaenoic or docosahexaenoic acid on growth and metastasis of breast cancer cells in nude mice. J Natl Cancer Inst 1995;87:587–592.

256 Rose DP, Connolly JM: Antiangiogenicity of docosahexaenoic acid and its role in the suppression of breast cancer cell growth in nude mice. Int J Oncol 1999;15:1011–1015.

257 Badawi AF, El-Sohemy A, Stephen LL, Ghoshal AK, Archer MC: The effect of dietary n–3 and n–6 polyunsaturated fatty acids on the expression of cyclooxygenase 1 and 2 and levels of p21ras in rat mammary glands. Carcinogenesis 1998;19:905–910.

258 Hamid R, Singh J, Reddy BS, Cohen LA: Inhibition by dietary menhaden oil of cyclooxygenase-1 and -2 in N-nitrosomethylurea-induced rat mammary tumors. Int J Oncol 1999;14:523–528.

259 Ayalasomayajula SP, Kompella UB: Celecoxib, a selective cyclooxygenase-2 inhibitor, inhibits retinal vascular endothelial growth factor expression and vascular leakage in a streptozotocin-induced diabetic rat model. Eur J Pharmacol 2003;458:283–289.

260 Ozaki NK, Beharry KD, Nishihara KC, Akmal Y, Ang JG, Sheikh R, Modanlou HD: Regulation of retinal vascular endothelial growth factor and receptors in rabbits exposed to hyperoxia. Invest Ophthalmol Vis Sci 2002;43:1546–1557.

261 Masferrer JL, Leahy KM, Koki AT, Zweifel BS, Settle SL, Woerner BM, Edwards DA, Flickinger AG, Moore RJ, Seibert K: Antiangiogenic and antitumor activities of cyclooxygenase-2 inhibitors. Cancer Res 2000;60:1306–1311.

262 Bicknell R, Vallee BL: Angiogenin stimulates endothelial cell prostacyclin secretion by activation of phospholipase A_2. Proc Natl Acad Sci USA 1989; 86:1573–1577.

263 Szymczak M, Murray M, Petrovic N: Modulation of angiogenesis by omega–3 polyunsaturated fatty acids is mediated by cyclooxygenases. Blood 2008; 111:3514–3521.

264 Pehowich DJ: Dietary n–3 fatty acids alter angiotensin-induced contraction and 1,2-diacylglycerol fatty acid composition in thoracic aortas from diabetic rats. Prostaglandins Leukot Essent Fatty Acids 1998;58:301–309.

265 Murota SI, Onodera M, Morita I: Regulation of angiogenesis by controlling VEGF receptor. Ann NY Acad Sci 2000;902:208–213.

266 Kanayasu T, Morita I, Nakao-Hayashi J, Ito H, Murota S: Enhancement of migration in bovine endothelial cells by eicosapentaenoic acid pretreatment. Atherosclerosis 1991;87:57–64.

267 Liu J, Vanttinen T, Hyden-Granskog C, Voutilainen R: Regulation of follistatin-related gene expression by protein kinase C and prostaglandin E_2 in cultured granulosa-luteal cells. Mol Hum Reprod 2002; 8:992–997.

268 Nakata H, Uemura Y, Kobayashi M, Harada R, Taguchi H: Cyclooxygenase-2 inhibitor NS-398 suppresses cell growth and constitutive production of granulocyte-colony stimulating factor and granulocyte macrophage-colony stimulating factor in lung cancer cells. Cancer Sci 2003;94:173–180.

269 Cammisotto PG, Gelinas Y, Deshaies Y, Bukowiecki LJ: Regulation of leptin secretion from white adipocytes by free fatty acids. Am J Physiol 2003;285: E521–E526.

270 Reseland JE, Haugen F, Hollung K, Solvoll K, Halvorsen B, Brude IR, Nenseter MS, Christiansen EN, Drevon CA: Reduction of leptin gene expression by dietary polyunsaturated fatty acids. J Lipid Res 2001;42:743–750.

271 Nitta K, Uchida K, Tsutsui T, Honda K, Kawashima A, Yumura W, Nihei H: Eicosapentaenoic acid inhibits mitogen-induced endothelin-1 production and DNA synthesis in cultured bovine mesangial cells. Am J Nephrol 1998;18:164–170.

272 Hida M, Fujita H, Ishikura K, Omori S, Hoshiya M, Awazu M: Eicosapentaenoic acid inhibits PDGF-induced mitogenesis and cyclin D1 expression via TGF-β in mesangial cells. J Cell Physiol 2003;196: 293–300.

273 Kohno M, Yasunari K, Minami M, Kano H, Maeda K, Yoshikawa J: Suppression by eicosapentaenoic acid of oxidized low-density lipoprotein and lysophosphatidylcholine-induced migration in cultured rat vascular smooth muscle cells. Metabolism 2000; 49:560–562.

274 Yu W, Murray NR, Weems C, Chen L, Guo H, Ethridge R, Ceci JD, Evers BM, Thompson EA, Fields AP: Role of cyclooxygenase-2 in protein kinase C β II-mediated colon carcinogenesis. J Biol Chem 2003;278:11167–11174.

275 Trebble T, Arden NK, Stroud MA, Wootton SA, Burdge GC, Miles EA, Ballinger AB, Thompson RL, Calder PC: Inhibition of tumour necrosis factor-α and interleukin-6 production by mononuclear cells following dietary fish-oil supplementation in healthy men and response to antioxidant co-supplementation. Br J Nutr 2003;90:405–412.

276 Mickleborough TD, Murray RL, Ionescu AA, Lindley MR: Fish oil supplementation reduces severity of exercise-induced bronchoconstriction in elite athletes. Am J Respir Crit Care Med 2003;168:1181–1189.

277 Babcock TA, Helton WS, Hong D, Espat NJ: Omega–3 fatty acid lipid emulsion reduces LPS-stimulated macrophage TNF-α production. Surg Infect (Larchmt) 2002;3:145–149.

278 Kielar ML, Jeyarajah DR, Zhou XJ, Lu CY: Docosahexaenoic acid ameliorates murine ischemic acute renal failure and prevents increases in MRNA abundance for both TNF-α and inducible nitric oxide synthase. J Am Soc Nephrol 2003;14:389–396.

279 Tsuji M, Murota SI, Morita I: Docosapentaenoic acid (22:5,n–3) suppressed tube-forming activity in endothelial cells induced by vascular endothelial growth factor. Prostaglandins Leukot Essent Fatty Acids 2003;68:337–342.

280 Zhang YW, Yao XS, Murota S, Morita I: Inhibitory effects of eicosapentaenoic acid on the hypoxia/reoxygenation-induced tyrosine kinase activation in cultured human umbilical vein endothelial cells. Prostaglandins Leukot Essent Fatty Acids 2002;67: 253–261.

281 Tevar R, Jho DH, Babcock T, Helton WS, Espat NJ: Omega–3 fatty acid supplementation reduces tumor growth and vascular endothelial growth factor expression in a model of progressive non-metastasizing malignancy. JPEN J Parenter Enteral Nutr 2002;26:285–289.

282 Rose DP, Connolly JM: Omega–3 fatty acids as cancer chemopreventive agents. Pharmacol Ther 1999; 83:217–244.

283 Yang SP, Morita I, Murota SI: Eicosapentaenoic acid attenuates vascular endothelial growth factor-induced proliferation via inhibiting Flk-1 receptor expression in bovine carotid artery endothelial cells. J Cell Physiol 1998;176:342–349.

284 Mukutmoni M, Hubbard NE, Erickson KL: Prostaglandin E_2 modulation of vascular endothelial growth factor production in murine macrophages. Prostaglandins Leukot Essent Fatty Acids 2001; 65: 123–131.

285 Aiello LP, Wong JS: Role of vascular endothelial growth factor in diabetic vascular complications. Kidney Int Suppl 2000;77:S113–S119.

286 Ferrara N, Davis-Smyth T: The biology of vascular endothelial growth factor. Endocr Rev 1997;18:4–25.

287 Smith LE: Pathogenesis of retinopathy of prematurity. Acta Paediatr Suppl 2002;91:26–28.

288 Lu M, Adamis AP: Vascular endothelial growth factor gene regulation and action in diabetic retinopathy. Ophthalmol Clin North Am 2002;15:69–79.

289 Aiello LP: Clinical implications of vascular growth factors in proliferative retinopathies. Curr Opin Ophthalmol 1997;8:19–31.

290 Kanayasu T, Morita I, Nakao-Hayashi J, Asuwa N, Fujisawa C, Ishii T, Ito H, Murota S: Eicosapentaenoic acid inhibits tube formation of vascular endothelial cells in vitro. Lipids 1991;26:271–276.

291 Von Knethen A, Callsen D, Brune B: Superoxide attenuates macrophage apoptosis by NF-κB and AP-1 activation that promotes cyclooxygenase-2 expression. J Immunol 1999;163:2858–2866.

292 Abribat T, Nedelec B, Jobin N, Garrel DR: Decreased serum insulin-like growth factor-1 in burn patients: relationship with serum insulin-like growth factor binding protein-3 proteolysis and the influence of lipid composition in nutritional support. Crit Care Med 2000;28:2366–2372.

293 Akbar M, Kim HY: Protective effects of docosahexaenoic acid in staurosporine-induced apoptosis: involvement of phosphatidylinositol-3 kinase pathway. J Neurochem 2002;82:655–665.

294 Hellstrom A, Perruzzi C, Ju M, Engstrom E, Hard AL, Liu JL, Albertsson-Wikland K, Carlsson B, Niklasson A, Sjodell L, LeRoith D, Senger DR, Smith LE: Low IGF-1 suppresses VEGF-survival signaling in retinal endothelial cells: direct correlation with clinical retinopathy of prematurity. Proc Natl Acad Sci USA 2001;98:5804–5808.

295 Kumar S, Boehm J, Lee JC: P38 MAP kinases: key signalling molecules as therapeutic targets for inflammatory diseases. Nat Rev Drug Discov 2003; 2:717–726.

296 Bogatcheva NV, Dudek SM, Garcia JG, Verin AD: Mitogen-activated protein kinases in endothelial pathophysiology. J Investig Med 2003;51:341–352.

297 Morita I, Zhang YW, Murota SI: Eicosapentaenoic acid protects endothelial cell function injured by hypoxia/reoxygenation. Ann NY Acad Sci 2001;947: 394–397.

298 Du Toit PJ, van Aswegen CH, du Plessis DJ: The effect of essential fatty acids on growth and urokinase-type plasminogen activator production in human prostate DU-145 cells. Prostaglandins Leukot Essent Fatty Acids 1996;55:173–177.

299 McGuire PG, Jones TR, Talarico N, Warren E, Das A: The urokinase/urokinase receptor system in retinal neovascularization: inhibition by A6 suggests a new therapeutic target. Invest Ophthalmol Vis Sci 2003;44:2736–2742.

300 Pakala R, Radcliffe JD, Benedict CR: Serotonin-induced endothelial cell proliferation is blocked by omega–3 fatty acids. Prostaglandins Leukot Essent Fatty Acids 1999;60:115–123.

301 Pakala R, Sheng WL, Benedict CR: Serotonin fails to induce proliferation of endothelial cells preloaded with eicosapentaenoic acid and docosahexaenoic acid. Atherosclerosis 1999;145:137–146.

302 Dominguez Z, Merhi-Soussi F, MacOvschi O, Nemoz G, Lagarde M, Prigent AF: Endothelial cell prostacyclin synthesis induced by lymphocytes is independent of the membrane fatty acid composition of both cell types and of E-selectin, VCAM-1 or ICAM-1-mediated adhesion. Br J Haematol 2001; 113:521–532.

303 Collie-Duguid ES, Wahle KW: Inhibitory effect of fish oil n–3 polyunsaturated fatty acids on the expression of endothelial cell adhesion molecules. Biochem Biophys Res Commun 1996;220:969–974.

304 Sivak JM, Fini ME: MMPS in the eye: emerging roles for matrix metalloproteinases in ocular physiology. Prog Retin Eye Res 2002;21:1–14.

305 Majka S, McGuire P, Colombo S, Das A: The balance between proteinases and inhibitors in a murine model of proliferative retinopathy. Invest Ophthalmol Vis Sci 2001;42:210–215.

306 Majka S, McGuire PG, Das A: Regulation of matrix metalloproteinase expression by tumor necrosis factor in a murine model of retinal neovascularization. Invest Ophthalmol Vis Sci 2002;43:260–266.

307 Harris MA, Hansen RA, Vidsudhiphan P, Koslo JL, Thomas JB, Watkins BA, Allen KG: Effects of conjugated linoleic acids and docosahexaenoic acid on rat liver and reproductive tissue fatty acids, prostaglandins and matrix metalloproteinase production. Prostaglandins Leukot Essent Fatty Acids 2001;65:23–29.

308 Suzuki I, Iigo M, Ishikawa C, Kuhara T, Asamoto M, Kunimoto T, Moore MA, Yazawa K, Araki E, Tsuda H: Inhibitory effects of oleic and docosahexaenoic acids on lung metastasis by colon-carcinoma-26 cells are associated with reduced matrix metalloproteinase-2 and -9 activities. Int J Cancer 1997;73:607–612.

309 Liu XH, Rose DP: Suppression of type IV collagenase in MDA-MB-435 human breast cancer cells by eicosapentaenoic acid in vitro and in vivo. Cancer Lett 1995;92:21–26.

310 Diep QN, Amiri F, Touyz RM, Cohn JS, Endemann D, Neves MF, Schiffrin EL: PPAR-α activator effects on Ang II-induced vascular oxidative stress and inflammation. Hypertension 2002;40:866–871.

311 Hirafuji M, Machida T, Hamaue N, Minami M: Cardiovascular protective effects of n–3 polyunsaturated fatty acids with special emphasis on docosahexaenoic acid. J Pharmacol Sci 2003;92:308–316.

312 Hirafuji M, Machida T, Tsunoda M, Miyamoto A, Minami M: Docosahexaenoic acid potentiates interleukin-1β induction of nitric oxide synthase through mechanism involving p44/42 MAPK activation in rat vascular smooth muscle cells. Br J Pharmacol 2002;136:613–619.

313 Curtis CL, Rees SG, Little CB, Flannery CR, Hughes CE, Wilson C, Dent CM, Otterness IG, Harwood JL, Caterson B: Pathologic indicators of degradation and inflammation in human osteoarthritic cartilage are abrogated by exposure to n–3 fatty acids. Arthritis Rheum 2002;46:1544–1553.

314 Grynberg A, Fournier A, Sergiel JP, Athias P: Membrane docosahexaenoic acid vs. eicosapentaenoic acid and the beating function of the cardiomyocyte and its regulation through the adrenergic receptors. Lipids 1996;31(suppl):S205–S210.

315 Kim HY, Akbar M, Kim KY: Inhibition of neuronal apoptosis by polyunsaturated fatty acids. J Mol Neurosci 2001;16:223–227, 279–284.

316 El-seweidy MM, El-swefy SE, Ameen RS, Hashem RM: Effect of age receptor blocker and/or anti-inflammatory coadministration in relation to glycation, oxidative stress and cytokine production in STZ diabetic rats. Pharmacol Res 2002;45:391–398.

317 Kaur M, Kaur J, Ojha S, Mahmood A: Dietary fat effects on brush border membrane composition and enzyme activities in rat intestine. Ann Nutr Metab 1996;40:269–276.

318 Klein RJ, Zeiss C, Chew EY, Tsai JY, Sackler RS, Haynes C, Henning AK, SanGiovanni JP, Mane SM, Mayne ST, Bracken MB, Ferris FL, Ott J, Barnstable C, Hoh J: Complement factor h polymorphism in age-related macular degeneration. Science 2005;308:385–389.

319 AREDS Research Group: The Age-Related Eye Disease Study (AREDS): Design implications. AREDS Report No 1. Control Clin Trials 1999;20:573–600.

320 Ross RJ, Verma V, Rosenberg KI, Chan CC, Tuo J: Genetic markers and biomarkers for age-related macular degeneration. Expert Rev Ophthalmol 2007;2:443–457.

321 Leveziel N, Souied EH, Richard F, Barbu V, Zourdani A, Morineau G, Zerbib J, Coscas G, Soubrane G, Benlian P: PLEKHA1-LOC387715-HTRA1 polymorphisms and exudative age-related macular degeneration in the French population. Mol Vis 2007;13:2153–2159.

322 Deangelis MM, Ji F, Adams S, Morrison MA, Harring AJ, Sweeney MO, Capone A Jr, Miller JW, Dryja TP, Ott J, Kim IK: Alleles in the HTRA serine peptidase 1 gene alter the risk of neovascular age-related macular degeneration. Ophthalmology 2008;115: 1209–1215.

323 Itoh T, Takenawa T: Phosphoinositide-binding domains: functional units for temporal and spatial regulation of intracellular signalling. Cell Signal 2002;14:733–743.

324 Lemmon MA: Pleckstrin homology domains and phosphoinositides. Biochem Soc Symp 2007:81–93.

325 Hawkins PT, Stephens LR: PI3kγ is a key regulator of inflammatory responses and cardiovascular homeostasis. Science 2007;318:64–66.

326 Akbar M, Calderon F, Wen Z, Kim HY: Docosahexaenoic acid: a positive modulator of Akt signaling in neuronal survival. Proc Natl Acad Sci USA 2005;102:10858–10863.

327 Szado T, Vanderheyden V, Parys JB, De Smedt H, Rietdorf K, Kotelevets L, Chastre E, Khan F, Landegren U, Soderberg O, Bootman MD, Roderick HL: Phosphorylation of inositol 1,4,5-trisphosphate receptors by protein kinase B/Akt inhibits Ca^{2+} release and apoptosis. Proc Natl Acad Sci USA 2008; 105:2427–2432.

328 Siddiqui RA, Harvey KA, Zaloga GP: Modulation of enzymatic activities by n–3 polyunsaturated fatty acids to support cardiovascular health. J Nutr Biochem 2008;19:417–437.

329 Jude S, Roger S, Martel E, Besson P, Richard S, Bougnoux P, Champeroux P, Le Guennec JY: Dietary long-chain omega–3 fatty acids of marine origin: a comparison of their protective effects on coronary heart disease and breast cancers. Prog Biophys Mol Biol 2006;90:299–325.

John Paul SanGiovanni, ScD
National Eye Institute, Clinical Trials Branch
National Institutes of Health, 10 Center Drive, MSC-1204
Building 10, CRC, Room 3-2521, Bethesda, MD 20892-1204 (USA)
Tel. +1 301 496 6583, Fax +1 301 496 7295, E-Mail jpsangio@nei.nih.gov

Author Index

Subject Index

Fish oil, *see* Docosahexaenoic acid; Eicosapentaenoic acid

Hill criteria, causality
consistency 19, 20
specificity 20, 21
strength 19
HTRA1, age-related macular degeneration susceptibility gene 139
Huntington's disease
clinical features 36, 37
eicosapentaenoic acid
mechanisms of action 39, 40
therapy 37–39
pathophysiology 37

Ischemia-reperfusion injury, docosahexaenoic acid mediation 52

Kennedy cycle, phosphatidylcholine synthesis 72–74

LA, *see* Linoleic acid
Linoleic acid (LA)
food sources 5
gene expression regulation 11, 12
metabolism 5, 6
α-Linolenic acid (ALA)
food sources 5
metabolism 5, 6
Lipoxins, formation and activities 7, 9, 10
5-Lipoxygenase (5-LOX), age-related macular degeneration role 116
5-LOX, *see* 5-Lipoxygenase

Magnetic resonance spectroscopy (MRS)
phosphorous-31 neurospectroscopy
depression 36
schizophrenia 42
principles 31–33
proton neurospectroscopy in myalgic encephalitis 40
registration 32, 33
MRS, *see* Magnetic resonance spectroscopy
Myalgic encephalitis
clinical features 40
fatty acid supplementation studies 41
proton neurospectroscopy 40
virus infection 40, 41

Neuroprotectin D1 (NPD1)

Alzheimer's disease neuroprotection 50, 61, 63
biosynthesis 46, 47, 55
ischemia-reperfusion injury mediation 52
mechanisms of action 55
prospects for study 52, 53
seizure induction 52
Nitric oxide (NO), age-related macular degeneration role and omega-3 fatty acid effects 132
NO, *see* Nitric oxide
NPD1, *see* Neuroprotectin D1

Omega-3 fatty acids, *see also specific fatty acids*
biological effects 7, 8
cost savings to healthcare systems 25
cultural symbolism of seafood 26
desaturase gene transfer studies 11
food sources 17
mental health studies
deficiency definition 18
depression studies
analogous deficiencies 24
biological gradient 21, 22
coherence 22, 23
meta-analysis of trials 23, 24
omega-6/omega-3 fatty acid ratio 12
plausibility 22
suicide risk, prevention, and treatment 24, 25
temporality 21
Hill criteria of causality
consistency 19, 20
specificity 20, 21
strength 19
Omega-6 fatty acids, *see also specific fatty acids*
biological effects 7, 8
Omega-6/omega-3 fatty acid ratio
eye disease studies 12, 13
gene transfer studies 11
mental health studies 12
metabolism 5–7
Paleolithic period 3, 4
population differences 5
Western diet 2, 4

PC, *see* Phosphatidylcholine
Phosphatidylcholine (PC)
biosynthesis
CDP-choline 1,2-diacylglycerol cholinephosphotransferase 78, 79